Emerging Technologies in Body Contouring

Emerging Technologies in Body Contouring

Edited by Alec Smith

STATES
ACADEMIC PRESS
www.statesacademicpress.com

States Academic Press,
109 South 5th Street,
Brooklyn, NY 11249, USA

Visit us on the World Wide Web at:
www.statesacademicpress.com

ISBN: 978-1-63989-177-1

Cataloging-in-Publication Data

Emerging technologies in body contouring / edited by Alec Smith.
p. cm.
Includes bibliographical references and index.
ISBN 978-1-63989-177-1
1. Surgery, Plastic. 2. Skin--Surgery. 3. Surgery, Plastic--Technological innovations. I. Smith, Alec.
RD118 .E44 2022
617.95--dc23

Table of Contents

Preface

Body contouring is a medical procedure where the appearance of skin and tissue is improved through surgery. Some of the prominent surgeries used for body contouring are liposuction, panniculectomy, abdominoplasty, buttock augmentation and breast augmentation. Liposuction involves the removal of fat from particular areas of the body through a suction technique. It can be performed on the arms, hips, thighs, abdomen, buttocks or neck. Individuals who have a stable body weight but have too much body fat in a particular part of the body are treated through this procedure. This surgery is usually performed under general anesthesia, however, in certain cases it can also be performed on an outpatient basis. This book traces the progress of research on body contouring and liposuction, and highlights some of its key concepts and applications. It elucidates new techniques and their applications in a multidisciplinary manner. The book will help the readers in keeping pace with the rapid changes in this field.

This book is a result of research of several months to collate the most relevant data in the field.

When I was approached with the idea of this book and the proposal to edit it, I was overwhelmed. It gave me an opportunity to reach out to all those who share a common interest with me in this field. I had 3 main parameters for editing this text:

1. Accuracy - The data and information provided in this book should be up-to-date and valuable to the readers.
2. Structure - The data must be presented in a structured format for easy understanding and better grasping of the readers.
3. Universal Approach - This book not only targets students but also experts and innovators in the field, thus my aim was to present topics which are of use to all.

Thus, it took me a couple of months to finish the editing of this book.

I would like to make a special mention of my publisher who considered me worthy of this opportunity and also supported me throughout the editing process. I would also like to thank the editing team at the back-end who extended their help whenever required.

Editor

1

Lower Body and Extremities Sculpting, Beautification, Changing of Proportions

Nikolay P. Serdev

Abstract

Creation of aesthetic proportions and volumes of the lower body and extremities is crucial for the beautification of a patient's body. In authors' hands, it includes ultrasonic-assisted liposuction (UAL) or VASER sculpting of abdomen, waist, buttocks, breeches, inner thighs, inner knees, and ankles for straightening and elongation of the leg form; UAL or VASER "knee form lift" for visible elongation of lower legs; Serdev Suture® lifting of the buttocks for leg elongation, changing the body-leg proportions and for buttocks projection. Important proportions are the equal width of shoulders to buttocks breadth, as well as the similarity of buttocks to breast volume in profile view. These proportions are important for European culture and most of the Caucasian and Asian patients. In many other cultures, an amphora-like sculpting of the lower body is desirable. Tiny ankles are a sophisticated addition to beauty. Strange augmented, unproportioned Brazilian buttocks are not everywhere accepted and not healthy in many cases. The author describes his techniques of UAL/VASER sculpting together with Serdev Suture® buttock lifts to lift and project buttocks; beautify, straighten and elongate lower extremities and change body proportions.

Keywords: lower body and leg contouring, better body proportions, buttock lift, Serdev suture buttock lift, VASER buttock lift, VASER knee lift, VASER leg elongation, VASER leg straightening, VASER ankle sculpting

1. Introduction

1.1. Ultrasonic-assisted liposculpture (UAL) and recently VASER

Ultrasonic-assisted liposculpture (UAL) and recently VASER are safe techniques that limit the trauma and blood loss [1]. They are used by the author to safely sculpture the lower face and whole body. Aesthetic proportions and volumes are important rules and are followed by the author as described in "History of Art". This multidisciplinary science describes the form and art to visualize the face and body aesthetics in human communication creating positive emotions and admirations. In the branch "Aesthetics", there has been a proliferation of the artistic acts and behavior of mankind [1, 2; http://www.visual-arts-cork.com/history-of-art.htm]. It became an important part of the Renaissance and influenced the philosophy and essence of beauty and its creation.

1.2. Buttock lifting using UAL/VASER for elongation of thighs

Buttocks are not an area to be treated by classic liposculpture, but they are easily treated by UAL/VASER [1]. Preferred areas are outer contours (in combination with outer thighs) and lateral lower buttocks. The skin perforation is located laterally. Using UAL/VASER, the infragluteal fold becomes 3–4 cm higher and gives visible elongation of thighs (**Figures 1** and **2**).

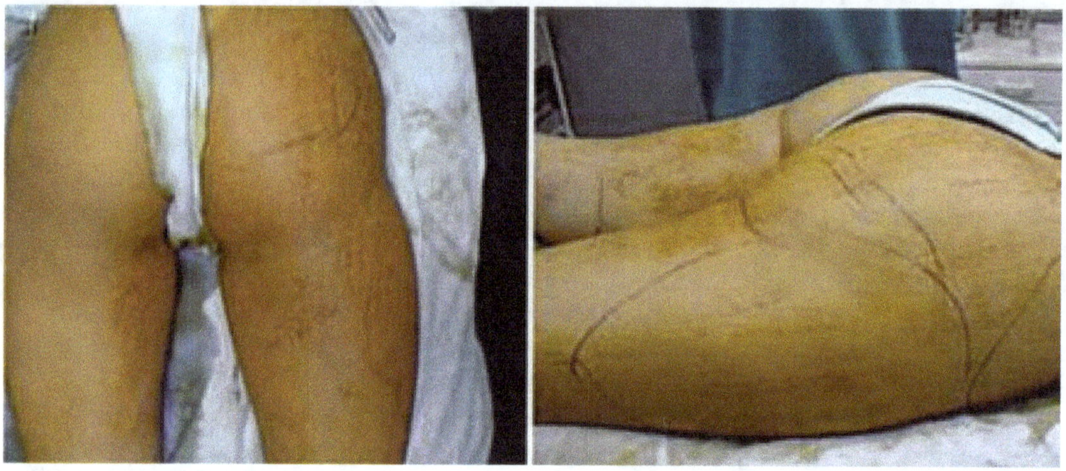

Figure 1. The left buttock is liposculptured. The left infragluteal line is much higher (3–4 cm) in comparison with the untreated right buttock.

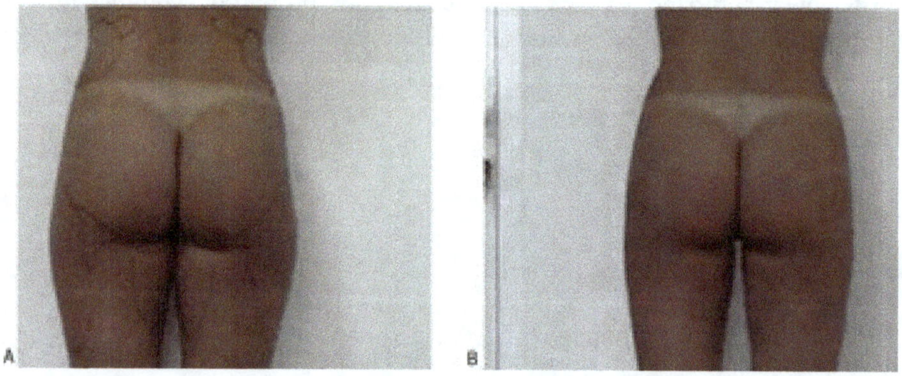

Figure 2. (A) Before (B) after UAL sculpting of waist, buttocks, outer and inner thighs to obtain correct Caucasian proportions with the effect of buttock lift and better body proportions.

1.3. Knee form lift using UAL/VASER for elongation of the lower legs

The knee lift is one of the most sophisticated liposculptures, because of the condyle contours. The technique aims to remove all the inner knee fat deposit on the inner surface of the tibial condyle and then higher only subdermal fat reduction until the nice form of the inner knee is reached. Deep liposuction in the area above the medial condyle is not recommended because it forms depressions and irregularities [1]. Following the above technique, the lower leg is transformed to a very nice symmetric form (patients characterize it as a "champagne bottle form"). The new form of the inner knee is formed much higher which elongates the lower leg visually and patients like it, because knee-long skirts and frocks give an imagination of long legs (**Figures 3** and **4**).

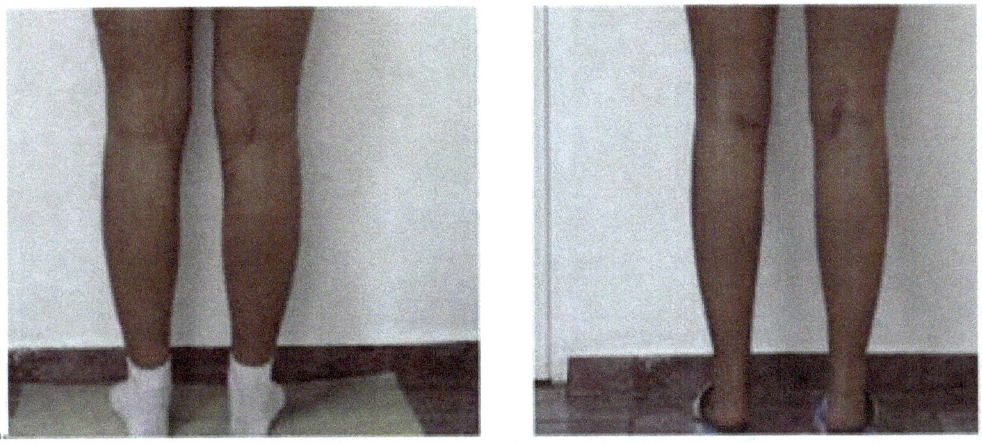

A. B.

Figure 3. (A) The lower extremities before. (B) Day one after UAL beautification of lower extremities and knee form lift for lower leg elongation and straightening. Minimal bruising and no irregularities.

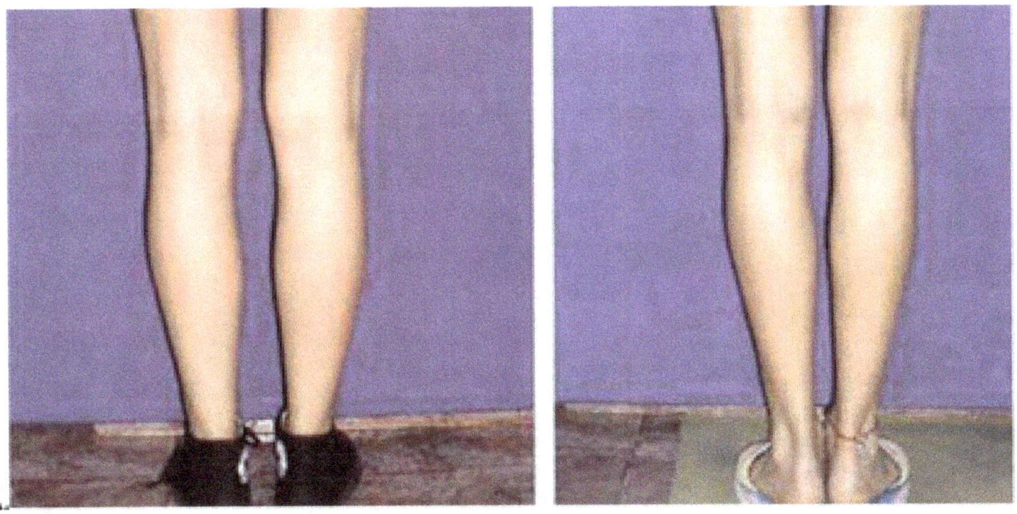

A. B.

Figure 4. UAL knee sculpting for knee lift and leg straightening. (A) Before (B) late result in a well-known model—mannequin. Lower legs in a straighten form, which will be clearly visible under a knee-level skirt or other type of dress. Whole legs are straightened with an elongated form. Ankles are sculptures to be thinner.

1.4. Thin ankles using UAL/VASER

Tiny ankles give noble appearance to ladies. There are four fat deposits on ankles: two lateral in front and two both sides of the Achilles tendon at the back. Four skin punctures using an 11-blade knife at the lowest place around the ankles give the best approach to all four fat deposits positioning the patient in prone position and the lower leg flexed in 90°. Using the tiniest probe and a 2 mm Mercedes cannula, the ankles can be formed thinner and as wanted (**Figures 5–7**).

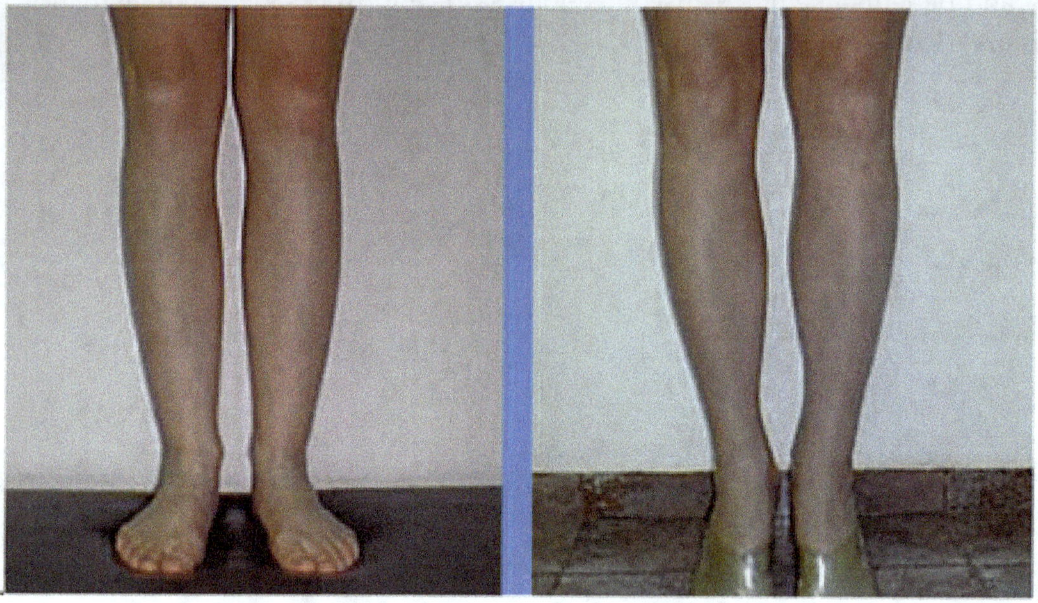

A. B.

Figure 5. (A) Before (B) 4 months after VASER liposculpting of ankles and inner knees.

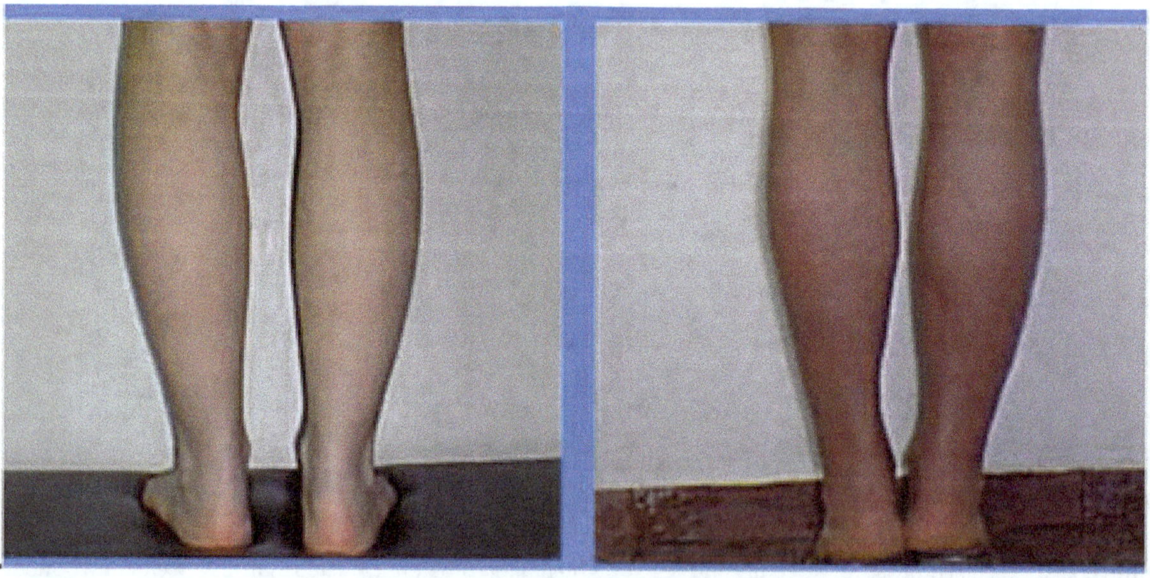

A. B.

Figure 6. (A) Before (B) 3 months after VASER liposculpting of ankles, lateral low legs, and inner knees.

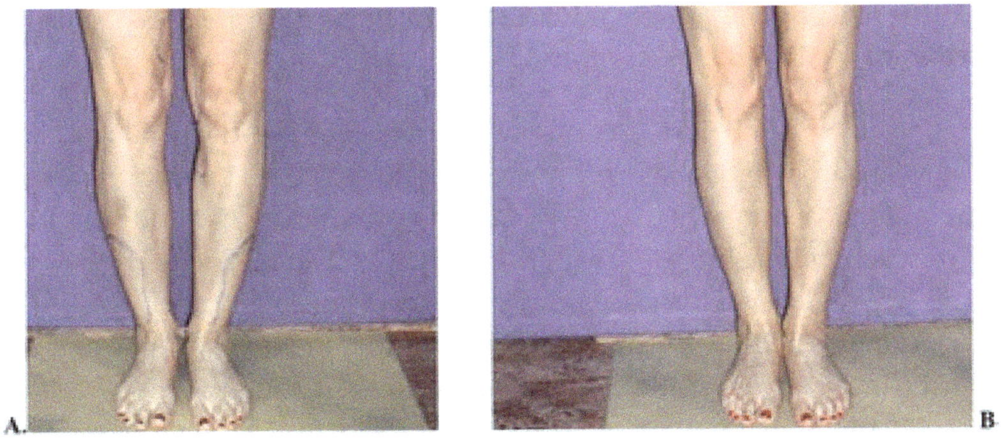

Figure 7. (A) Before (B) 6 months after VASER liposculpting of ankles, lateral low legs, and inner knees plus fat transfer to inner lower leg.

1.5. Sculpting the waist, abdomen, outer buttocks, outer thighs, inner thighs, inner knees and ankles using UAL/VASER for leg straightening and elongation

Caucasian body structure is easily sculptured to finest, because of good body construction with marked fat deposits. The author uses UAL since 1994 and recently VASER, removing only deep fat collections, leaving superficial subdermal fat layer untouched. Such approach permits removal of the total deep fat deposits, smooth results without irregularities even in skinny patients and models, which is the finest fat sculpture for leg straightening and elongating [1] (**Figure 8**).

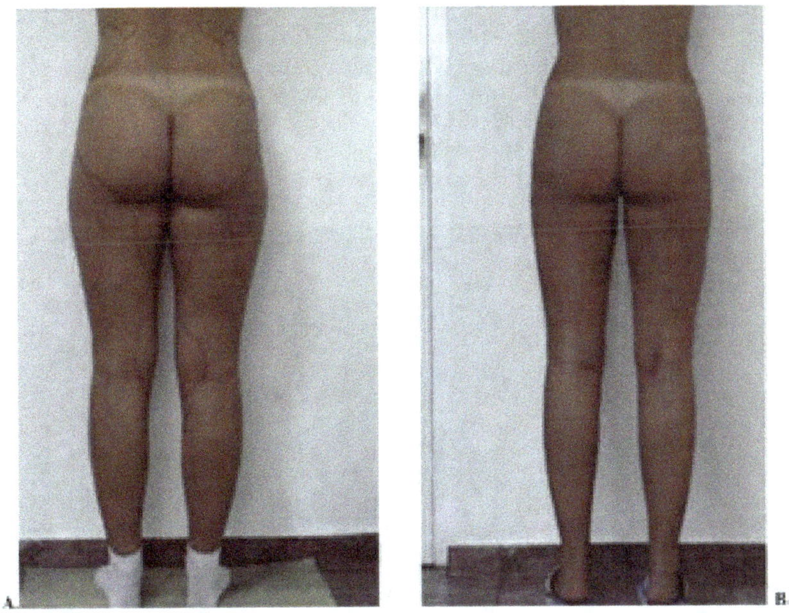

Figure 8. (A) The lower body and extremities before. (B) Day one after UAL beautification of lower body and extremities, UAL buttock lift, leg elongation and straightening. Elongation of the lower leg and thighs is visible. Minimal bruising is presented thanks to the atraumatic work using UAL. No irregularities due to deep liposculpting technique.

1.6. Buttock lifting using the scarless transcutaneous Serdev Suture® technique for leg elongation and changing of body proportions

The transcutaneous Serdev Suture® technique is a sewing of the mobile fibrotic buttock soft tissue higher to the strong immobile Serdev sacrocutaneus fascia. This fascia is connecting the lateral borders of the sacrum with the overlying skin and is located each side in a line between the Venera dimples and the highest point of the intragluteal fold. Each Serdev suture® uses three skin perforations: lateral, medial—just above the anus and upper—between the two Serdev fascias (**Figures 9–11**). The idea is to tie the buttock trabecular system and the soft tissue fibrosis like a bucket to project it and in the same time hang it higher on the Serdev fascia. The suture should be round in order to perform equal pressure in each point. Thus, the buttocks are projected, rounded, and lifted. The equal pressure around the suture prevents from tissue trauma and cutting trough [3–5].

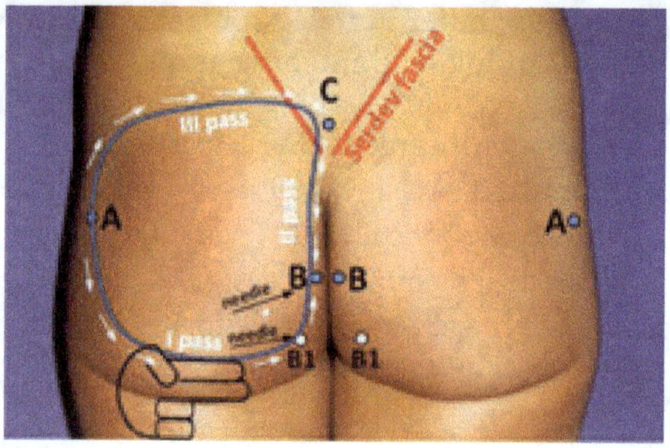

Figure 9. The skin perforations are marked with A, B and C. Point C is one for both sides. The suture is located deep in the soft tissue, but above the gluteus maximus fascia. It forms a round circle to prevent from unequal pressure and cutting through the tissue. The upper part of the suture is fixed above the Serdev sacrococcygeal fascia. After tying the suture, the buttocks will be projected and lifted.

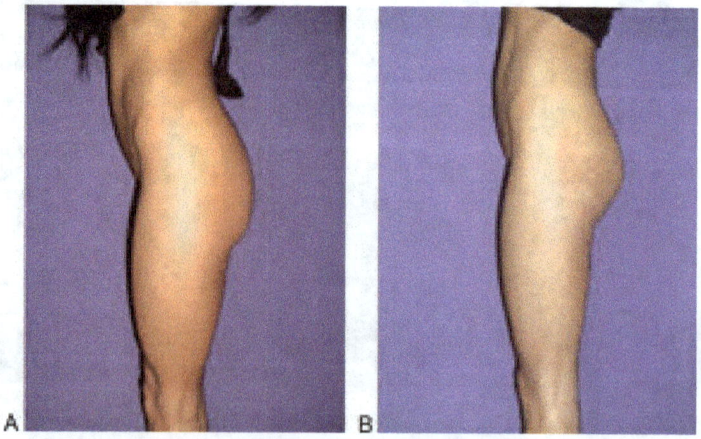

Figure 10. (A) Before (B) after a Serdev Suture® buttock lift in a dancer. Visible elongation of the thigh and better, higher projection of the buttocks.

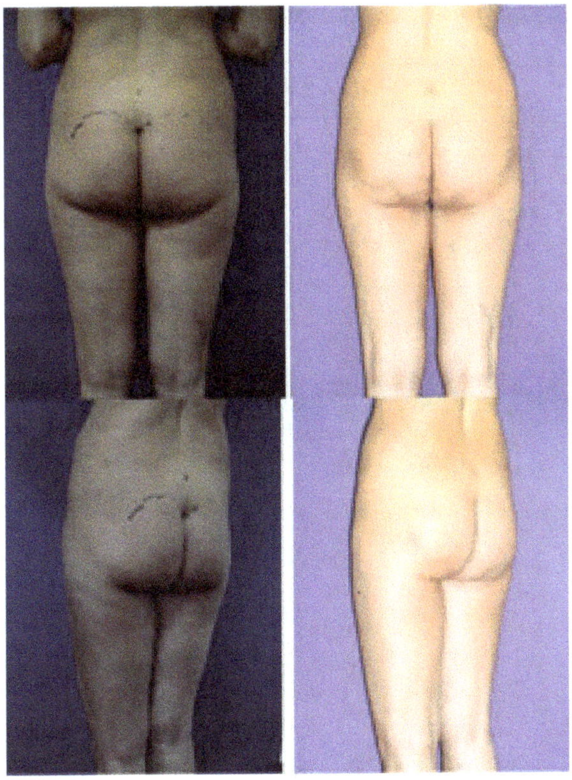

Figure 11. Left: Before, right: after buttock lift using Serdev Suture® in a 62-year-old patient. Lifting with elongation of the thighs is visible as well as better texture of the skin.

Blunt semielastic Serdev® needles and Bulgarian polycaproamide threads 4, 6 and 8 are used for buttock lift suture (**Figure 12**).

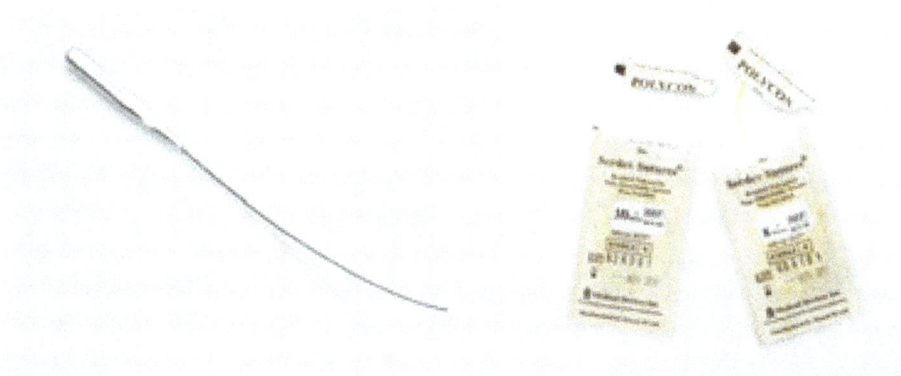

Figure 12. Serdev® needle, blunt, semielastic, and Polycon braided absorbable (in 2 years) threads for Serdev Suture®.

1.7. Simultaneous UAL/VASER lower body and extremities contouring and sculpting with Serdev Suture® buttock lift

The author uses simultaneous combination of the UAL/VASER and Serdev Suture® buttock lift technique [3–5] to obtain a correctly contoured and sculpted lower body and extremities with elongation of the legs, higher and projected buttocks as well as better body proportions (**Figures 13–15**).

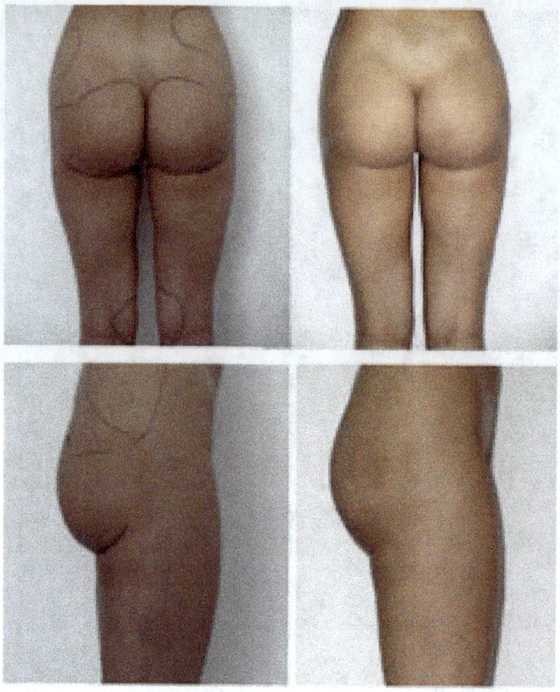

Figure 13. Left: before, right: after simultaneous UAL contouring and sculpting of the lower body and extremities and Serdev Suture® buttock lift.

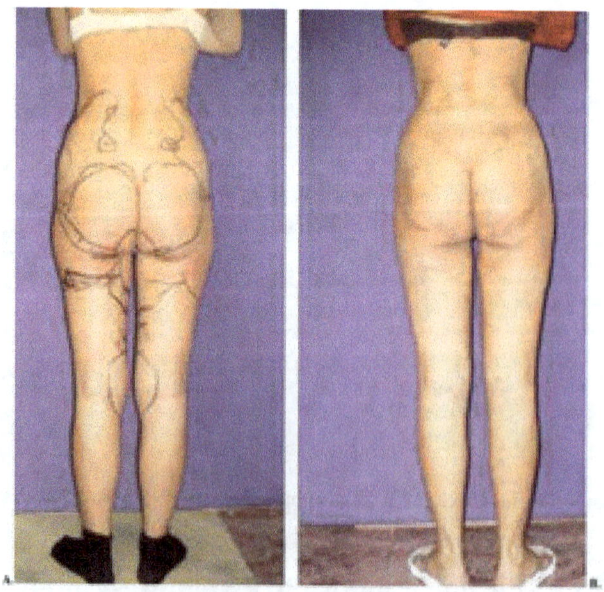

Figure 14. (A) Before (B) day one after the total VASER liposculpting of lower body and lower extremities, and simultaneous Serdev Suture® buttock lift in a 52-year-old patient. Pre-op marking is still visible. Correct proportions are present, the leg form is elongated and straightened and buttocks are smaller and proportional to Caucasian body, rounded lifted and projected. Younger appearance and beautification with better body proportions are presented.

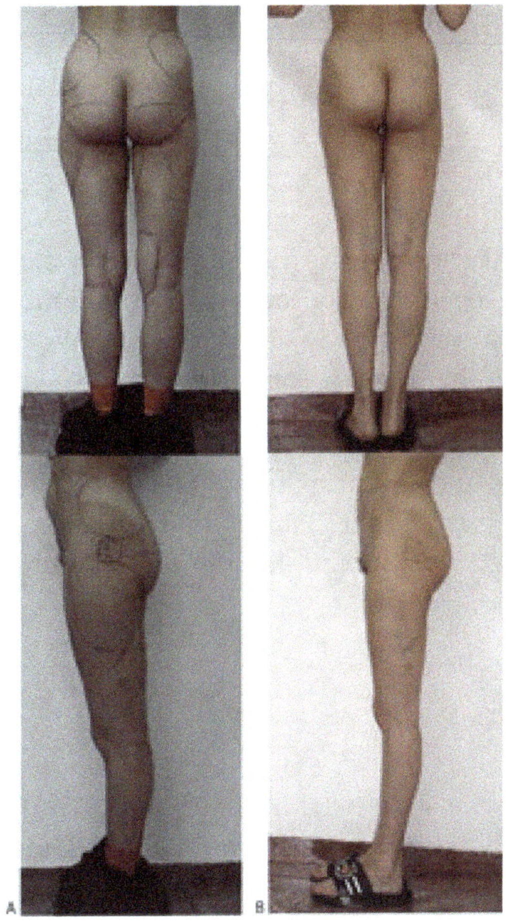

Figure 15. (A) Before (B) day one after the total VASER liposculpting of abdomen, lower body and lower extremities, and simultaneous buttock lift in a 33-year-old patient. Correct proportions are present, the lower legs and the total leg form are elongated and straightened and buttocks are smaller and proportional to Caucasian body, rounded lifted and projected. Younger appearance and beautification with better body proportions are presented.

2. Results

No complications have been seen in thousands of UAL (1994–2006) and VASER afterwards. The author does not use skin protection, because the ultrasound does not work lateral on the length of the probe. To prevent from any early post-op period complications, we follow our patients' day-by-day until there is wound drainage—usually 4–7 days, mostly from the inner knee skin perforation.

Buttock lift using Serdev Suture® gave only one complication of infiltration in the first patient because of the use of nylon threads that are rigid. In this technique, the Bulgarian threads are used instead of nylon, which are semielastic and absorbable in 2 years permitted the author to perform thousands of buttock lifts with a sole complication of single infection of one of the skin perforations in five patients, which was treated easily in 2–3 days. We follow patients with buttock lift for 5–7 days to help them with taking shower, cleaning and dressing of wounds.

Elastic garments are used for a month and a half.

3. Discussion

UAL/VASER contouring and sculpting are a safer and nearly bloodless procedure in comparison with other liposuction techniques, because they both liquefy the total deep fat deposit, need lower aspiration pressure and give a very effective results saving the vessels and nerves. Blood loss and bruising are minimal as represented in figures given in the chapter.

Buttock lift using the Serdev Suture® technique is also atraumatic due to the blunt semielastic needles, semielastic threads and the principle of a round suture to prevent from irregular tension and cutting through the tissue. Pain is limited and patients work after 4–5 days. Bandages are used for some days until the skin punctures drain.

4. Conclusion

Both UAL/VASER (keeping the superficial fat layer untouched) and Serdev Suture® techniques alone or in their combination give perfect results in the hands of the author. Perfection in contouring and sculpting the lower body and extremities with higher and projected buttocks, elongated and straight lower extremities and lower legs gives good body proportions and beautify our patients.

Author details

Nikolay P. Serdev

Address all correspondence to: serdev@gmail.com

1 New Bulgarian University, Sofia, Bulgaria

2 Medical Center "Aesthetic Surgery, Aesthetic Medicine", New Bulgarian University, Sofia, Bulgaria

References

[1] Serdev NP, Ultrasound Assisted Liposculpture – UAL: A Simplified Safe Body Sculpturing and Aesthetic Beautification Technique. Advanced Techniques in Liposuction

and Fat Transfer, Ed. Serdev NP, ISBN 978-953-307-668-3, InTech, September 9, 2011, DOI: 10.5772/25146

[2] Serdev NP, Year 1994, Suture Suspensions for Lifting or Volume Augmentation in Face and Body (English Version), International Journal of Cosmetic Surgery, 2000, 1: 2561–2568.

[3] Serdev NP, Miniinvasive Face and Body Lifts – Closed Suture Lifts or Barbed Thread Lifts. Ed. Serdev NP, 1012, October 02, 2013 under CC BY 3.0 license, DOI: 10.5772/2654

[4] Serdev NP, Serdev Sutures® Face and Body Lifts and/or Volumizing Marllor Ed. 2013.

[5] Serdev NP, Serdev Sutures® Lifts in Body Areas, Miniinvasive Face and Body Lifts – Closed Suture Lifts or Barbed Thread Lifts. Ed. Serdev NP, 1012, ISBN 978-953-51-1196-2, Published: October 2, 2013, DOI: 10.5772/55672

2

Circular Abdominoplasty (Belt Lipectomy) in Obese Patients

Hossam ElKafrawy and Sherif Wasief

Abstract

Circular abdominoplasty, belt lipectomy, 360° abdominoplasty and lower body lift are all synonyms of a body contouring procedure with the aim of sculpting the torso, modifying abdominal contour, loins and lower back contours. Apart from buttock lifting and affecting lateral thighs, these procedures tremendously affect patients' waist size and body image. In the literature, different incision levels, different dissection extents according to the sex of the patient, with different areas of anatomical adherence and different modifications like buttock enhancement by de-epithelialized lower back flaps are described. Most of these operations target post-weight reduction patients. Still these procedures can be performed in obese patients, either after failed diet control, failed bariatric surgery or patients refusing GIT operations though seeking lifestyle modification through body contouring. A group of patients with obesity affecting pre-, intra- and post-operative course, with increased complication rate, when performed with a knowing what-to-do team takes about 3–4 hours. However, with the help of anaesthetists accustomed to this risky group of patients, it could be executed safely and efficiently.

Keywords: abdominoplasty, circular abdominoplasty, 360° abdominoplasty, belt lipectomy, lower body lift

1. Introduction

Abdominoplasty has evolved since a simple dermo-lipectomy was satisfactory for the patient and the plastic surgeon. Nowadays, it may be performed for a very demanding patient. Concealing the final scars became an important goal. With the advent of suction-assisted liposuction, remodelling of the entire trunk in a single operation became possible with superior aesthetic results [1].

The methodology of the plastic surgeon has evolved from a simple dermo-lipectomy to various combinations and techniques targeting aesthetic remodelling of the abdominal wall and waist re-creation [1].

Circular abdominoplasty, belt lipectomy, 360° abdominoplasty and lower body lift are all synonyms of body contouring procedures with the aim of sculpting the torso, modifying abdomen, loins and lower back contour, lifting buttocks and affecting anterior and lateral thighs. These procedures tremendously affect the patient waist size and overall body image [2].

Originally, these procedures were performed on patients who wanted to lose weight by a great extent after successful diet management and lifestyle remodelling, or in bariatric surgery patients.

A good share in the literature described different incision levels, different dissection extents according to the sex of the patient, with different areas of anatomical adherence, and different modifications like buttock enhancement by de-epithelialized back flaps [3–6].

Still these operations can be performed in the waist of locally obese patients. These procedures can also be performed in patients with failed diet control, failed bariatric surgery, weight gain after years of bariatric operations, border-line obese patients which are not recommended for bariatric surgery and patients refusing GIT operations though seeking lifestyle modification through body contouring.

2. Anatomy

The anatomical area of concern extends to include anterior abdomen, lateral abdomen, mons pubis, anterior thighs, lateral thighs, lower back and buttocks.

Aesthetic thinking of the whole area as a unit, which is divided into further sub-units, is more convenient and gives better aesthetic outcomes.

2.1. Layers of the abdominal wall

The anterolateral abdominal wall consists, from the outside in, of the skin, superficial fascia, deep fascia, external and internal abdominal oblique, transverse abdominis and associated aponeuroses, rectus abdominis and pyramidalis and the transversalis fascia [7].

The skin has average thickness and loosely attaches to the underlying tissue. It exhibits certain surface markings such as the umbilicus, linea alba and linea semilunaris [7].

The superficial fascia comprises a variably fatty superficial layer known as Camper's fascia [7]. In the lower wall of the anterior abdomen, a deeper membranous layer known as Scarpa's fascia becomes more evident [7]. This layer remains connected, though loosely, to the deep fascia that covers the aponeurosis of the external abdominal oblique muscle. The strength of the Scarpa's fascia can stabilize sutures placed when closing incisions of the abdominal wall [8].

3. Patient consultation

3.1. Abdominoplasty classification and patient selection

A lot of techniques are used for different types of patients as follows:

(1) Liposuction only (suction, laser, ultrasound and power assisted).

(2) Mini abdominoplasty (with or without liposuction).

(3) Conventional abdominoplasty (with or without liposuction).

(4) High lateral tension abdominoplasty (after Lockwood) [9, 10].

(5) Circular abdominoplasty (belt lipectomy/lower body left): When excess tissues (skin and/or adipose tissue) are present at the lateral abdomen and lower back (**Figure 1**), circular abdominoplasty is proposed as one surgical option.

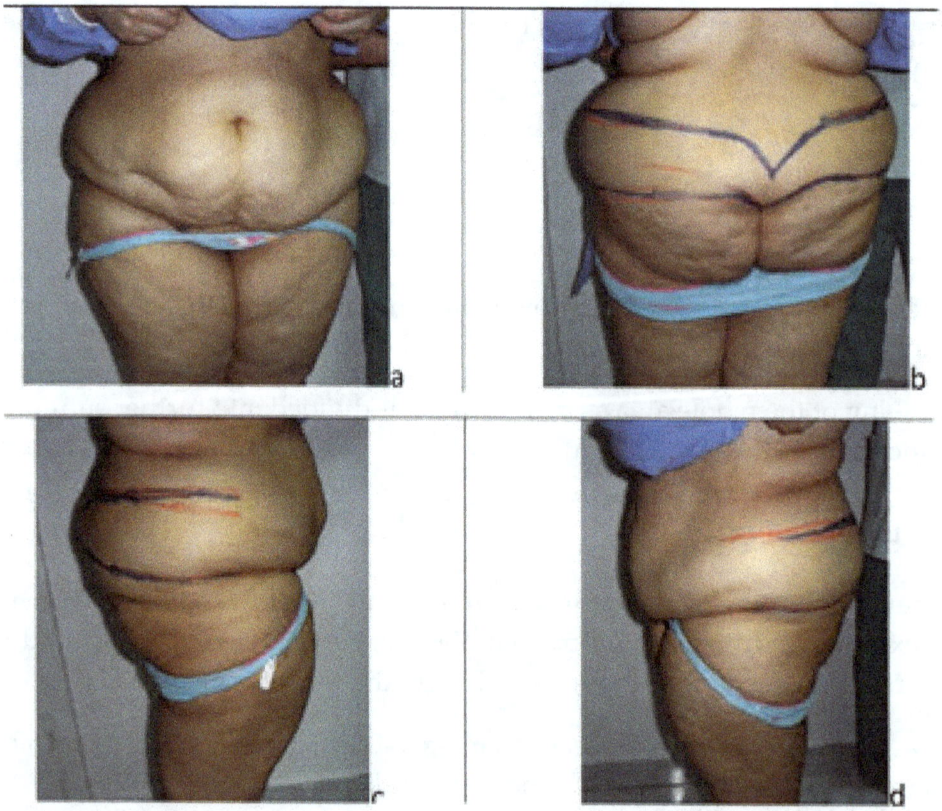

Figure 1. 29 years old, female patient, 97 kg, showing lower abdominal obesity, anterior lateral and posterior areas are all affected. (a) Anterior view, (b) posterior view, (c) right lateral view and (d) left lateral view.

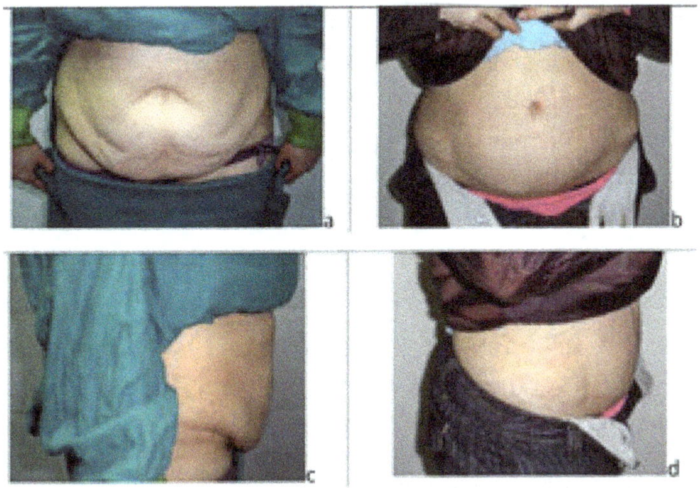

Figure 2. 31 years old female patient undergone abdominoplasty operation, (a) pre-operative anterior view, (b) post-operative anterior view, (c) pre-operative right lateral view and (d) post-operative right lateral view.

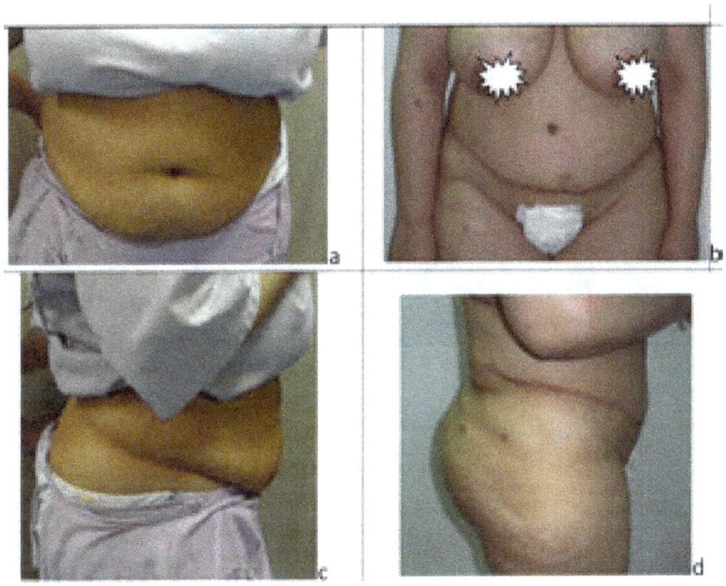

Figure 3. 28 years old female patient undergone an abdominoplasty operation with extended wound attacking lateral abdominal obesity, (a) pre-operative anterior view, (b) post-operative anterior view, (c) pre-operative right lateral view and (d) post-operative right lateral view.

3.2. Main problem

Abdominoplasty is a very common procedure in plastic surgery (**Figure 2**). It is very effective in managing anterior contour problems, especially lower part of the abdomen, and to a lesser extent lateral and upper areas, which improve a lot but to a lesser extent than the lower part.

In most of obese patients, lateral abdomen remains a problem for the plastic surgeon. If left, it certainly affects the aesthetic result, and if managed in the supine position, it could be controlled but the most lateral part of the procedure is actually on the posterior surface of the body, very uncomfortable during wound closure (**Figure 3**).

4. Surgical technique

4.1. Patient marking

While standing the patient, back markings are done first; a very important beginning landmark is the upper limit of the natal cleft. Noting the buttock length is variable in-between different sex, ethnic groups and patient body length.

The tissues are pulled superiorly by an assistant to mimic the effect of our surgery—expecting the end scar position, putting in mind the effect of liposuction (if done) in increasing tissue laxity in the lower (buttock) flap.

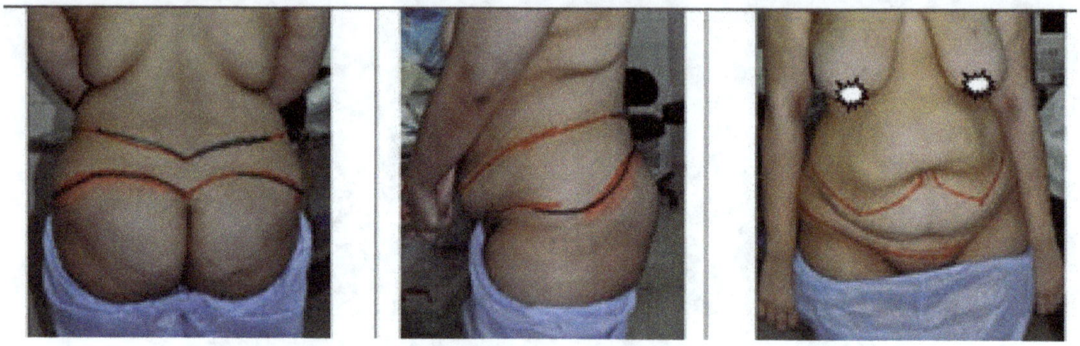

Figure 4. Patient marked for upper and lower incision lines.

The mid-scapular line meets the maximum convexity in the lower marking; then, the lateral down shift of the line is designed to meet the cellulite correction design of lateral high tension abdominoplasty proposed by Lockwood T [11].

The main target is ending in a nicely placed seagull wing scar on the back easily concealed by undergarments.

El-kafrawy H. technique implies estimation of the tissue excess and marking of the upper excision limit from the start (**Figure 4**). Wasief Sh. technique implies a cut as you go method after tissue dissection and intraoperative estimation of tissue excess before final determination of upper incision (**Figure 5**). Both methods target a closure with least tension especially at the natal cleft line and central parts with adherent tissues; with least tissue mobility.

Then, the patient turns to face the operator with right side, tissue pull by the assistant to abolish the lateral thigh laxity (cellulite) and the lower limit of the excision is marked. It is designed as a continuation of the back markings. The left side in turn is marked in a similar manner.

The abdominoplasty marking is done while the patient is lying supine, 6–8 cm from anterior fourchette is marked after surgeon assessment of the particular tissue proportions and patient consultation about self-image in the mons area. Low abdominoplasty incision is marked at the mid-clavicular line, 2–3 cm from the thigh crease, which is an important landmark in such an area with minimal tissue laxity. Then, the markings meet the lateral marking according to lateral tissue laxity.

Liposuction will increase tissue laxity and should be estimated in markings for the upper incision in the pre-operative markings proposed by El-Kafrawy H.

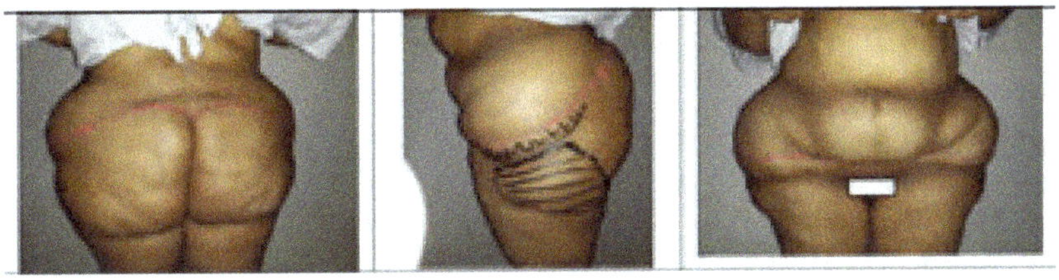

Figure 5. Patient marked for the lower incision only as proposed by Wasief Sh.

4.2. Anaesthesia

Operations were done under general anaesthesia.

4.3. Positioning

Patients were anaesthetized on patient trolley, airway secured and then transmitted by our team into prone position on the operating table.

4.4. Sterilization and draping

4.4.1. Tumescent injection

1:100,000 adrenaline solution in saline injected sub-dermally all over the markings to decrease blood loss during skin incision.

1:1,000,000 tumescent solution is used all over the liposuction and excision area.

4.5. Surgery

Skin incised at lower markings till the deep dermis by scalpel, mono-bolar diathermy is used through the fatty tissue and fascia of the back. Thin layer of fat is left covering the muscles of the back. At the lower incision, fat modulation is done according to the body proportions. Slight cephalic sloping dissection is done if no volume is needed for the buttocks and large degree of sloping is done if volume is needed for buttocks, up to de-epithelialisation only in patients with deflated buttocks seeking augmentation gluteoplasty.

El-kafrawy H. technique implies cutting on the upper marking with tissues excised en-block beginning on the right side.

Wasief Sh. technique implies intra-operative skin marking for the upper limit by methylene blue, followed by excision according to tissue laxity.

Closure of back incision in three layers, superficial fascia closed by absorbable size 0 sutures, sub-dermal 3-0 or 2-0 absorbable and sub-cuticular skin closure by 3-0 absorbable or non-absorbable sutures. Stay sutures at the most lateral parts are advised allowing tissue modulation when the abdominoplasty flap is cut.

Temporary dressing is done, changed at the end of procedure after it gets soaked with fluids during the anterior part of the operation.

Patient is repositioned on trolley in the supine position and then transferred to the operating table in the supine position.

Prepped and draped, tumescent fluid is injected; low abdominoplasty incision is chosen by the authors. Skin incised till dermis by scalpel, and then mono-polar diathermy is used.

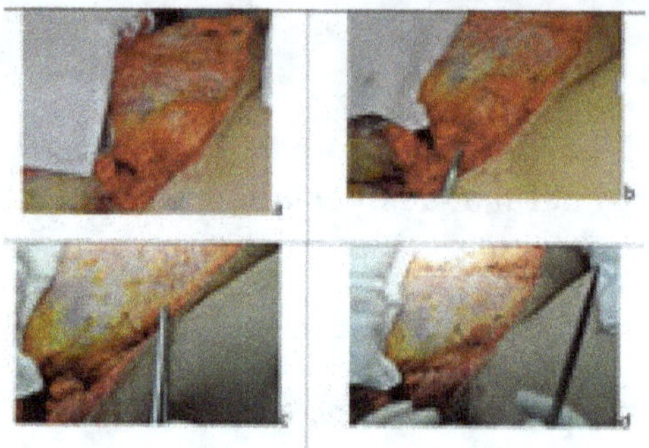

Figure 6. (a) An intra-operative view showing lateral area with fat left to obliterate dead space. (b–d) Intra-operative view showing superficial fascia sutures to iliac crest.

Fatty layers are preserved in the lower part containing lymphatics; superficial fascia is left in a more extended fashion, used to bear fascial suspension sutures to iliac crest (**Figure 6**). One raw suture line by 1 poly prolene or 0 non-absorbable multifilament suture is used routinely by El-kafrawy H. Two row suspension lines to distribute tension were proposed by Wasief Sh. after patients complained feeling sutures cutting through tissues during trunk movement 5 days post-operatively.

5. Results

From February 2009 till April 2016, 37 patients were included in this series, ages 23–54 years old, 12 patients (32.4%) with co-morbidities (DM and hypertension), BMI 27–33, four patients (10.8%) were smokers and stopped smoking 4 weeks before surgery, seven patients (18.9%) with previous failed bariatric interventions, two lap band and five sleeve gastrectomy, 18 patients (48.6%) refused to undergo bariatric surgeries after failure to reduce weight with nutrition control regimens and 12 patients (32.4%) were over-weight in the range of BMI 27–30.

Eleven patients (29.7%) were not satisfied with the long 360° scar in the first 6 months, reduced to seven patients (18.9%) after scar maturation, two patients (5.4%) were not satisfied with the high position of the back scar and all 37 patients (100%) were satisfied with the waist creation with the hour glass body transformation; all patients were satisfied with the buttock cellulite left, lateral thigh cellulite lift.

Sixteen patients (43.2%) had minor delayed wound healing along with incision line managed conservatively, 11 patients (29.7%) had blood constituent transfusions, hospital admission ranged 2–4 days and one patient admitted to ICU post-operatively.

Surgeon assessment of patients after surgery resulted in 100% satisfaction for the waist creation, buttock lift and lateral thigh lift, anterior thigh improvement noticed but not corrected totally, two patients (5.4%) had higher incisions than planned, hypertrophic back scars notices in eight patients (21.6%) managed by topical silicon products application, CO_2 fractional laser drilling and five fluro-uracil injections (see **Figures 7–12**).

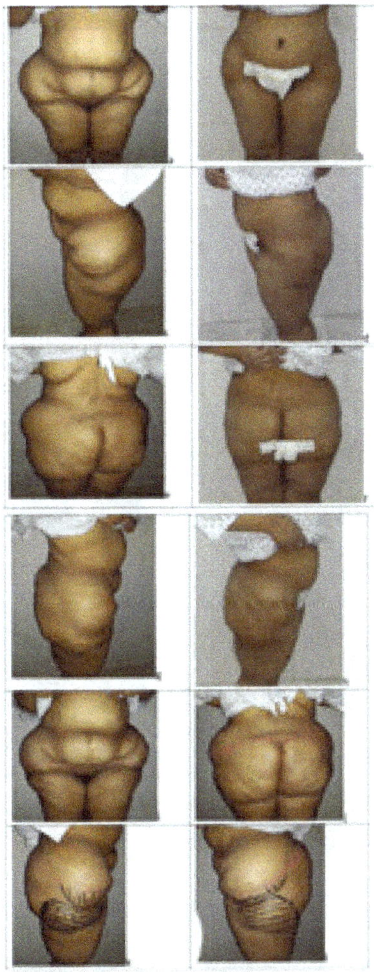

Figure 7. 42 years old obese patient with superadded localized obesity in lateral abdomen and trochanteric area. a,c,e,g,I,k pre-operative views b,d,f,h,l post-operative views.

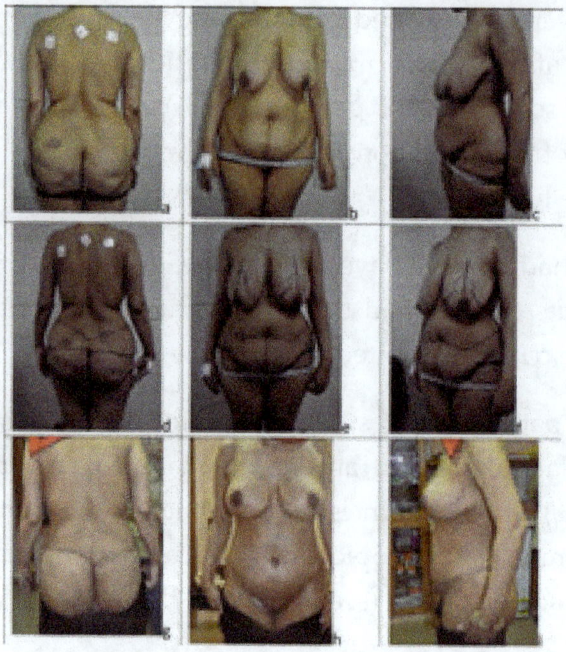

Figure 8. 36 years old patient undergone combined circular abdominoplasty with breast reduction mastopexy. (a–f) Pre-operative view and (g–i) post-operative view.

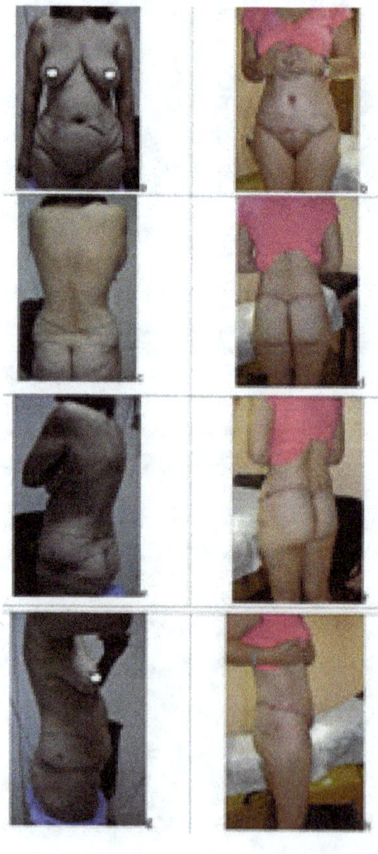

Figure 9. 28 years old patient. (a, c, e, g) Pre-operative view. (b, d, f, h) Post-operative view.

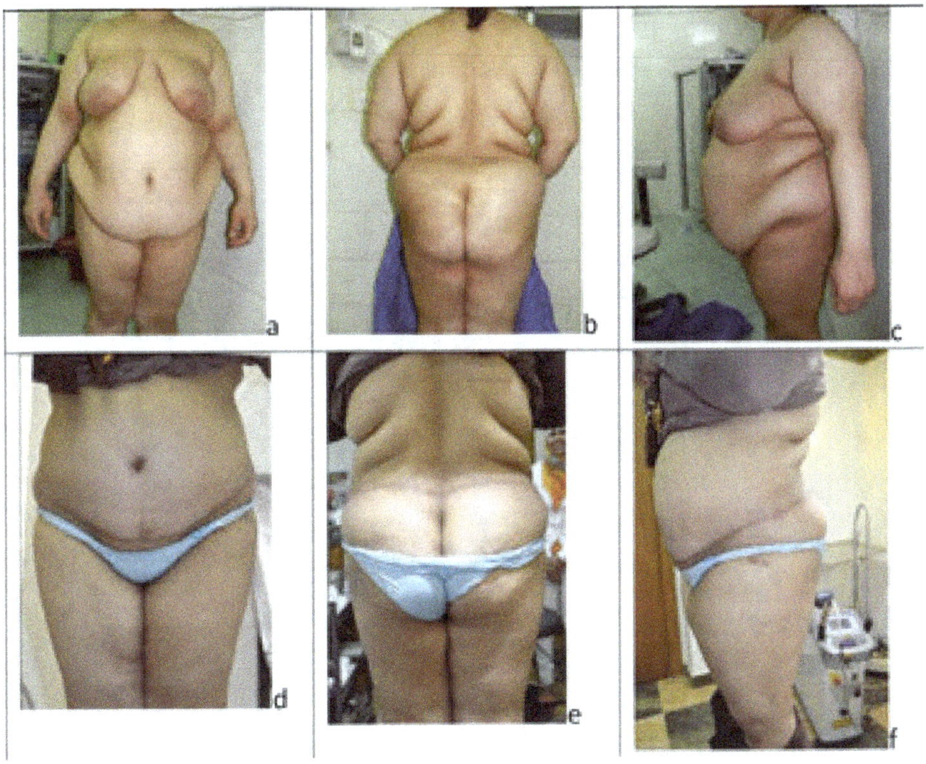

Figure 10. 36 years old patient undergone circular abdominoplasty. (a) Pre-operative anterior view, (b) pre-operative posterior view, (c) pre-operative left lateral view, (d) post-operative anterior view, (e) post-operative posterior view and (f) post-operative left lateral view.

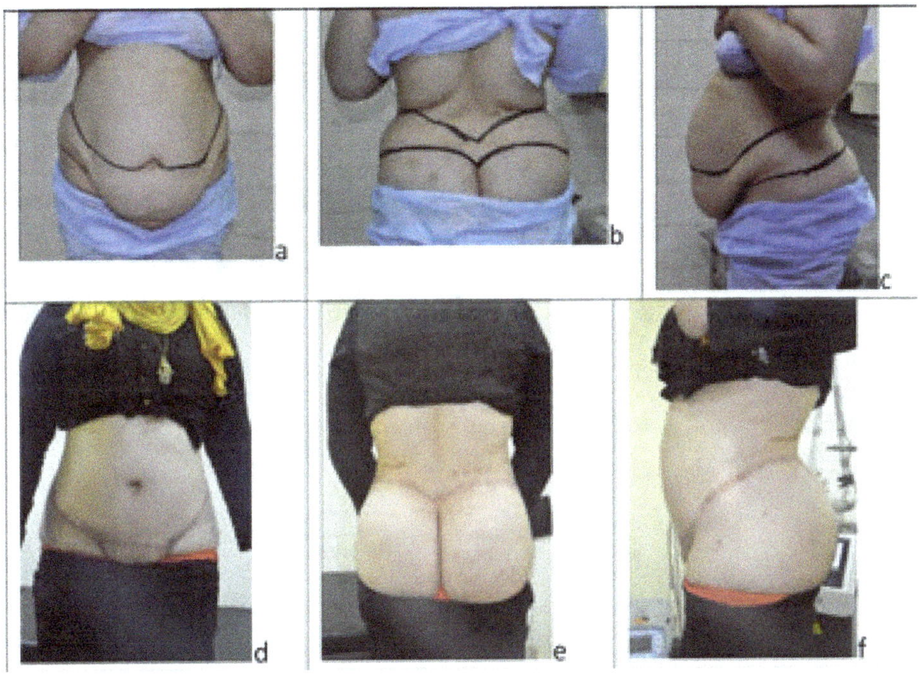

Figure 11. (a) Pre-operative anterior view, (b) pre-operative posterior view, (c) pre-operative left lateral view, (d) post-operative anterior view, (e) post-operative posterior view and (f) post-operative left lateral view.

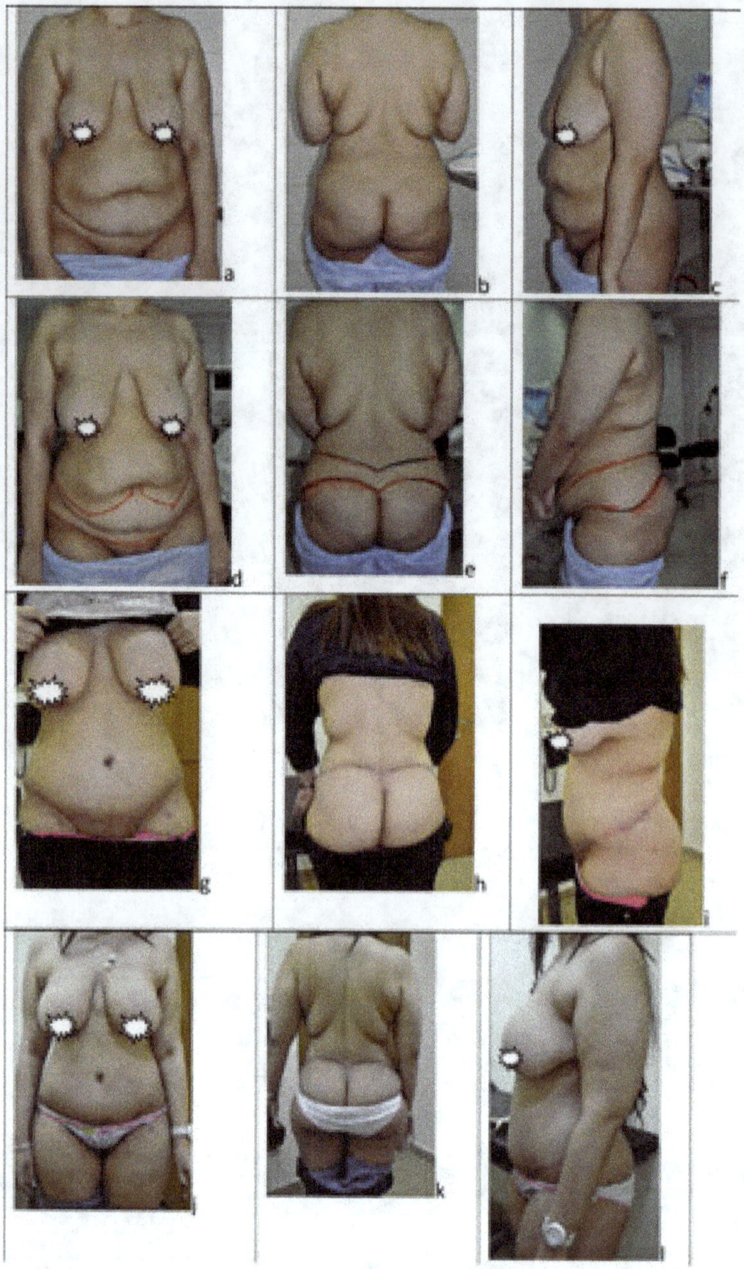

Figure 12. 38 years old patient undergone circular abdominoplasty operation. (a) Pre-operative anterior view, (b) pre-operative posterior view, (c) pre-operative left lateral view, (d) pre-operative anterior view, (e) pre-operative posterior view and (f) pre-operative left lateral view. (g) post-operative anterior view, (h) post-operative posterior view, (i) post-operative left lateral view, (j) post-operative anterior view, (k) post-operative posterior view and (l) post-operative left lateral view.

6. Discussion

Obese patients are at risk of developing various health-related problems [10]. However, they have a myriad of options such as diet control, practicing physical activities and surgical interventions to reach a normal body mass index, thus, decreasing the life time risk of co-morbidities.

Some patients may have difficulties in weight reduction, failed diet control, failed bariatric surgeries and refusal to undergo surgical gastrointestinal interventions. In this group of patients, circular abdominoplasty may be an option with the following advantages and disadvantages:

Advantages:

1. Abdominoplasty with aesthetic remodelling of antero-lateral abdominal wall.
2. Creation of a defined waist.
3. Decreasing cellulite in anterior thighs, lateral thighs and buttocks.
4. Defining the aesthetic angle between lower back and buttocks.

Disadvantages:

1. Operating on a riskier group of patients with higher BMI.
2. Longer operation time and increased operation risk.
3. Nearly double the scar length and double the time for wound healing.
4. Longer convalescence period.

The operative time in the beginning took about 4–5 h which was reduced to 3–4 h in our centre with a trained team accustomed to this type of patients and operation. In the event of two-team approach, working on both sides simultaneously may reduce the time to 2:30 h.

In our practice using a post-operative questionnaire, consulted patients who refused the idea of circular abdominoplasty and ended with long abdominoplasty scars may substantially say that 'we should have circular abdominoplasty if we expected such long scars'.

Prevention and management of abdominoplasty complications is very important in this group of patients.

Thrombo-embolism protection is very important in this patient group because of increased risk of obesity and increased operative time.

7. Conclusion

Circular abdominoplasty is an option in obese patients, provided that the surgical environment is prepared to commence on a smooth fast track surgery to decrease the operative risk. The procedure gives a better defined waist and a better body contouring of the whole area. However, when liposuction is done in the same operation, the risk of bleeding increases.

Acknowledgements

"I am honored to have professor Hossam El-Kafrawy as my mentor in plastic surgery. Working in his team for years till we became partners." Sherif Wasief.

Author details

Hossam ElKafrawy[1] and Sherif Wasief[2*]

*Address all correspondence to: sherif_wasief@yahoo.com

1 Department of Plastic Surgery, Alexandria University, Alexandria, Egypt

2 Plastic Surgery Unit, Shark El Madina Hospital, Alexandria, Egypt

References

[1] Shiffman MA, Mirrafati S. *Aesthetic surgery of the abdominal wall.* Berlin: Springer, 2005, pp. 5–6.

[2] Gonzalez R. Buttocks lifting: how and when to use medial, lateral, lower, and upper lifting techniques. Clin Plast Surg 2006;33:467–478.

[3] Centeno RF. Autologous gluteal augmentation with circumferential body lift in the massive weight loss and aesthetic patient. Clin Plast Surg 2006;33:479–496.

[4] Colwell AS, Borud LJ. Autologous gluteal augmentation after massive weight loss: aesthetic analysis and role of the superior gluteal artery perforator flap. Plast Reconstr Surg 2007;119:345–56.

[5] Raposo-Amaral CE, Cetrulo CL Jr, Guidi Mde C, Ferreira DM, RaposoAmaral CM. Bilateral lumbar hip dermal fat rotation flaps: a novel technique for autologous augmentation gluteoplasty. Plast Reconstr Surg 2006;117:1781–1788.

[6] Sozer SO, Agullo FJ, Wolf C. Autoprosthesis buttock augmentation during lower body lift. Aesthetic Plast Surg 2005;29:133–137; discussion 138–140.

[7] Shiffman MA, Mirrafati S. *Aesthetic surgery of the abdominal wall.* Berlin: Springer, 2005, pp. 11–14.

[8] Del Valle GO, Combs P, Qualls C, Curet LB. Does closure of Camper Fascia reduce the incidence of post-cesarean superficial wound disruption? Obstet Gynecol 1992;80:1013–1016.

[9] Pascal JF, Le Louarn C. Remodeling body lift with high lateral tension. Aesthetic Plast Surg 2002;26:223–230.

[10] Melanson KJ, Mcinnis KJ, Rippe JM, Blackburn G, Wilson PF. Obesity and cardiovascular disease risk: research update. Cardiol Rev 2001;9(4):202–207. doi: 10.1097/00045415-200107000-00005

[11] Lockwood T. High-lateral-tension abdominoplasty with superficial fascial system suspension. Plast Reconstr Sur 1995;96(3):603–615. doi: 10.1097/00006534-199509000-00012

3

Assessment of Postoperative Venous Thromboembolism Risk in Body Sculpting Procedures

Alexandro Aguilera Salgado,
Johnatan Figueroa Padilla and José Cortés Arreguín

Abstract

Venous thromboembolism is a common complication following surgical procedures. It is imperative for us to identify which risks factors are present in our patients, not only because body sculpting procedures are elective, but also to help us perform an individualized assignment of venous thromboembolism risk. Once we have identified the risk, we can select a method of venous thromboembolism prophylaxis based on the guidelines by the American College of Chest Physicians and the other individualized risk scales presented in this chapter. Our main goal is to keep as low as possible the incidence of venous thromboembolism and its complications.

Keywords: venous, thromboembolism, risk, body, sculpting, postoperative

1. Introduction

Body sculpting procedures can be associated to postoperative venous thromboembolism in patients with certain characteristics. This entity can lead to fatal consequences, like pulmonary embolism and death, that is why it is important for us to clearly assess the risk for each individual in the preoperative setting, in order to establish certain procedures and prophylaxis, which may help us lower or diminish these risks to the minimum. Given these are elective procedures, it should be our main concern that our patients are well prepared before the surgery with a complete preoperatory analysis of the risks both the patient and the surgery per se represent.

2. Background

Venous thromboembolism represents a wide spectrum of disease, ranging from deep venous thrombosis to pulmonary embolism, a very relevant complication following body sculpting procedures, especially those who combine two or three procedures in one surgery. Some studies have reported that each year 350,000–600,000 Americans suffer from deep venous thrombosis and pulmonary embolism and that at least 100,000 deaths are directly or indirectly related to venous thromboembolism [1]. These numbers represent the incidence in general population, not specifically following body sculpting procedures, nevertheless some studies in the last few years have discussed this matter.

Some data collected from a worldwide survey among certificated plastic surgeons revealed pulmonary embolism as the main cause of death following a liposuction, which represented the 23% of all deaths [2]. Another study that included all the procedures performed inside an operating room reported that 63.6% of the postoperative deaths were secondary to thromboembolism [3]. Considering large-volume liposuction procedures, Albin and de Campo reported an incidence of venous thromboembolism of 1.7% in patients where the aspirated volume was larger than 5 L [4]. Grazer and Goldwyn cited a 1.9% incidence of venous thromboembolism in a series of abdominoplasty patients [5]. Finally, in combined procedures and with longer surgical times as belt lipectomies, there is a higher incidence of thromboembolism, as reported by Aly and colleagues with a 9.4% incidence in this group of patients [6].

Given these high rates of mortality following venous thromboembolism complicated with pulmonary embolism after body sculpting procedures, it should be logic for us to think that the surgeons performing these procedures would establish a prophylaxis protocol in all their patients in order to lower the risk of the development of venous thromboembolism. Nevertheless, some worldwide studies have reported that only 43.7% of the surgeons performing liposuction procedures and 60.8% of the surgeons performing a combined body sculpting procedure use thromboembolism prophylaxis [7]. This can be secondary to the belief that venous thromboembolism has a low incidence, or because of the fear to have bleeding complications and postoperative hematomas, with dehiscence of wound and infection.

3. Risk factors

In order to develop a venous thromboembolism, two variables must be present interacting between them: first, the individual patient's risk factors which cannot be modified and are usually permanent and second, the circumstances surrounding the time and place where the thromboembolism occurs, being transient in nature, with the possibility to be modified most of the times.

Risk factors inherent to the patient include age, active malignancy, history of venous thromboembolism, other chronic diseases such as heart or respiratory failure, spinal cord injury, multiple trauma, myocardial infarction, congenital or acquired coagulation disorders (antithrombin deficiency, Protein C and Protein S deficiency, elevated coagulation factors), hormone replacement therapy, and oral contraception. Critically ill patients receiving intensive care are also considered to be a population at risk for developing venous thromboembolism.

According to the British Thoracic Society, patient risk factors are traditionally classified into major and minor categories (**Table 1**) [8]. Remember, these predisposing factors cannot be modified, so the seldom presence of them justifies the use of prophylaxis. The important thing here is not only to be able to identify those factors, but also to assess the overall risk of venous thromboembolism in each patient and to establish the appropriate prophylaxis regimen in each case [9].

Major risk factors (RR = 5–20)	**Minor risk factors (RR = 2–4)**
Postoperative state: major abdominal/pelvic surgery, hip/knee joint replacement, postoperative intensive care	Cardiovascular: congenital heart disease, heart failure, hypertension, superficial venous thrombosis, central venous catheter
Obstetrics: late pregnancy, caesarian section, puerperium	Humoral: estrogen use: oral contraception, hormone replacement therapy
Lower limb affections: fractures, extensive varicosities	Miscellaneous: chronic obstructive lung disease, neurological impairment, latent malignancy, thrombotic defects, long-distance travel in the sitting position, obesity
Malignancies: abdominal/pelvic, advanced/ metastatic stage	
Limited mobility: hospitalization geriatric care	Other: inflammatory bowel disease, nephrotic syndrome, chronic dialysis, myeloproliferative disease, paroxysmal nocturnal hemoglobinuria
Miscellaneous: history of previous venous thromboembolism	

Table 1. Risk factor of venous thromboembolism, according to the British Thoracic Society [8].

Besides these risk factors inherent to the patient, the surgical procedure per se represents also a risk factor to the patient. General anesthesia, supine position as well as immobilization produce blood stasis. Decreased venous return also diminishes the clearance of activated clotting factors, which in turn augments the hypercoagulable state. Finally, intimal injury is secondary to venous traction and to the vasodilatory effect of anesthesia, which favors platelets deposits in the sites of vascular injury, initiating the coagulation cascade.

4. Natural history of venous thromboembolism

As described earlier in this chapter, venous thromboembolism includes various stages of complex developments, which can be fatal as they lead the patient to a pulmonary embolism. Regardless of the patient's risk factors, the surgery alone is one of the most important risk factors we will face. During surgery, the patient will be prone to stasis, hypercoagulability and endothelial injury, which in turn can explain how 50% of deep vein thrombosis associated with surgery start intraoperatively. The first affected veins will be the most distal ones, located at the calf region. Of these affected cases, approximately 50% may resolve spontaneously within 72 h with the use of adequate venous thromboprophylaxis, which will help in the lysis of thrombi and prevent the formation of new ones. When the deep vein thrombosis is isolated to the calf, it will rarely cause leg symptoms or clinically important pulmonary embolisms [10].

Of the untreated symptomatic calf deep vein thromboses, approximately 25% will extend to more proximal veins as late as 1 week after the surgery, and subsequently break free to cause pulmonary embolism in the late stages. Each of these stages may or may not be associated with symptoms. The development of symptoms depends on the extent of thrombosis, the adequacy of collateral vessels, and the severity of associated vascular occlusion and inflammation.

In those cases where the thrombi moves in a more proximal direction toward the inguinal region and it is symptomatic but without chest symptoms, approximately 50% of the patients will have a pulmonary embolism on lung scan [11]. From day 3 to day 7 of the postoperative period the patient will be at the highest risk of the development of fatal pulmonary embolism, being fatal around 10% of symptomatic pulmonary embolisms within one hour of first symptoms. Furthermore, the patient will be at the highest risk of developing symptomatic venous thromboembolism within 2 weeks of surgery, but that risk will remain elevated for 2–3 months [12].

The severity of acute pulmonary embolism is determined primarily by its hemodynamic impact, presenting as sudden pulmonary hypertension. In healthy patients, it is known that a pulmonary bed obstruction of 30–50% is needed in order to develop pulmonary hypertension [13]. In the other hand, patients with a previous history of lung or heart disease will develop pulmonary hypertension with even a minor obstruction in the pulmonary circulation. The acutely developing pulmonary hypertension in pulmonary embolism leads to an increase in right ventricular after load, morphologically presenting as right ventricular dilation and may eventually cause right heart failure, which results in decreasing of left ventricular filling, and deteriorated diastolic left ventricular function due to right ventricular dilation. After a diagnosed pulmonary embolism, 50% of patients have right ventricular dysfunction on echocardiography. These events can lead to a fall in blood pressure and present as syncope, hypotension or carcinogenic shock, resulting in sudden death [14]. After a symptomatic deep vein thrombosis, there is an approximately 10% cumulative incidence of severe postthrombotic syndrome after 5 years.

5. Assessment of postoperative venous thromboembolism risk

In each patient to undergo a surgical body contouring procedure should be implemented a strategic scheme of risk assessment, planning and establish measures to reduce morbidity and mortality [15]. We must identify the preventive management of hypercoagulable states. Risk stratification will allow us to make good decisions, especially in patients at high risk.

Over the past two decades, thromboprophylaxis has taken greater importance, given the increase in the number of surgical procedures performed in the body contour area. Because of this, there have been designed, applied, and evaluated various risk models for venous thromboembolism [16–19]. The most widely known and validated model is the one developed by Caprini et al.

This model was initially published in 1991 [20], which with the passage of time has been modified and refined. In the published version of 2005, plastic and reconstructive surgery patients were included, predicting the risk of venous thromboembolism within 30 or 60 days (**Figure 1**) [21]. As a result of these validation studies, strata have been identified to report level of risk and response to prophylaxis based on risk level [22–23].

Choose All That Apply

Each Risk Factor Represents 1 Point

- ❑ Age 41-60 years
- ❑ Minor surgery planned
- ❑ History of prior major surgery (< 1 month)
- ❑ Varicose veins
- ❑ History of inflammatory bowel disease
- ❑ Swollen legs (current)
- ❑ Obesity (BMI > 25)
- ❑ Acute myocardial infarction
- ❑ Congestive heart failure (< 1 month)
- ❑ Sepsis (< 1 month)
- ❑ Serious lung disease incl. pneumonia (< 1 month)
- ❑ Abnormal pulmonary function (COPD)
- ❑ Medical patient currently at bed rest
- ❑ Other risk factors____________________

Each Risk Factor Represents 2 Points

- ❑ Age 60-74 years
- ❑ Arthroscopic surgery
- ❑ Malignancy (present or previous)
- ❑ Major surgery (> 45 minutes)
- ❑ Laparoscopic surgery (> 45 minutes)
- ❑ Patient confined to bed (> 72 hours)
- ❑ Immobilizing plaster cast (< 1 month)
- ❑ Central venous access

Each Risk Factor Represents 3 Points

- ❑ Age over 75 years
- ❑ History of DVT/PE
- ❑ **Family history of thrombosis***
- ❑ Positive factor V Leiden
- ❑ Positive prothrombin 20210A
- ❑ Elevated serum homocysteine
- ❑ Positive lupus anticoagulant
- ❑ Elevated anticardiolipin antibodies
- ❑ Heparin-induced thrombocytopenia (HIT)
- ❑ Other congenital or acquired thrombophilia If yes:

Type____________________

***most frequently missed risk factor**

Each Risk Factor Represents 5 Points

- ❑ Elective major lower extremity arthroplasty
- ❑ Hip, pelvis or leg fracture (< 1 month)
- ❑ Stroke (< 1 month)
- ❑ Multiple trauma (< 1 month)
- ❑ Acute spinal cord injury (paralysis)(< 1 month)

For Women Only (Each Represents 1 Point)

- ❑ Oral contraceptives or hormone replacement therapy
- ❑ Pregnancy or postpartum (<1 month)
- ❑ History of unexplained stillborn infant, recurrent spontaneous abortion (≥ 3), premature birth with toxemia or growth-restricted infant

Total Risk Factor Score ☐

Figure 1. The 2005 Caprini risk assessment model. COPD, chronic obstructive pulmonary disease; DVT, deep venous thrombosis; PE, pulmonary embolism. Caprini, Thrombosis risk assessment as a guide to quality patient care. 2005.

The most recent version of the Caprini Risk Assessment Model was published in 2010 (**Figure 2**) [24]. When compared with the 2005 Risk Assessment Model, the 2010 Risk Assessment Model has four distinct, data-driven changes, including addition of new risk factors or reweighting of old risk factors. Some studies have shown that Caprini 2010 model gives an altered estimate of the risk of thromboembolism with consequent inappropriate application of preventive measures, so what right now the evidence does not support is its use in patient stratification until it is validated more widely [25].

A1: Each risk factor represents 1 point

- ○ Age 40–59 years
- ○ Minor surgery planned
- ○ History of prior major surgery
- ○ Varicose veins
- ○ History of inflammatory bowel disease
- ○ Swollen legs (current)
- ○ Obesity (BMI > 30)
- ○ Acute myocardial infarction (< 1 month)
- ○ Congestive heart failure (< 1 month)
- ○ Sepsis (< 1 month)
- ○ Serious lung disease incl. pneumonia (< 1 month)
- ○ Abnormal pulmonary function (chronic obstructive pulmonary disease)
- ○ Medical patient currently at bed rest
- ○ Leg plaster cast or brace
- ○ Central venous access
- ○ Blood transfusion (< 1 month)
- ○ Other risk factor/s________________ ____________________________

A2: For women only (each represents 1 point)

- ○ Oral contraceptives or hormone replacement therapy
- ○ Pregnancy or postpartum (< 1 month)
- ○ History of unexplained stillborn infant, recurrent spontaneous abortion (≥ 3), premature birth with toxemia of pregnancy or growth restricted infant

B: Each risk factor represents 2 points

- ○ Age 60–74 years
- ○ Major surgery (< 60 minutes)*
- ○ Arthroscopic surgery (> 60 minutes)*
- ○ Laparoscopic surgery (> 60 minutes)*
- ○ Previous malignancy
- ○ Morbid obesity (BMI > 40)

C: Each risk factor represents 3 points

- ○ Age 75 years or more
- ○ Major surgery lasting 2–3 hours*
- ○ BMI > 50 (venous stasis syndrome)
- ○ History of SVT, DVT/PE
- ○ Family history of DVT/PE
- ○ Present cancer or chemotherapy
- ○ Present factor V Leiden
- ○ Positive prothrombin 20210A
- ○ Elevated serum homocysteine
- ○ Positive lupus anticoagulant
- ○ Elevated anticardiolipin antibodies
- ○ Heparin-induced thrombocytopenia (HIT)
- ○ Other thrombophilia-type______________

D: Each risk factor represents 5 points

- ○ Elective major lower extremity arthroplasty
- ○ Hip, pelvis or leg fracture (< 1 month)
- ○ Stroke (< 1 month)
- ○ Multiple trauma (< 1 month)
- ○ Acute spinal cord injury (paralysis)(< 1 month)
- ○ Major surgery lasting over 3 hours*

Total risk factor score:

Figure 2. The 2010 Caprini risk assessment model. Risk assessment as a guide to thrombosis prophylaxis. *Curr Opin Pulm Med*. 2010.

The 2012 American College of Chest Physicians guidelines note that at any level of 2005 Caprini score, plastic and reconstructive surgery patients are at decreased risk of venous thromboembolism compared with patients undergoing abdominal and pelvic surgery [26]. Prior validation studies of the 2005 Caprini score in plastic and reconstructive surgery patients [27] and the head and neck surgery population [28] showed that 70–80% of patients in the overall population are classified as lower risk (2005 Caprini scores of 3–4 or 5–6). Thus, only a small proportion of patients fall into the highest risk strata.

We recommend that all plastic and reconstructive surgery patients should be risk-stratified for perioperative venous thromboembolism risk using a 2005 Caprini score and that surgeons consider chemoprophylaxis on a case-by-case basis in patients with Caprini score >8.

6. Thrombosis and venous thromboembolism prophylaxis

Venous stasis is a recognized venous thromboembolism risk factor. Stasis, along with hypercoagulability and intimal damage, constitutes the central tenets of Virchow's triad for thrombosis. Stasis also promotes venous dilation, resulting in intimal microtears. This exposes subendothelial collagen and initiates the clotting cascade. Venous dilation is known to predict deep venous thrombosis in other surgical subspecialties [29].

In recent years there has been consensus in plastic surgery looking forward to find the best available evidence on prevention, taking into account the best scientific articles of all specialties related to venous thrombosis. The most important aspects for a surgeon about this issue are enlisted.

7. Type of anesthesia

General anesthesia, paralysis, or both eliminate calf muscle pump action in the lower extremities. The calf muscle pump propels venous blood cranially and, in concert with the venous valve system, mitigates venous stasis and venous dilation. A recent study of 200 patients having elective plastic surgery under spontaneous breathing, avoid gas, face up, extremities mobile (SAFE) anesthesia with postoperative duplex ultrasound screening showed an asymptomatic deep venous thrombosis rate of 0.5%. This rate is similar to symptomatic venous thromboembolism rates among low-risk (2005 Caprini score of 3 or 4) plastic surgery in patients undergoing surgery under general anesthesia [21, 30]. The recommendation on this issue is limited by the fact that some operations require general anesthesia, and thus this recommendation is not applicable to all patients.

Pannucci et al. [25] recommend using non-general anesthesia when appropriate. When possible, consideration should be given to using monitored anesthesia care, local anesthesia with sedation, or neuraxial anesthesia instead of general anesthesia with a grade 1C level of evidence (**Table 2**) [31].

Grade	Description	Benefit vs risk and burdens	Quality of supporting evidence	Implications
1A	Strong recommendation, high-quality evidence	Benefits clearly outweigh risks and burdens, or vice versa	RCTs without important limitations or overwhelming evidence from observational studies	Strong recommendation and can apply to most patients in most circumstances without reservation
1B	Strong recommendation, moderate-quality evidence	Benefits clearly outweigh risks and burdens, or vice versa	RCTs with important limitations or exceptionally strong evidence from observational studies	Strong recommendation and can apply to most patients in most circumstances without reservation
1C	Strong recommendation low- or very low-quality	Benefits clearly outweigh risks and burdens, or vice versa	Observational studies or case series	Strong recommendation but may change when higher quality evidence becomes available

Grade	Description	Benefit vs risk and burdens	Quality of supporting evidence	Implications
	evidence			
2A	Weak recommendation, high-quality evidence	Benefits closely balanced with risks and burden	RCTs without important limitations or overwhelming evidence from observational studies	Weak recommendation, best action may differ depending on circumstances or patient's or societal values
2B	Strong recommendation moderate-quality evidence	Benefits closely balanced with risks and burden	RCTs with important limitations or exceptionally strong evidence from observational studies	Weak recommendation, best action may differ depending on circumstances or patient's or societal values
2C	Weak recommendation low- or very low-quality evidence	Uncertainty in the estimated of benefits risks, and burden; benefits, risk, and burden may be closely balanced	Observational studies or case series	Very weak recommendation; other alternatives may be equally reasonable

Reproduced from Guyatt et al. [31].

Table 2. RCTs (randomized controlled trials).

8. Use of pneumatic compression and/or elastic stockings

Elastic stockings (also known as graduated compression stockings) may preferentially shunt venous blood from the superficial to the deep venous system through perforating veins.

Shunting augments the volume and velocity within the deep venous system, theoretically decreasing stasis and the likelihood of thrombosis [32, 33]. Elastic stockings are significantly more effective than no stockings for both deep venous thrombosis and pulmonary embolus prevention in general and orthopedic surgery patients [33].

Intermittent pneumatic compression devices (also known as sequential compression devices) work by means of multiple mechanisms. The sequential compression serially "pumps" blood from caudal to cranial, using the venous valve system to facilitate egress of venous blood and minimizing venous stasis and venous dilation. Intermittent pneumatic compression also stimulates the body's endogenous fibrinolytic mechanism. Blood samples taken distant from the intermittent pneumatic compression site show stimulation of bloodborne fibrinolytic activity when intermittent pneumatic compression is applied. Thus, intermittent pneumatic compression applied to a single leg can provide deep venous thrombosis risk reduction by means of both a direct and an indirect mechanism [34]. A meta-analysis by Ho and Tan shows that intermittent pneumatic compression is superior to elastic compression stockings for deep venous thrombosis risk reduction [35].

The latest recommendations about this are using intermittent pneumatic compression to prevent perioperative venous thromboembolism events in plastic surgery patients [25]. In the absence of rigorous publications in plastic surgery, this recommendation was derived largely from meta-analyses in other specialties (Grade 1B). Same recommendation applies for elastic compression stockings, but most meta-analyses recommend the intermittent pneumatic compression over the compression stockings (Grade 1B).

9. Effectiveness of chemoprophylaxis and bleeding risk

When we refer to chemoprophylaxis, we are referring to unfractionated heparin or low molecular weight heparin provided at prophylactic doses. The 2012 American College of Chest Physicians guidelines on deep venous thrombosis and pulmonary embolus prevention for nonorthopedic surgical patients do not recommend low-dose aspirin as first-line venous thromboembolism prophylaxis; as a result, experts do not recommend aspirin as first-line venous thromboembolism prophylaxis for plastic surgery patients.

Low-dose aspirin is recommended as prophylaxis only when unfractionated heparin and low molecular weight heparin are contraindicated or not available [26]. Only one study that compared aspirin to low molecular weight heparin in 505 free flap patients showed no difference in postoperative venous thromboembolism or bleeding. However, based on a relative paucity of data, we could not make recommendations specific to plastic surgery patients [36].

The oral factor Xa inhibitor "apixaban" has U.S. Food and Drug Administration approval for stroke reduction in nonvalvular atrial fibrillation, deep venous thrombosis, and pulmonary embolism prophylaxis after adult hip or knee replacement [37]. The oral factor Xa inhibitor "rivaroxaban" has U.S. Food and Drug Administration approval for stroke prophylaxis in nonvalvular atrial fibrillation, deep venous thrombosis and pulmonary embolism prophylaxis after adult hip and knee replacement, and for treatment of deep venous thrombosis or pulmonary embolism events [38]. Neither drug is U.S. Food and Drug Administration approved for venous thromboembolism prophylaxis in the general surgery population.

Prior studies of patients undergoing abdominal and pelvic surgery have shown significant venous thromboembolism risk reduction with a combination of chemoprophylaxis plus intermittent pneumatic compression versus intermittent pneumatic compression alone [39, 40]. Meta-analyses in high-risk surgical patients, including a Cochrane review, showed that combination prophylaxis significantly decreased the risk of symptomatic pulmonary embolism and symptomatic deep venous thrombosis [41, 42].

Population level data in plastic surgery did not show a significant venous thromboembolism risk reduction with chemoprophylaxis. In addition, there was evidence of harm in the overall population with increased rates of reoperative hematoma. These findings, paired with the known low venous thromboembolism risk among many plastic surgery patients, suggest that chemoprophylaxis should not routinely be provided to all plastic surgery patients [21].

Bleeding risk with chemoprophylaxis did not show a clear trend in the risk-stratified analysis. As 2005 Caprini score increased, estimates became less precise, as evidenced by the wider confidence intervals. This finding has face validity, as the 2005 Caprini score has been validated to predict risk of venous thromboembolism but not risk of bleeding. In other studies, plastic surgery patients with 2005 Caprini scores of >8 had a 60-day venous thromboembolism rate of 11.3% when no prophylaxis was provided, whereas chemoprophylaxis is reported to decrease 60-day venous thromboembolism risk by 50% [43].

When plastic surgeons choose to use chemoprophylaxis, there are minimal data to support an evidence-based recommendation for the appropriate duration of chemoprophylaxis. However, as length of inpatient stay was variable, patients received different durations of chemoprophylaxis. Prior work in plastic surgery has shown that among super high-risk patients (2005 Caprini score >8), venous thromboembolism events occur with the same frequency at postoperative weeks 3–8 as they do at weeks 1–2. The expert panel of 2015 does not recommend adding routine chemoprophylaxis to intermittent pneumatic compression for venous thromboembolism prophylaxis in the general non-risk-stratified plastic surgery population. They recommend that all plastic and reconstructive surgery patients should be risk-stratified for perioperative venous thromboembolism risk using a 2005 Caprini score and that surgeons consider chemoprophylaxis on a case-by-case basis in patients with Caprini score >8 (Grade 1C).

10. Timing of chemoprophylaxis administration

Ultimately, the surgeon must balance the relative risks of venous thromboembolism with chemoprophylaxis-associated venous thromboembolism risk reduction and bleeding risk in their decision to provide chemoprophylaxis. Davison and Massoumi [44] said: "An hematoma is a medical stress, an inconvenience, an embarrassment, or an additional procedure, but rarely does it kill a patient. Thromboembolism that progresses to a pulmonary embolism kills the patient 50% of the time." The classic teaching has been that deep venous thrombosis forms in the operating table, in response to induction of hypotension and vasodilation. Thus, initiation of preoperative mechanical and chemoprophylaxis are conceptually appealing for venous thromboembolism risk reduction.

The 1999 American Society of Plastic Surgeons consensus statement on deep venous thrombosis prophylaxis by McDevitt recommended that "thromboprophylaxis for the surgical patient should begin before the operative procedure. All such measures are directed toward enhancing venous flow, decreasing serum thrombogenic factors, and stabilizing the vascular endothelium." As such, low molecular weight heparin administered at least 2 h before surgery was recommended for moderate-and high-risk patients, "when dissection will not be extensive" [45]. However, there are insufficient data to recommend preoperative over postoperative chemoprophylaxis for venous thromboembolism prevention in the non-risk-stratified plastic surgery population. Also preoperative chemoprophylaxis was not associated with an increased risk of hematoma compared to postoperative chemoprophylaxis in the non-risk-stratified plastic surgery population (Grade 2C).

11. Unfractionated heparin versus low molecular weight heparin

Many studies had very wide confidence intervals, and their aggregate effect may have skewed data for this clinical question. There is a meta-analysis that included 16 randomized controlled trials and nearly 13,000 patients showed no significant difference in postoperative venous thromboembolism, major bleeding, or minor bleeding for cancer patients who received preoperative unfractionated heparin versus low molecular weight heparin [46].

In a single-center study of breast surgery patients, low molecular weight heparin was suggested to have a higher risk of preoperative hematoma compared with unfractionated heparin [47]. The data presented in the various studies are ambiguous, but there are some suggestions based on exhaustive reviews. In conclusion, neither subtype of heparin (low molecular weight or unfractionated) conferred an advantage over mechanical prophylaxis alone for venous thromboembolism risk reduction in the non-risk-stratified plastic surgery population. Low molecular weight but not unfractionated heparin conferred an increased risk of reoperative hematoma in the non-risk-stratified plastic surgery population [25] (Grade 2C).

12. Effectiveness and bleeding risk for chemoprophylaxis by surgery type

There are special situations in plastic surgery, for example, complex reconstructions with free flaps for breast or head and neck cancer. An analysis of transverse rectus abdominis musculocutaneous (TRAM) flap patients was unable to separate pedicled TRAM flap from free TRAM flap breast reconstructions. Thus, these results are difficult for interpretation, as the extent of surgery, duration of surgery, and tightness of abdominal wall closure are substantially different between the two groups [48–50].

Patient group	Intervention	Recommended?	Grade
All plastic surgery patients	Non-general anesthesia	Yes	1C
All plastic surgery patients	Intermittent pneumatic compression	Yes	1B
All plastic surgery patients	Chemoprophylaxis	No	1C
All plastic surgery patients	Preoperative risk stratification (Caprini)	Yes	1C
Caprini score >8	Chemoprophylaxis	Individualized	1C
All plastic surgery patients	Preoperative vs. postoperative chemoprophylaxis	Insufficient data for recommendation	2C
All plastic surgery patients	Low molecular weight vs. unfractioned heparin	No recommendation on medication type	2C
TRAM, body contouring, general head and neck	Chemoprophylaxis	No	2C
Head and neck free flaps	Chemoprophylaxis	Individualized	2C

Reproduced from Pannucci et al. [25].

Table 3. Recommendations and GRADE level.

Head and neck reconstruction using a free flap showed a significant venous thromboembolism risk reduction with chemoprophylaxis but also a significant increase in a composite bleeding endpoint. Bleeding within the neck or adjacent to the airway can be life threatening and thus has a different risk profile than prior recommendations. Surgeons must consider chemoprophylaxis on a case-by-case basis. After an exhaustive review of the existing literature, a consensus recommendation was created and is summarized in **Table 3**.

The risk of venous thromboembolism in esthetic or reconstructive plastic surgery is real, and complications may range from minor to life threatening. In the setting of elective surgery, all these considerations should be strongly considered and weighed against the potential for postoperative bleeding and secondary monitoring or interventions.

13. Conclusion

Given the morbidity and mortality associated with venous thromboembolism and the inaccuracy of screening modalities, prevention should be the goal in this group of patients. We recommend an individualized assessment of risk in each patient and according to the scales presented, determine the individual risks, and the best prophylaxis to be applied before and after the surgery.

Author details

Alexandro Aguilera Salgado[1*], Johnatan Figueroa Padilla[2] and José Cortés Arreguín[3]

*Address all correspondence to: alexandruss@hotmail.com

1 National Institute of Pediatrics, Mexico City, Mexico

2 National Institute of Cancerology, Mexico City, Mexico

3 Moreno Valle Traumatology and Orthopedics Hospital, Mexico City, Mexico

References

[1] U.S. Department of Health and Human Services. The Surgeon General's call to action to prevent deep vein thrombosis and pulmonary embolism. 2008. Available at: http://www.surgeongeneral.gov/topics/deepvein/calltoaction/call-to-action-on-dvt-2008.pdf.

[2] Grazer FM, de Jong RH. Fatal outcomes from liposuction: census survey of cosmetic surgeons. Plast Reconstr Surg. 2000; 105:436.

[3] Clayman MA, Caffee HH. Office surgery safety and the Florida moratoria. Ann Plast Surg. 2006; 56:78.

[4] Albin R, de Campo T. Large-volume liposuction in 181 patients. Aesthetic Plast Surg 1999; 23:5.

[5] Grazer FM, Goldwyn RM. Abdominoplasty assessed by survey, with emphasis on complications. Plast Reconstr Surg. 1977; 59:513.

[6] Aly AS, Cram AE, Chao M, Pang J, McKeon M. Belt lipectomy for circumferential truncal excess: The University of lowa experience. Plast Reconstr Surg. 2003; 111:398.

[7] Broughton G, II, Rios JL, Rohrich RJ, Brown SA. Deep venous thrombosis prophylaxis practice and treatment strategies among plastic surgeons: survey results. Plast Reconstr Surg. 2007; 119:157.

[8] British Thoracic Society Standards of Care Committee Pulmonary Embolism Guideline Development Group. British Thoracic Society guidelines for the management of suspected acute pulmonary embolism. Thorax 2003; 58:470–83.

[9] Anderson FA, Spencer FA. Risk factors for venous thromboembolism. Circulation. 2003; 107:I9–I16.

[10] Seruya M. MOC-PS CME: venous thromboembolism prophylaxis in plastic surgery patients.. Plast Reconstr Surg. September 2008; 122(3), 1701–1708.

[11] Moser KM, Fedullo PF, et al. Frequent asymptomatic pulmonary embolism in patients with deep venous thrombosis. JAMA. 1994; 27:223–225.

[12] Kearon C. Natural history of venous thromboembolism. Circulation. 2003; 107:I22.

[13] McIntyre KM, Sasahara AA. The hemodynamic response to pulmonary embolism in patients without prior cardiopulmonary disease. Am J Cardiol. 1971; 28:288–94.

[14] Bělohlávek J, Dytrych V, Linhart A. Pulmonary embolism: epidemiology, risk factors and risk stratification, pathophysiology, clinical presentation, diagnosis and nonthrombotic pulmonary embolism. Exp Clin Cardiol. 2013; 18(2), 129–138.

[15] Poponick, Bosker. The current challenge of venous thromboembolism in the hospitalized patient: Optimizing recognition, evaluation, and prophylaxis of deep venous thrombosis and pulmonary embolism. Part I: Patient identification, risk factor assessment, and diagnostic strategies. Hosp Med Consensus Rep. Available at: www.clinicalconsensusreports.com. Accessed November 28, 2007.

[16] Kucher N, Koo S, Quiroz R, Cooper JM, Paterno MD, Soukonnikov B, Goldhaber SZ. Electronic alerts to prevent venous thromboembolism among hospitalized patients. N Engl J Med. 2005; 352:969–977.

[17] Pannucci CJ, Shanks A, Moote MJ, Bahl V, Cederna PS, Naughton NN, Wakefield TW, Henke PK, Campbell DA, Kheterpal S. Identifying patients at high risk for venous thromboembolism requiring treatment after outpatient surgery. *Ann Surg*. 2012; 255:1093–1099.

[18] Yale SH, Medlin SC, Liang H, Peters T, Glurich I, Mazza JJ. Risk assessment model for venothromboembolism in posthospitalized patients. Int Angiol. 2005; 24:250–254.

[19] Rogers SO, Kilaru RK, Hosokawa P, Henderson WG, Zinner MJ, Khuri SF. Multivariable predictors of postoperative venous thromboembolic events after general and vascular surgery: results from the patient safety in surgery study. *J Am Coll Surg*. 2007; 204:1211–1221.

[20] Arcelus JI, Candocia S, Traverso CI, Fabrega F, Caprini JA, Hasty JH. Venous thromboembolism prophylaxis and risk assessment in medical patients. Semin Thromb Hemost. 1991; 17(Suppl 3):313–318.

[21] Pannucci CJ, Bailey SH, Dreszer G, Fisher Wachtman C, Zumsteg JW, Jaber RM, Hamill JB, Hume KM, Rubin JP, Neligan PC, Kalliainen LK, Hoxworth RE, Pusic AL, Wilkins EG. Validation of the Caprini risk assessment model in plastic and reconstructive surgery patients. J Am Coll Surg. 2011; 212:105–112.

[22] Caprini JA. Thrombosis risk assessment as a guide to quality patient care. Dis Mon. 2005; 51:70–78.

[23] Motykie GD, Zebala LP, Caprini JA, Lee CE, Arcelus JI, Reyna JJ, Cohen EB. A guide to venous thromboembolism risk factor assessment. J Thromb Thrombolysis. 2000; 9:253–262.

[24] Caprini JA. Risk assessment as a guide to thrombosis prophylaxis. Curr Opin Pulm Med. 2010; 16:448–452.

[25] Pannucci CJ, MacDonald JK, Ariyan S, Gutowski KA, Kerrigan CL, Kim JY, Chung KC. Benefits and risks of prophylaxis for deep venous thrombosis and pulmonary embolus in plastic surgery: a systematic review and meta-analysis of controlled trials and consensus conference. Plast Reconstr Surg. February 2016; 137(2):709–30.

[26] Gould MK, Garcia DA, Wren SM, Karanicolas PJ, Arcelus JI, Heit JA, Samama CM, American College of Chest Physicians. Prevention of VTE in nonorthopedic surgical patients: antithrombotic therapy and prevention of thrombosis: American College of Chest Physicians Evidence-Based Clinical Practice Guidelines. Chest. 2012; 141(Suppl):e227S–e277S.

[27] Sellam P, Trevidic P. The thromboembolic risk in abdominal plastic surgery: a randomized statistical study. Ann Chir Plast Esthet. 1999; 44:545–548.

[28] Shuman AG, Hu HM, Pannucci CJ, Jackson CR, Bradford CR, Bahl V. Stratifying the risk of venous thromboembolism in otolaryngology. Otolaryngol Head Neck Surg. 2012; 146:719–724.

[29] Comerota AJ, Stewart GJ, Alburger PD, Smalley K, White JV. Operative venodilation: a previously unsuspected factor in the cause of postoperative deep vein thrombosis. Surgery. 1989; 106:301–308; discussion 308.

[30] Swanson E. Ultrasound screening for deep venous thrombosis detection: a prospective evaluation of 200 plastic surgery outpatients. Plast Reconstr Surg Glob Open. 2015; 3:e332.

[31] Guyatt G, GuttermanD, Baumann MH, et al. Grading strength of recommendations and quality of evidence in clinical guidelines: report from an American College of Chest Physicians task force. Chest. 2006; 129:174–181.

[32] Benkö T, Cooke EA, McNally MA, Mollan RA. Graduated compression stockings: knee length or thigh length. Clin Orthop Relat Res. 2001; 383:197–203.

[33] Sachdeva A, Dalton M, Amaragiri SV, Lees T. Elastic compression stockings for prevention of deep vein thrombosis. Cochrane Database Syst Rev. 2010; 7:CD001484.

[34] Comerota AJ, Chouhan V, Harada RN, et al. The fibrinolytic effects of intermittent pneumatic compression: mechanism of enhanced fibrinolysis. Ann Surg. 1997; 226:306–313; discussion 313.

[35] Ho KM, Tan JA. Stratified meta-analysis of intermittent pneumatic compression of the lower limbs to prevent venous thromboembolism in hospitalized patients. Circulation 2013; 128:1003–1020.

[36] Gavriel H, Thompson E, Kleid S, Chan S, Sizeland A. Safety of thromboprophylaxis after oncologic head and neck surgery: study of 1018 patients. Head Neck 2013; 35:1410–1414.

[37] Bristol Meyers Squibb. U.S. FDA approves Eliquis (apixaban) to reduce the risk of blood clots following hip or knee replacement surgery. March 14, 2014. Available at: http://news.bms.com/pressrelease/us-fda-approves-eliquis-apixaban-reduce-risk-blood-clots-following-hip-or-knee-replace. Accessed April 27, 2015.

[38] Bayer HealthCare. Rivaroxaban (Web). Available at: www.xareltohcp.com. Accessed April 27, 2015.

[39] Turpie AG, Bauer KA, Caprini JA, Comp PC, Gent M, Muntz JE; Apollo Investigators. Fondaparinux combined with intermittent pneumatic compression vs. intermittent pneumatic compression alone for prevention of venous thromboembolism after abdominal surgery: a randomized, double-blind comparison. J Thromb Haemost. 2007; 5:1854–1861.

[40] Henke PK, Arya S, Pannucci C, et al. Procedure-specific venous thromboembolism prophylaxis: a paradigm from colectomy surgery. Surgery. 2012; 152:528–534; discussion 534.

[41] Kakkos SK, Caprini JA, Geroulakos G, Nicolaides AN, Stansby GP, Reddy DJ. Combined intermittent pneumatic leg compression and pharmacological prophylaxis for

prevention of venous thromboembolism in high-risk patients. Cochrane Database Syst Rev. 2008; 4:CD005258.

[42] Kakkos SK, Caprini JA, Geroulakos G, et al. Can combined (mechanical and pharmacological) modalities prevent fatal VTE? Int Angiol. 2011; 30:115–122.

[43] Pannucci CJ, Dreszer G, Wachtman CF, et al. Postoperative enoxaparin prevents symptomatic venous thromboembolism in high-risk plastic surgery patients. Plast Reconstr Surg. 2011; 128:1093–1103.

[44] Davison SP, Massoumi W. Our complication, your problem. Plast Reconstr Surg. 2007; 120:1428–1429.

[45] McDevitt NB. Deep vein thrombosis prophylaxis. American Society of Plastic and Reconstructive Surgeons. Plast Reconstr Surg. 1999; 104:1923–1928.

[46] Akl EA, Kahale L, Sperati F, et al. Low molecular weight heparin versus unfractionated heparin for perioperative thromboprophylaxis in patients with cancer. Cochrane Database Syst Rev. 2014; 6:CD009447.

[47] Hardy RG, Williams L, Dixon JM. Use of enoxaparin results in more haemorrhagic complications after breast surgery than unfractionated heparin. Br J Surg. 2008; 95:834–836.

[48] Losken A, Carlson GW, Culbertson JH, et al. Omental free flap reconstruction in complex head and neck deformities. Head Neck. 2002; 24:326–331.

[49] Losken A, Carlson GW, Tyrone JW, et al. The significance of intraabdominal compartment pressure after free versus pedicled TRAM flap breast reconstruction. Plast Reconstr Surg. 2005; 115:261–263.

[50] Pannucci CJ, Alderman AK, Brown SL, Wakefield TW, Wilkins EG. The effect of abdominal wall plication on intraabdominal pressure and lower extremity venous flow: a case report. J Plast Reconstr Aesthet Surg. 2012; 65:392–394.

4

Axillary Breast: Contouring the Axilla

Medha A. Bhave (Khair)

Abstract

Commonest cause of disturbed axillary aesthetics is aberrant breast tissue. Our study presents 24 consecutive patients with axillary breast or lipomas, treated with liposuction alone or excision with limited liposuction of axillary folds and dog ears; between 2005 and 2015. Optimum aesthetic outcome was due to i) Pre-op marking in maximum abduction ii) Elliptical excision of apical, hairy skin in the direction of maximum laxity irrespective of location of axillary breast iii) Raising thick flaps to avoid tethering of the scar iv) Meticulous dissection to preserve nerves, axillary pad of fat and lymph nodes, v) Limited liposuction under vision to sculpt axillary folds and dog ears, vi) Suturing in position of maximum abduction, vi) Stretchable tape for dressing instead of pressure garment suitable for unique shape of axilla.

First patient treated with liposuction alone required removal of residual mass whereas patients undergoing axillaplasty had no major complications, had acceptable scars and were happy to have reduction in hair bearing axillary skin. Thereafter only two more patients were treated with liposuction alone. (5 axillae) 21 patients (42 axillae) underwent excisional sculpting of axilla with limited liposuction. Complications were minor and axillary scars were imperceptible and acceptable. We prefer excisional axillaplasty with limited liposuction after the excision. Liposuction alone cannot address the problem satisfactorily and safely.

Keywords: axillary breast, axillary aesthetics, excisional axillaplasty, limited liposuction in axilla, accessory breast

1. Introduction

Axilla can be the seat of many deforming swellings but the commonest malady that compromises appearance and causes concern is axillary breast. Other benign conditions such as lipoma, lymphadenopathy, hidradenitis suppurativa and vascular malformations must be kept in mind nevertheless.

Peri-pubertal and peri-partum increase in the size of axillary breast causes not only aesthetic concerns but discomfort due to poor arm posture, sweating, and stickiness; not to mention the limitation of choice in apparels that can be worn.

2. Surgical anatomy of the axilla

Axilla is a pyramidal structure—with a concave floor made up of skin and subcutaneous fat—facing laterally and inferiorly [1].

The four borders are

A—anterior axillary fold comprising of free border of pectoralis major,

B—posterior axillary fold comprising of free border of latissimus dorsi muscle,

C and D—the anterior and posterior lines defining the upper, medial arm.

The medial and lateral faces of pyramid comprise of convex upper rib cage medially and inter-tubercular sulcus of humerus laterally. The anterior and posterior faces are free. The apex of

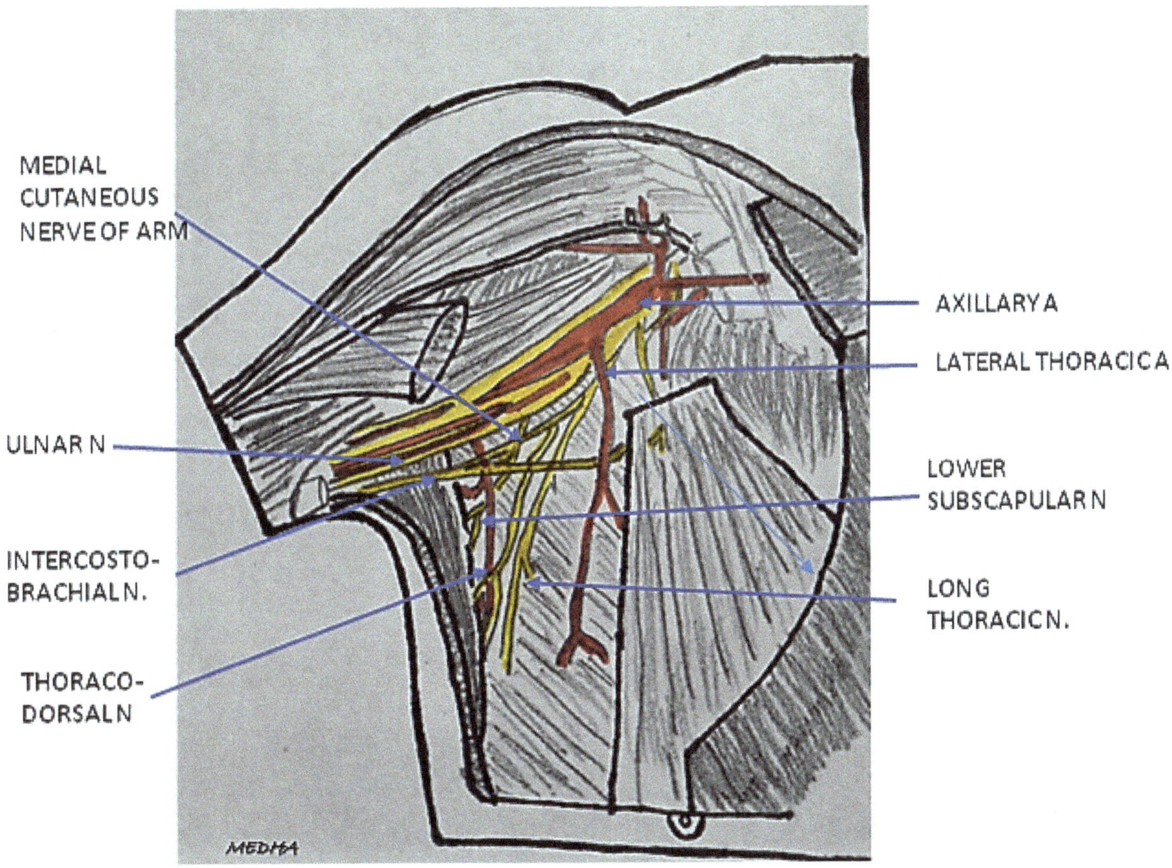

Figure 1. Surgical anatomy of axilla.

the axilla harbors axillary pad of fat, lymph-nodes and lymphatics draining Upper limb as well as the neuro-vascular structures. The latter include intercosto-brachial nerve, medial cutaneous nerve of the arm and the cephalic vein. The apex has axillary artery and vein, invested in layer of fascia. Spencer's foramen is an opening in the pectoral fascia which allows passage of axillary tail of the breast. **Figure 1** illustrates the anatomy in detail.

3. Aesthetic considerations in axilla

3.1. Aesthetic landmarks and their anatomy: physiology of axillary skin

The anterior and posterior axillary folds and the concave floor are key features to consider in order to improve aesthetics of the axilla. The anterior and posterior axillary folds smoothly curving to medial arm can be termed anterior and posterior axillary aesthetic lines respectively, akin to dorsal aesthetic lines of the nose (**Figure 2**).

A fatty fold rolls over into axilla filling it and reducing the definition. A scar crossing the fold of axilla interrupting its smooth transition into medial line of arm violates the aesthetic

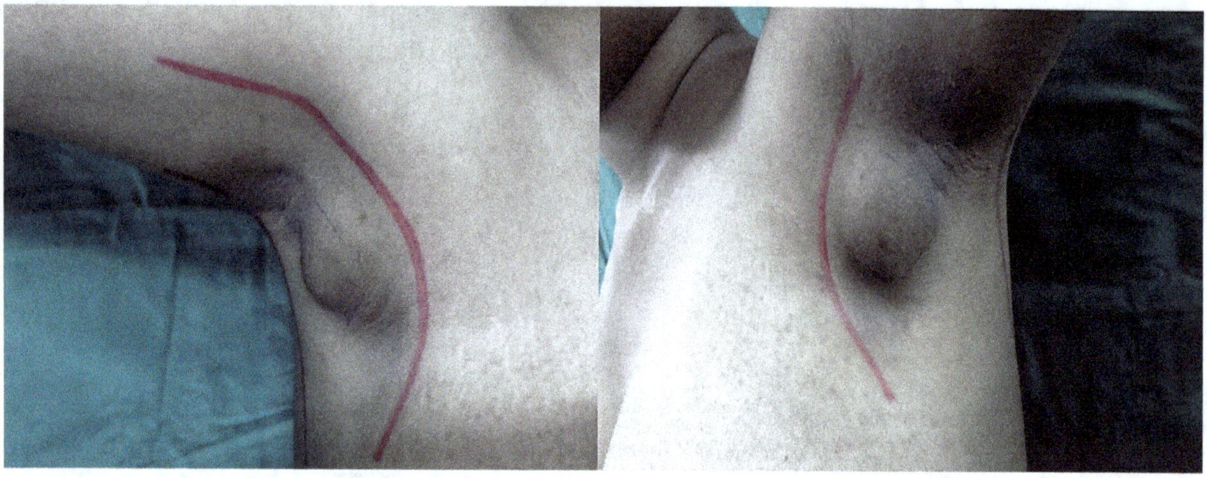

Figure 2. Anterior and posterior axillary aesthetic lines.

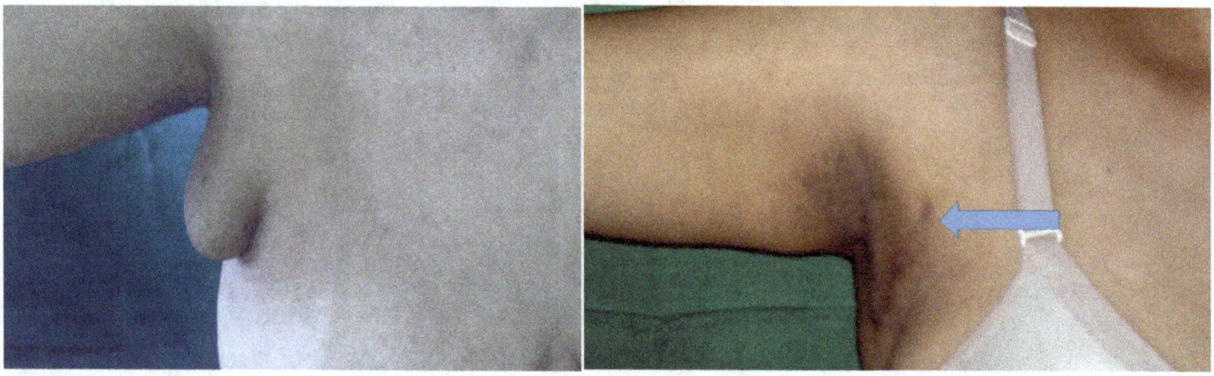

Figure 3. A scar crossing the anterior axillary fold compromises outcome.

landmarks, as illustrated in **Figure 3** which shows pre-operative and post-operative photographs of a patient.

Full and convex floor makes it appear unattractive; as also when the floor is irregular, scarred and tethered.

The axillary skin is hairy and rich in apocrine type of sweat glands that open into the piliary canal of the hair follicle. They are larger (800 μm) and secrete a substance that is thicker than that secreted by eccrine glands distributed over rest of the body. The substance is oily, odorless and rich in proteins, lipids and steroids. This nurtures the bacteria on the skin leading to peculiar odor. The apocrine sweat contains pheromone-like substances. The axillary apocrine glands are active during sexual excitement and under stress [2, 3].

It is a common practice to shave axilla in women who wear sleeveless tops as well as in metrosexual men. In tropical countries like India, men often wear sleeveless apparel due to hot climate.

4. Embryology: mammary ridge

4.1. Accessory breast and Kajava classification

4.1.1. Definition of axillary breast

*4.1.1.1. Classification of axillary breast**

The mammary ridge in fetal life extends from axilla to groin. Incomplete involution can lead to accessory breast anywhere along this milk line.

Accessory breast tissue is defined as the presence of extra breast tissue in ***addition*** to normal breast tissue [4]. About 2–6% women have this condition and 20% of all accessory breasts occur in axilla [5, 6]. The accessory breast was classified by Kajava et al. in 1915; based on composition of the aberrant tissue [6, 7]. The diagrammatic representation shown in **Figure 4** can be useful for diagrammatic representation, though the classification is rather cumbersome for practical use.

The axillary breast is a type of accessory breast, located in the axilla. It can be of any Kajava type though we have seen only type 4 in axilla. If there is a connection through spencer's foramen, it can be considered as axillary tail of the breast. In the absence of connection, it is simply an accessory breast tissue in the axilla. Though the management remains the same, ligation of the tail is an important maneuver in case of axillary tail—as it may contain a vessel.

An anatomical sub-classification of axillary breast was proposed by Bhave, according to location [8].

1. Central axillary
2. Para-mammary
3. Medial arm.

Figure 5 shows clinical illustration of the same.

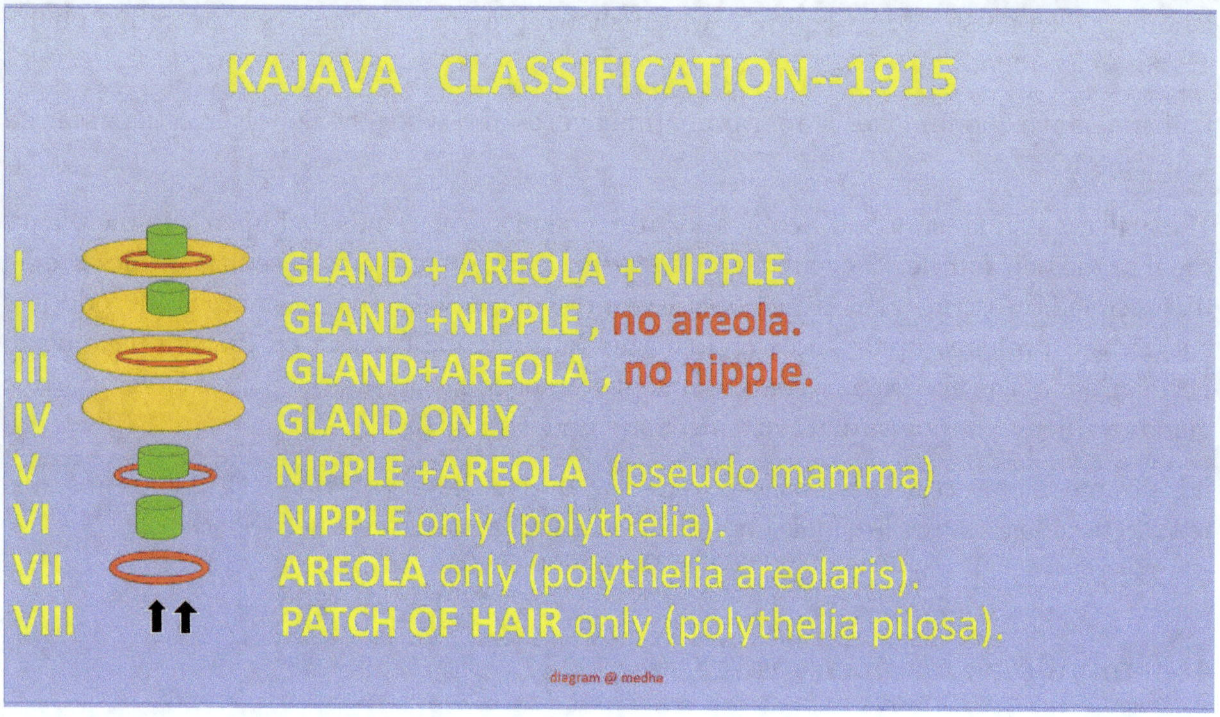

Figure 4. Diagrammatic representation of Kajava classification based on composition of accessory breast. Solid oval = breast tissue, hollow oval = areola, rod = nipple, arrows = hair.

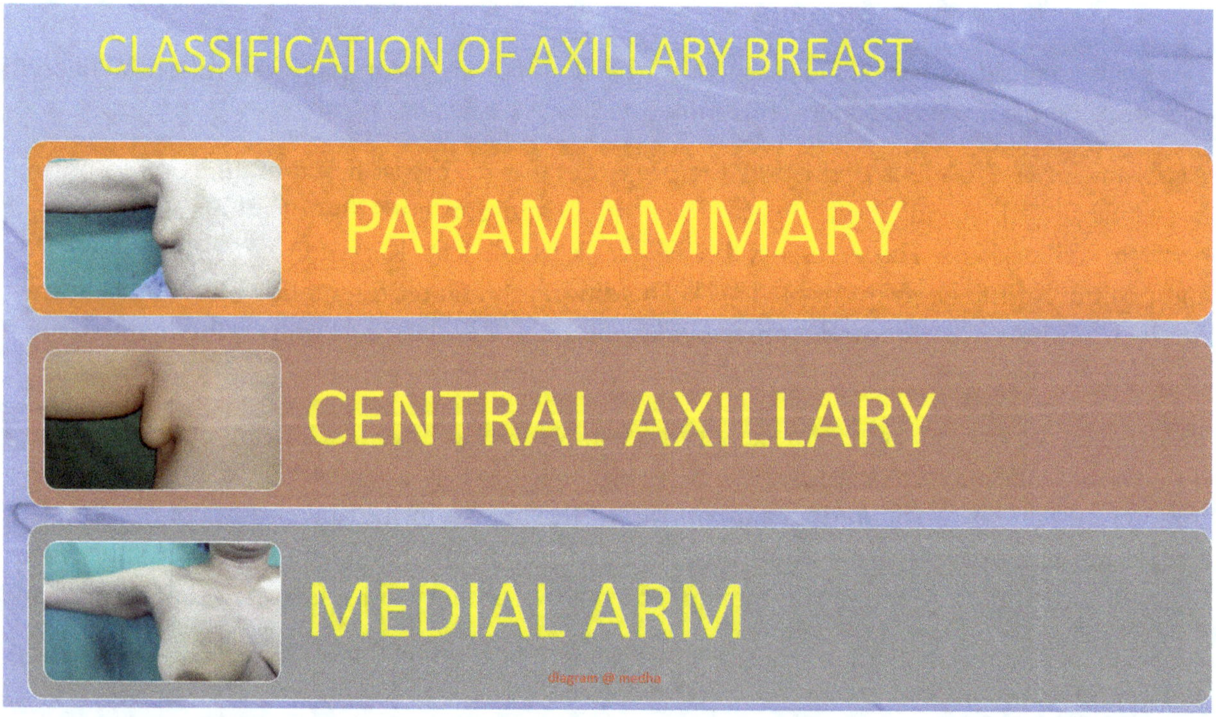

Figure 5. Classification of axillary breast—Bhave Medha.

The classification has diagnostic significance, as many type 2 and 3 breasts can be misdiagnosed as other pathology, which may lead to inferior choice of incision and poor cosmetic outcome.

5. Clinical presentation: symptoms

5.1. Expectations from surgeon

5.1.1. Philosophy of interpretation of a woman's symptoms

Table 1 summarizes the common symptoms in our series. Most of other reports in the literature are by radiologists. Hence the commonest presentation in their series is asymptomatic. There is lack of awareness of the available modes of treatment and fear of scar, which leads to under-reporting. Even if the condition is congenital, most women develop the swelling during hormonal surges such as menarche or pregnancy. The presentation may be at any age, since this is not a pressing complaint unless the patient is worried about cancer.

The reason why treatment is sought is often said to be inability to wear sleeveless tops. In fact, Laurence Kirwan has included this in definition.

Inability to wear proper clothes	23/24
Inability to maintain proper arm posture	20/24
Sweating, sticky skin and discomfort	20/24
Cosmetic concern	18/24
Pain in the lump	11/24
Fear of malignancy- voiced by older patients	2/24
Pain along the medial arm	1/24

Table 1. Symptomatology.

In our series, most of the women felt sweaty, sticky and malodorous due to the presence of mass in the axilla. Fear of cancer, inability to maintain arms in proper posture, pain along the medial arm were the other symptoms. Inability to wear proper clothes was a secondary reason in most women.

A woman needs not only to be heard but also listened to. A surgeon should consider the functional aspects of body contouring surgery before aesthetic as most of the women, especially from India are not seeking to wear exposing attire, but simply want to be comfortable and efficient in daily life.

6. Differential diagnosis

Every structure in the axilla can cause swelling and be confused with axillary breast [8].

A. Lymphadenopathy—tubercular is the commonest in India. **Figure 6**.

B. Hidradenitis suppurativa—very common in tropical countries.

C. Lipoma.

D. Malignancy.

E. Sebaceous cyst.

F. Vascular malformation.

In our series, we have encountered everything except vascular malformation.

It must be noted that the axillary breast can be seat of every benign and malignant disease that can occur in mammary tissue.

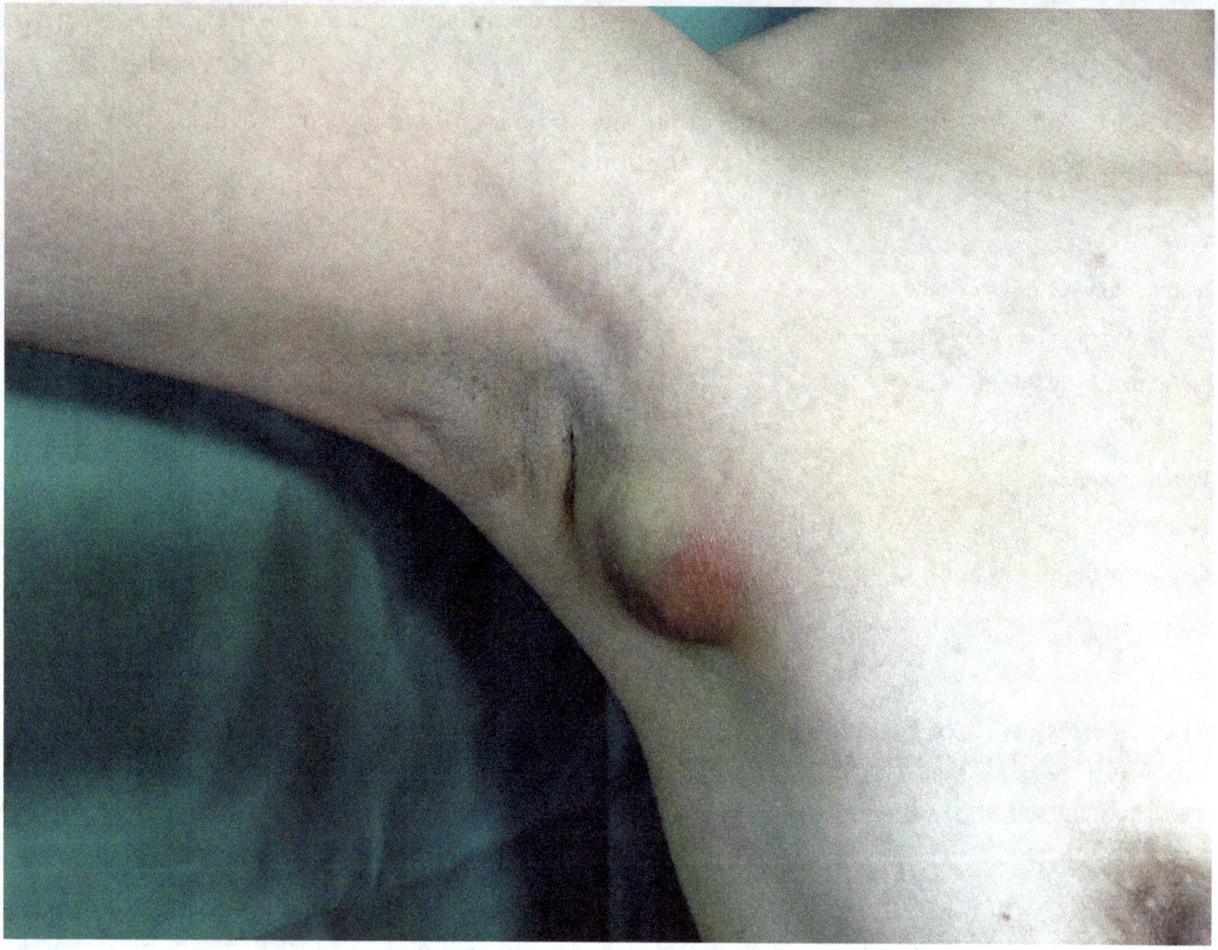

Figure 6. Tubercular lymphadenopathy. Patient presented 2 days prior to this cellulitis as axillary breast.

7. Investigations

It follows from the above discussion that ultrasonography of the axilla is the primary modality to diagnose the nature of the swelling, define its contents and establish or rule out vascular connection.

Color Doppler should be done in case of vascular swellings as and when required. Mammography is routinely done to rule out any associated breast pathology.

MRI may be required in some cases where additional pathology like tubercular lymphadenopathy or malignancy is suspected.

8. Treatment modalities and logical choice

The various treatment modalities include [9, 10]

A—open excision,

B—liposuction,

C—non surgical methods like injection lipolysis, high intensity focalised ultrasound (HIFU), etc.

D—combination of excision and suction—axillaplasty.

A—Open Excision.—This can be undertaken in a small mass. But for a large mass this may result in long scars that may cross aesthetic landmarks of axilla.

B—liposuction alone—following hazards of closed procedures in axilla are encountered.

Axilla in abduction—as required for the operation—brings important neuro-vascular structures to the floor and thus makes them prone to injury by the cannula. In adduction, these structures remain at the apex but one cannot operate in such a position. Hence, liposuction alone is a hazardous choice as a primary modality.

Usually, the axillary breast tissue contains fair number of glandular structures, making it difficult to produce satisfactory result with liposuction alone. The use of sharp cannula—as used in male gynaecomastia by some surgeons—is not advisable, due to proximity of important structures. Leaving behind residue of the gland—and suctioning only to produce contouring—is against the principles of surgery. The residue can re-enlarge later. Thus, even if closed liposuction has advantages like minimal scar; the dead space and non-retraction of skin are major deterrents to wide use of this method. Though tumescent liposuction is strongly advocated by some authors [9, 10], it may be hazardous for aforementioned reasons.

C—non surgical procedures like injection lipolysis cannot be used as the agents can cause venous thrombosis and fibrosis in the axilla leading to peri-neural inflammation, fibrosis and pain.

D—axillaplasty—definition and concept.

The term axillaplasty was introduced by Laurence Kirwan in 2009. He defines axillaplasty as follows—axillaplasty is a procedure to correct the overhang of fat and skin above the bra at the armpit, which limits tops that women can wear. The fat is suctioned and excess skin is removed creating a neat thin line scar hidden in the apex of the axilla. The wound is closed with a knotless absorbable barbed 2-0 and 3-0 barbed suture, which aids in the healing [11].

He presented the procedure in 2009 at Las Vegas aesthetic meeting.

We adopted the procedure for management of the axillary breast. Open excision of the breast tissue and skin is done first, reserving the liposuction only to contour the axilla suction the anterior and posterior axillary folds, minimize the dog ears and reduce the length of the axillary scar.

Documentation—sonography report stating the percentage of breast stroma and fatty tissue.

Photographs—frame—mid neck to nipple level

Views—"spread wing" view with arms at right angle—both sides, Rt axilla, Lt axilla.

—Arms abducted above the head—both sides—depicts relation with pectoralis major

—Arms by side—both sides.

8.1. The detailed procedure of excisional axillaplasty

General anaesthesia is used after proper medical fitness is evaluated [8]. Marking is done with arm in abduction—the lax skin is pinched and marked as an ellipse in the direction of maximum laxity. This skin is to be excised (**Figure 7**).

Palpable extent of the gland is marked with dotted lines. The axillary folds may be marked if too bulky [8].

Infiltration is done in a deep plane with 1 in 200,000 adrenaline with, 1% lignocaine in saline. Subdermal infiltration is used only for the incision. If simultaneous liposuction of the back is planned, it is marked pre-operatively and infiltrated after completion of axillaplasty. Skin incision is deepened till superficial fascia as depicted in **Figure 8**. Thick flaps are elevated on either sides to define the axillary breast [8].

Meticulous dissection to separate the breast, preserving every nerve going through the mass, is undertaken. Pectoral border medially, cephalic vein superiorly and the lateral edge of the mass laterally are the limits of dissection. Intercostobrachial nerve is invariably found to be passing through the mass and needs to be preserved as shown in **Figure 9**. The medial cutaneous nerve of arm if encountered, axillary pad of fat and lymph nodes is preserved. The mass usually separates well. If connection with the mammary tissue is identified through foramen of spence, it should be ligated and haemostasis achieved. Excision is essential because there is no other way to safely remove the tough breast tissue with suction. The sharp cannula used sometimes in gynaecomastia cannot be used for fear of damage to nerves.

8.2. Limited liposuction of dog ears, axillary folds and back

Arm is then abducted and temporary staplers are used to secure best position for suturing with minimum dog ears. The dog ears are then thoroughly suctioned. Chasing the dog ear lengthens the scar and if it crosses any anatomical land-mark, the aesthetic outcome suffers. If required, the thick flaps can now be suctioned to contour the floor. Flaps that are too thin will tether to the floor and give unnatural appearance. Moreover, this suction is well away from the important neurovascular structures. It must be noted that liposuction alone is not enough to produce the desired result due to invariable presence of firm breast tissue in the mass.

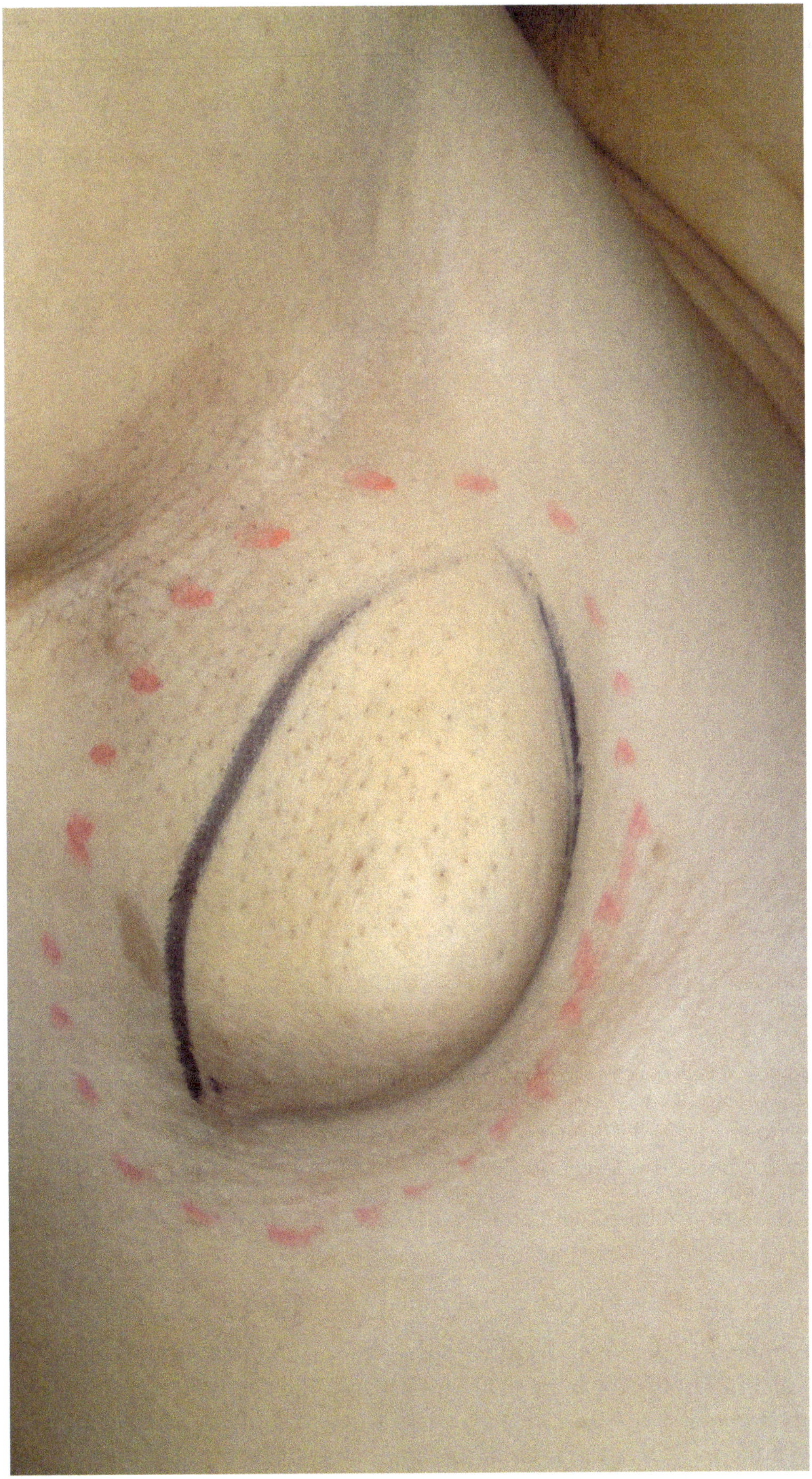

Figure 7. Marking the incision in direction of maximum laxity. Dotted lines mark the margin of the palpable mass.

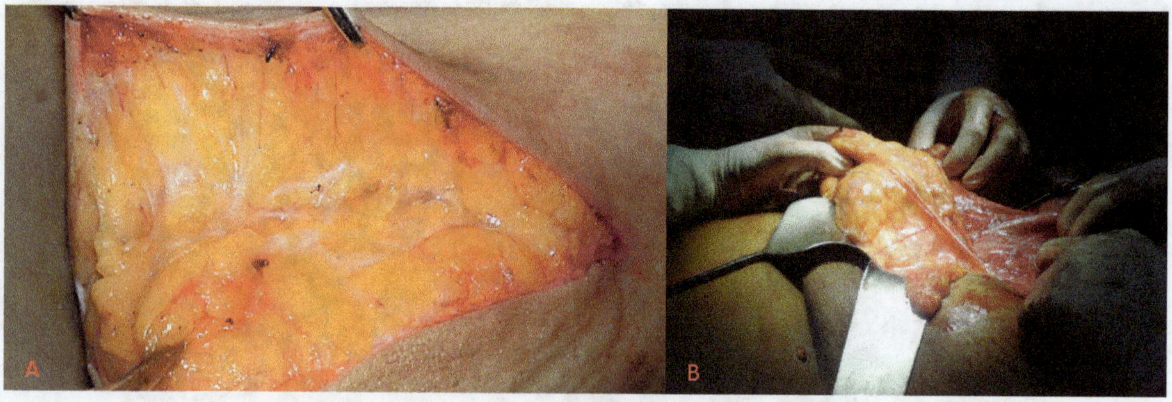

Figure 8. (A) Flaps at level of superficial fascia. (B) Well demarcated mass.

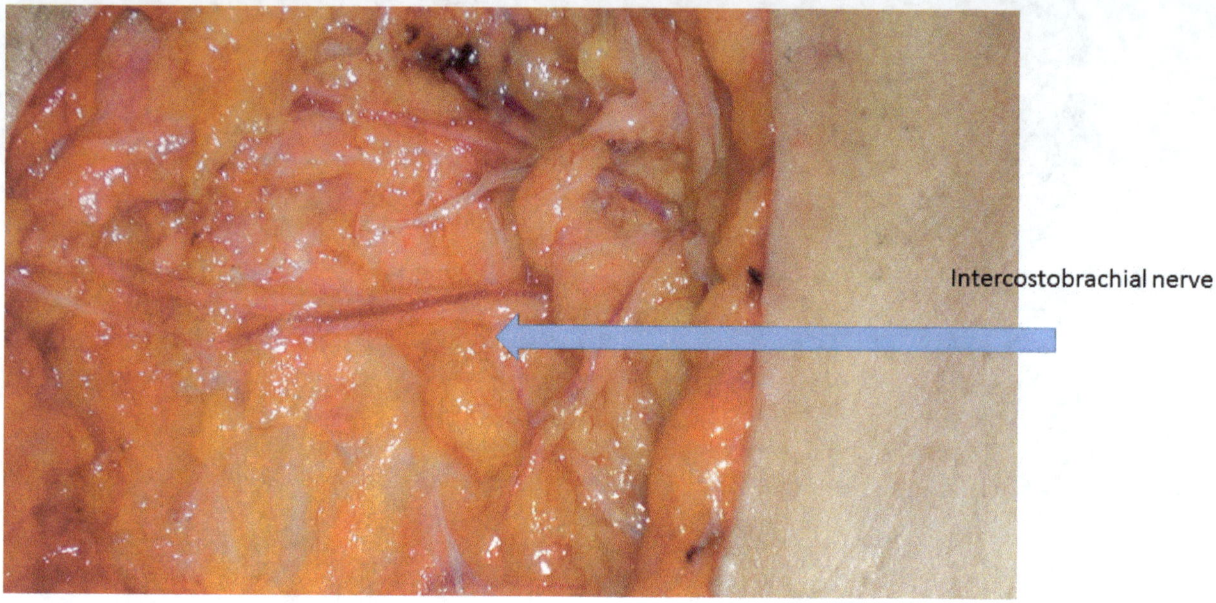

Figure 9. Meticulous dissection of nerves and vessels involved in the swelling is needed to avoid post-operative neuralgia.

8.3. Drains

Suturing is done with 3-0 PDS in two layers. We never needed drains in any of our patients, but they should be used when in doubt.

Axillaplasty can be combined with breast reduction [12].

8.4. Properties of hair bearing skin and advantages of reduction

The hair bearing skin does not retract well after liposuction [8]. Thus, skin excess cannot be taken care of as addressed in abdominal liposuctions. The overhang remains if liposuction is used alone and necessitates excision. Thus, it is wiser to combine the two at the outset. The axillary sweating and hair are matters of concern for most women, and they are happy to have this skin reduced. Despite presence of hair, the scars are imperceptible and often better accepted in exchange of reduction in hair bearing skin.

9. Post-operative program: dressings

9.1. Problem of pressure garments

9.1.1. Problems of compressive dressing

The dressing is done with a thick gauze and cotton pad secured with stretchable many tailed tape as depicted in **Figure 10**. Hypo allergic tape can be used but one may not be able to obtain adequate pressure. Pressure garments are not reliable due to the peculiar shape of the axilla. They can also cause compression of the nerves and veins in the arms due to tight sleeves resulting in edema of the dorsi of the hands. The very first patient in

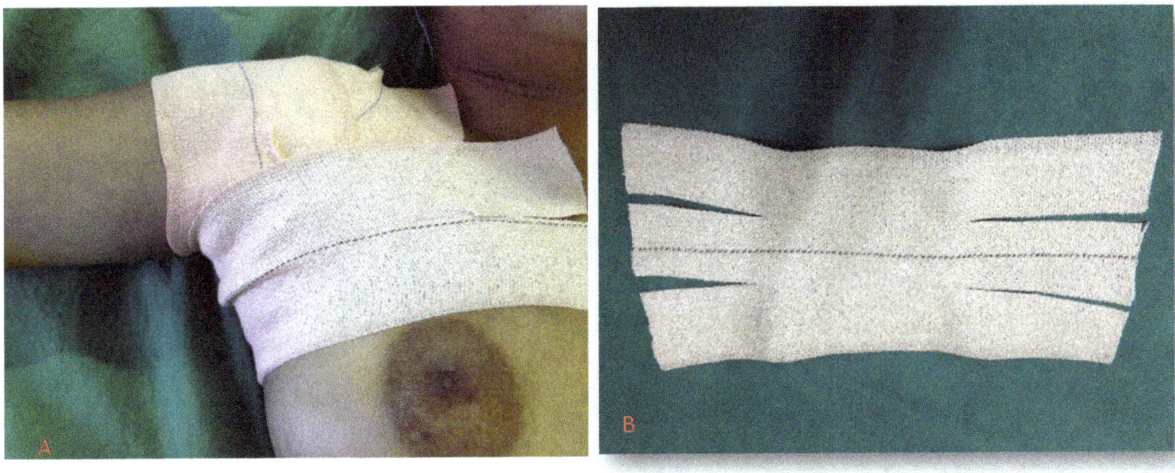

Figure 10. (A) Many tailed dressing drapes well around axilla with concave floor. (B) Way to cut the tape.

our series had come for minimal access surgery. She found it extremely difficult to wear the garment during post-op period due to tingling numbness in the forearms and hands due to excessive pressure on the arms due to tight sleeves. Even after releasing that pressure, we realized that more pressure was at the junction of sleeves and body of the garment than on axilla. Figure of eight dressing—like a clavicular brace—was tried but was found to be inefficient. We have found the many-tailed elastic tape very useful as it goes around the contours of shoulder and chest wall to provide sufficient compression without nerve compression and distal edema. One patient in our series developed severe allergy and blisters due to the tape. Careful monitoring is required, and the tape has to be removed if patient complains of itching without waiting for blisters to develop.

10. Results of excisional axillaplasty with limited liposuction

Our study comprises 24 patients presenting with axillary masses.

The result of surgery upon our initial patient, who insisted on liposuction alone, paved the way to our current method of choice-excisional sculpting with limited liposuction. After her

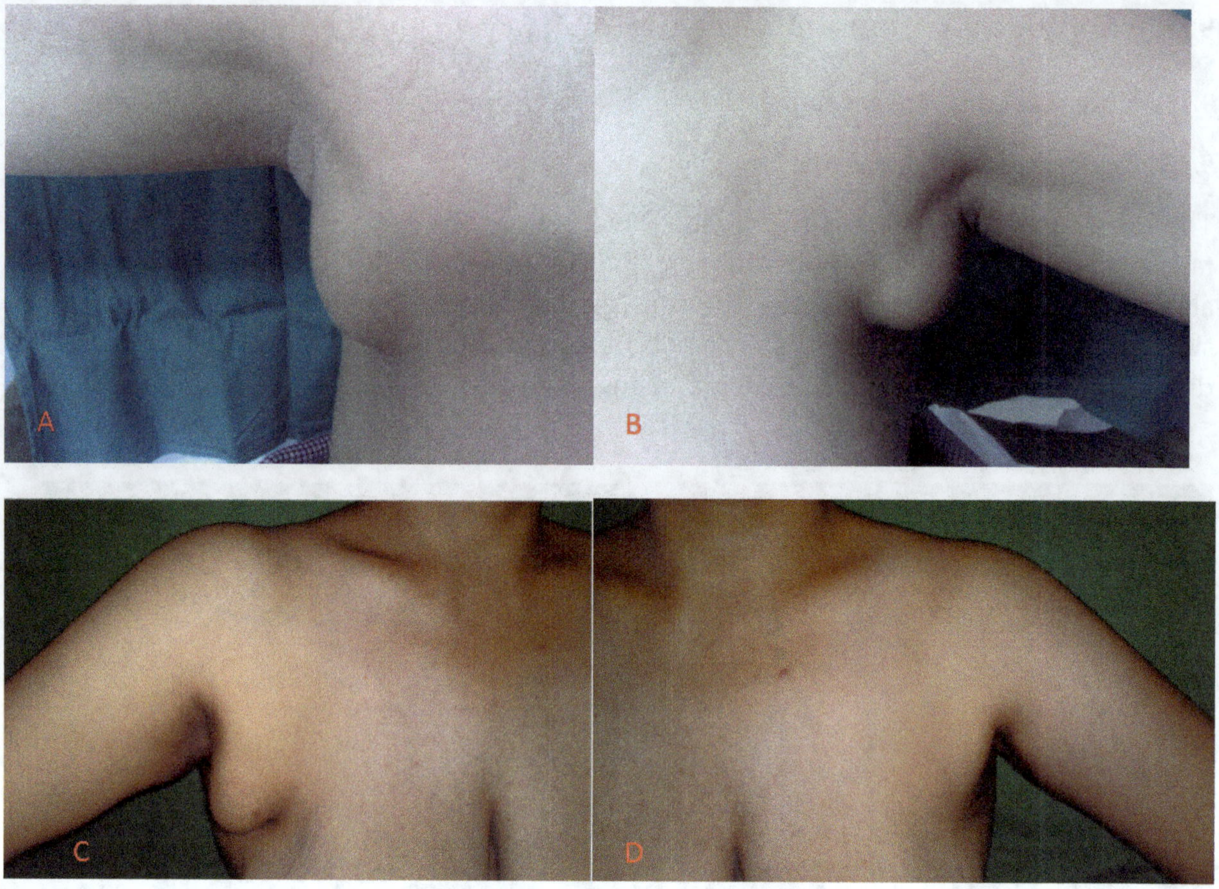

Figure 11. (A and B) Pre-op of 24 year old air-hostess. (C and D) After closed liposuction. Note residual gland in Rt axilla. Glabrous skin appears to be in excess but non retraction of hairy skin has resulted in excess.

liposuction of both axillary breasts, she had residual mass on right side with solid breast tissue. She had burning of medial arms possibly due to nerve injury. She could not wear garment in post-op period due to distal swelling and tingling numbness. She had to undergo revision surgery on right side to remove residual mass and excess hair bearing skin, which did not retract after surgery as shown in **Figure 11C**.

Thereafter, only one patient underwent liposuction, but she had predominantly fatty tissue. She was lost to follow-up after 1 month.

The rest of the patients was treated by axillaplasty as described above. All patients were photographed pre-operatively, 1 and 6 months post-operatively. They were evaluated for scar quality and aesthetic outcome. **Figure 12** shows a routine result of open axillaplasty.

The rest of the results are tabulated in **Table 2**.

Most of the patients who appeared to have dog ears and mildly hypertrophic scar were found to have total diminution of the scar and resolution of dog ears at the end of 6 months (**Figure 13**).

One patient who had a lipoma in the axilla had previously undergone injection lipolysis outside. She was found to have thrombosis of all the veins in the field as illustrated in

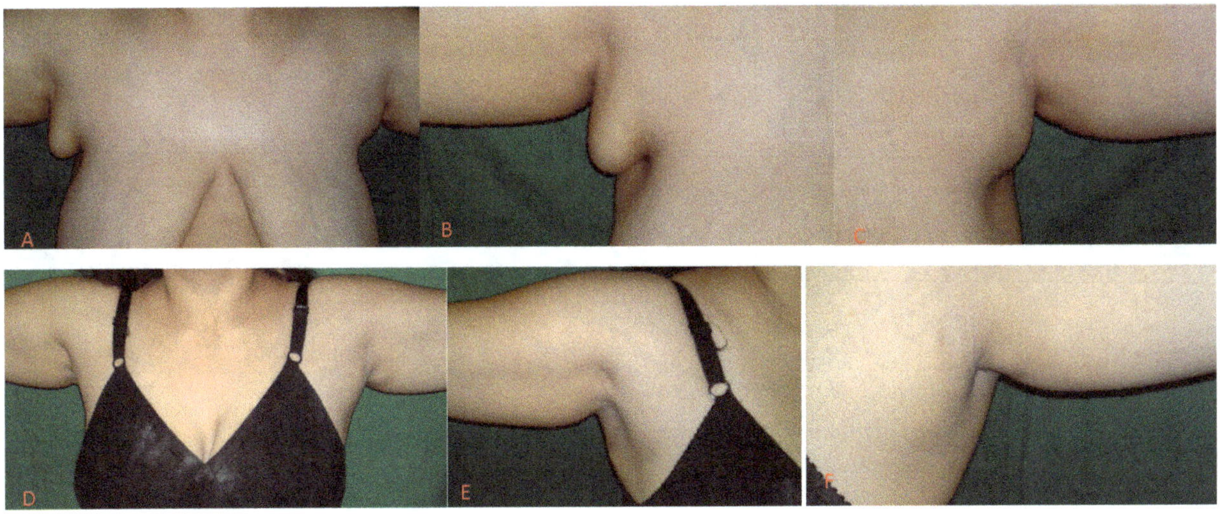

Figure 12. (A–C) Pre-op views Rt side axillaplasty, Lt-liposuction alone. (D–F) 6 months post-op.

Figure 14. This patient had severe medial arm burning pain, both locally and in the medial arm, for about 9 months and needed pregabalin therapy for the same.

The results clearly show that excisional sculpting of axilla is far safer and also an effective method to manage fatty axillary swellings [8, 9, 12]. **Figure 15** shows results of axillaplasty on medial arm type of axillary breast.

The well-maintained axillary aesthetic lines are demonstrated in another patient with central type of axillary breast are shown in **Figure 16**.

Method	No. of patients treated	Complications	Comment
Liposuction alone	Three patients, five axillae(One patient underwent excision on the other side)	One axilla, residual mass, nerve pain	Open surgery required
Axillaplasty with limited liposuction	21 Patients, 44 axillae	As in **Table 3**	As assessed at 6 months post-op

Table 2. Results.

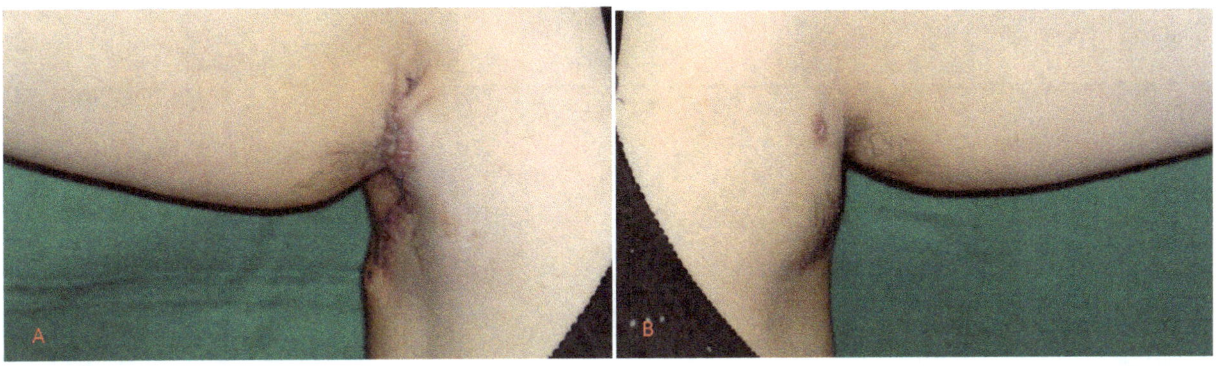

Figure 13. Interim status of patient in **figure 12**, taken at 1 month post-op, A-rt axilla, B-lt axilla. [The scars settled after 6 months as shown in **figure 12 (D-F)**].

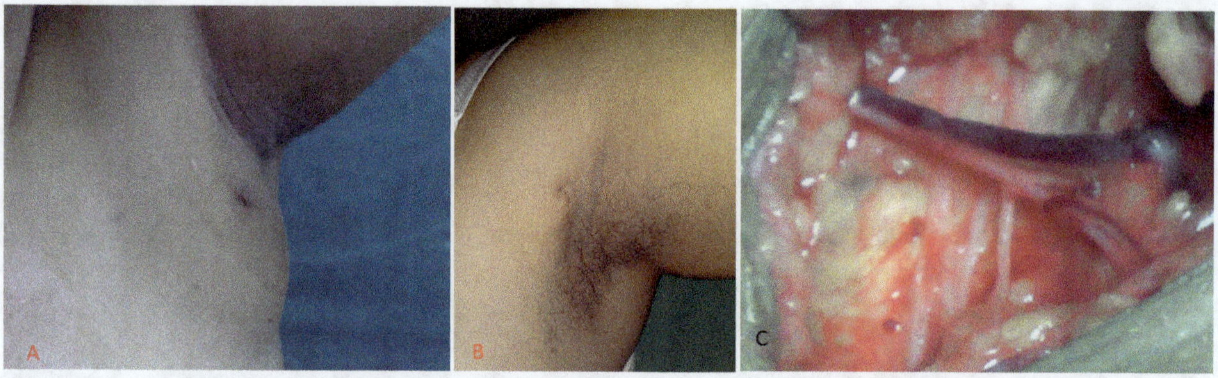

Figure 14. (A) Axillary lipoma with history of injection lipolysis done elsewhere. (B) 6 months after axillaplasty, scar is imperceptible. (C) Intra-op view showing thrombosed veins.

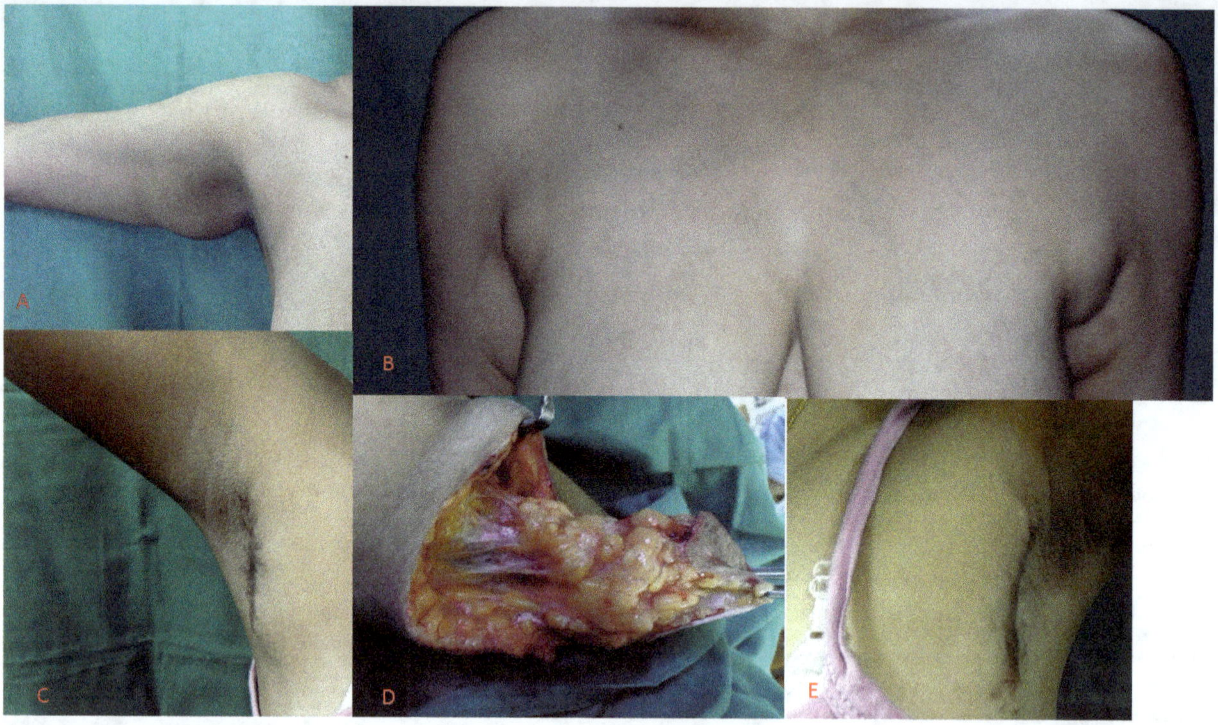

Figure 15. (A and B) Show pre-op views of medial arm type of axillary breast. All skin could be recruited to axilla to avoid a scar on inner arm. (D) Shows communication through foramen of Spencer. (C and E) Show post-op results with mild scar hypertrophy.

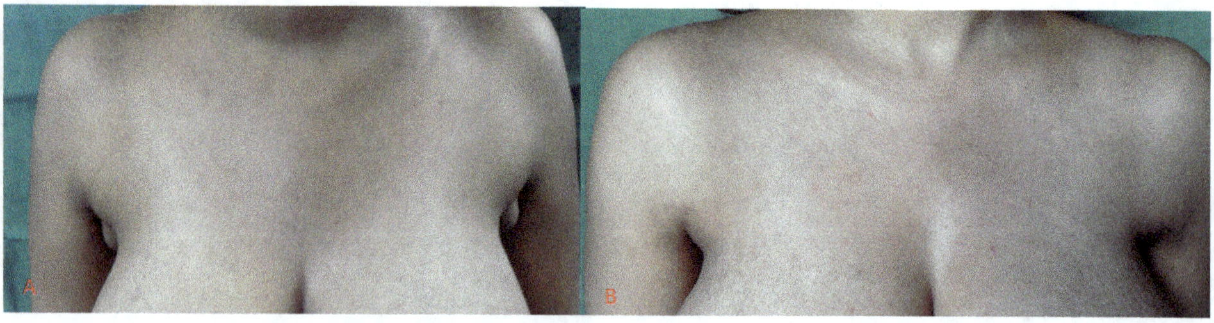

Figure 16. Well maintained axillary aesthetic lines after axilla plasty. 6 months post-op. A—pre-op, B—post-op.

11. Complications

The complications in our series are listed in **Tables 2** and **3** [8].

Bleeding due to vascular injury was not seen in our series. Excessive mobilization in post-op period can sometimes result in late hematoma. This occurred in one axilla of one of our patients on 8th post-op day. It responded to evacuation and pressure with many tailed elastic tape dressing.

Pain—post-operative shoulder stiffness and pain occurs in all patients. Injury to medial cutaneous nerve of arm and Intercostobrachial nerve can cause burning pain in the respective territory. This resolves in 1–6 months but may need neuro-regulators temporarily.

Infection—never occurred in our series. A pre-op cleansing schedule with surgical scrub solution is a part of our protocol.

Nerve injury—every small cutaneous twig in the field that does not lead to the skin being excised needs to be preserved. Else the area of supply would be seat of burning pain.

Seroma—never occurred in our series. Inadequate pressure can cause hematoma and seroma.

Dog ear—minor dog ears always settle with time.

Scars—hypertrophy.

Contracture.

Proper direction of incision in alignment with maximum laxity helps prevent contractures. Limited skin excision and closure without tension prevents hypertrophy. Some patients having

Complications	No. of patients	Comments
Mild scar hypertrophy	3	In one patient, scar crossed the anterior axillary fold but was not hypertrophic
Medial arm pain	2	Pain despite preservation of nerves Resolved with long-term pregabalin therapy
Allergy to sticking plaster	2	One required deroofing of blisters and collagen cover
Infection, seroma	Nil	
Haematoma	1	Developed due to forced passive exercise by a relative on 10th post-op. day. Responded to evacuation and pressure dressing
Dog ear	Nil	
Residual mass	Nil	
Axillary contracture	Nil	

Table 3. Complications of open axillaplasty with axillary sculpting in our series.

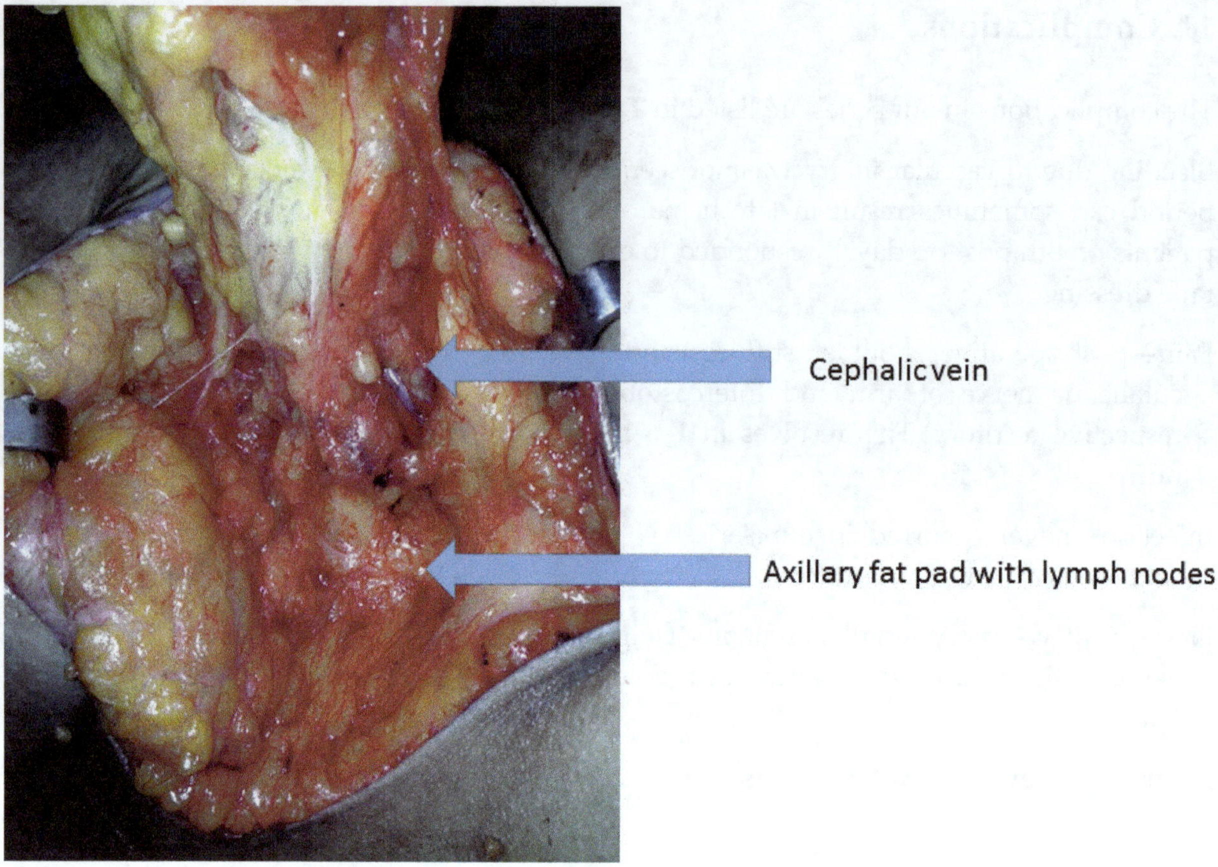

Figure 17. Lymphedema can be avoided by careful preservation of fat pad and nodes. Large nodes if any should be sent for histopathology.

tendency to hypertrophy can have problem, which can be managed with standard intralesional kenacort injections and silicon-based scar products.

Theoretically, lymphedema is possible complication, but preservation of axillary pad of fat and lymph nodes if any, limiting dissection below cephalic vein, helps to prevent it as shown in **Figure 17**. We have not encountered a single case so far.

12. Conclusion

Commonest disfiguring mass in axilla is axillary breast. Traditional liposuction for management incurs risk of nerve and vascular injury. Liposuction as sole modality of treatment is neither efficient nor sufficient for complete removal of axillary mass. Only excision results in ugly scars that violate the aesthetic landmarks of axilla. Excisional axillaplasty inclusive of excisional sculpting with limited liposuction for dog ears and axillary folds is safer choice. Scars in axilla heal exceptionally well despite being in the hair-bearing skin, if limited excision is planned, in the direction of maximum laxity. Other variants of axillary breast like paramammary and medial arm must be diagnosed correctly so that incision for removal can be placed in the axilla for better aesthetic outcome.

Acknowledgements

Dr. Anand Bhave, M. D., Staff at Param hospital and ICU, Thane.

Author details

Medha A. Bhave (Khair)

Address all correspondence to: bhavemedha@yahoo.co.in

Param Hospital and ICU, Thane, Maharashtra, India

References

[1] Warwick R, Williams P. Gray's Anatomy. 35th edition: Longman Group Ltd; 1973. p. 648.

[2] Wilke K., Martin A., Terstegen L., Biel S.S. A short history of sweat gland biology. International Journal of Cosmetic Science. 2007;**29**(November):169–179.

[3] Shelley J.D., Hurley H.J. The physiology of human axillary apocrine sweat gland. Journal of Investigative Dermatology. 1953;**20**(4):285–297.

[4] Lesavoy M.A., Gomez-Garcia A., Nejdi R., Yospur G., Syjau T.J., Chang P. Axillary breast tissue: clinical presentation and surgical treatment. Annals of Plastic Surgery. 1995;**35** (4):356–360.

[5] Owen Kang, R. Accessory Breast Tissue [Internet]. Available from: http://radiopaedia.org/articles/accessory-breast-tissue [Accessed: 1/06/2016]

[6] Patel P.P., Ibrahim A.M., Zhang J, et al. Accessory breast tissue. Eplasty. 2012;**2**:iC5. PMCID:PMC3336208.

[7] Sahu S., Hussain M., Sachan P. Bilateral accessory breast. Internet Journal of Surgery. 2007;**17**(2).

[8] Bhave M.A. Axillary breast: navigating uncharted Terrain. Indian Journal of Plastic Surgery. 2015;**48**(September–December):283–287.

[9] Bartsich S.A., Ofodile F.A. Accessory breast tissue in the axilla: classification and treatment. Plastic and Reconstructive Surgery; 2011;**128**(1):35e–36e.

[10] Fan J. Removal of accessory breasts, a novel tumescent liposuction approach. Aesthetic Plastic Surgery. 2009;**33**(6):809–813. doi:10.1007/s00266-009-9373-5.

[11] Kirwan L. drkirwan.com [Internet]. Available from: http://drkirwan.com/procedures/breast/axilla-plasty/ [Accessed: 1/06/2016]

[12] Aydogan F., Baghaki S., Celik V., Kocael A., Gokcal F., Cetinkale O., Unal H. Surgical treatment of axillary accessory breasts. The American Surgeon. 2010;**77**(3):270–272, PMID:20349654.

5

The History of Body Contouring Surgery

Balkovic Marija and Jankovic Irena

Abstract

Body contouring surgery is a rapidly evolving field in plastic surgery. In accordance with improvements in abdominal contour surgery, procedures to improve redundant skin elsewhere on the body were being devised. Initial attempts to correct the anomalies were made in the 1920s by Thorek and his contemporaries and consisted primarily of elliptical excisions of skin. All of the advances made in body contouring, from the original work of Kelly and his contemporaries to the modifications seen every decade, have contributed to a dynamic and evolving specialty. Currently, there is no field within the domain of plastic surgery growing with the same rapidity, and with worldwide obesity continually on the rise, the growth of this field is unlikely to abate in the near future. The contributions of Thorek, Passot, Pitanguy, Baroudi, Grazer, Wise, Regnault, Lassus, Illouz, Klein, Lockwood, and others have provided the necessary armamentarium to approach the post-weight loss patient knowingly, intently, and adequately equipped to restore pleasing contour to the patients we as surgeons care for. The combination of regional dermolipectomies, lifts, and suction lipoplasty has the potential to restore the elegant human form, to recreate gesture, and to restore appropriate structure.

Keywords: history, body contouring, surgery

1. History of body contouring

Physical look has always been very important to majority of people [1]. Unaesthetic fat deposits or loose skin, especially the ones without response to diet or physical exercise, has always been some of the major issues of modern age aesthetic surgery patients [2]. There are, however, differences in the distribution of the body fat between male and female patients. Men have less body fat around the waist, especially in the abdominal area; women generally have a higher percentage of body fat than men, especially around their thighs and buttocks, which is called gynoid fat. In overweight women, normally, the deposition of fat is mainly found below the waist. Patients with the extra amount of fat can feel uneasy, anxious, or embarrassed. Plastic and aesthetic surgery, through abdominoplasty and liposuction, has solved this problem, in order to achieve pleasant cosmetic results, i.e., to deliver an improved aesthetical image to the patients [2].

Evolving together with weight loss surgery, the field of body contouring surgery has assayed to sculpt a satisfying form surgically. Operative interventions of this type, where surgeons remove large amounts of fat and excess skin, are not something new, although they are growing rapidly with quite accessible treatment.

2. History of abdominal procedures

First, there were functional panniculectomies with various approaches concerning the scar shape and its location [2]. Over a century ago, in 1880, in France, Demars and Marx reported a large resection of skin and fat from the abdominal wall. In 1899, Dr. Kelly performed a panniculectomy with an elliptical transversal incision around the umbilicus [3]. In 1901, Peters described a similar surgery extracting 7450 g from a patient, including the umbilicus, without the undermining [4]. Gaudet and Morestin extracted fat and skin with correction of an umbilical hernia while preserving the umbilicus. Eventually, Babcock in 1916 described dermolipectomies using vertical incision [5].

Most authors would agree that the earliest work by these pioneers and others generally represented truly functional panniculectomies. There was tremendous variation in scar location and morphology, but the basic approach was exactly the same, simple dermolipectomy [6].

Thorek is the one to be praised for the contour surgery's first major aesthetic accomplishment. He performed the first umbilicus-preserving abdominoplasty in 1924 [7]. The significant contribution of Passot would need to be mentioned here—he used undermining as a modification of Kelly's technique [8]. Vernon in the 1950s developed a novel concept by combining extensive undermining with the umbilical transposition and relocation, which is a procedure still in use today. Callia described aponeurotic suturing as an important piece of his procedure in 1967, which involved an infrainguinal incision [9]. The famous Pitanguy in the same year published a series of 300 abdominal lipectomies with infrainguinal incision [10]. Previously, the published literature consisted mostly of case reports or a few number of patients. In the 1970s, Regnault modified the Pitanguy's incision into the "W" incision [11]. In 1973, Grazer championed the "bikini line" incision used frequently today [9]. An observation in 1977 by Grazer and Goldwyn that abdominoplasty decreased anterior projection of the abdomen but did little to change waist diameter led to Psillakis' assertion in 1978 that muscular aponeurotic suturing was an underutilized tool to decrease waistline dimensions [12]. Pregnancy produces changes in the body contours due to skeletal modification and flaccidity of the cutaneous and musculoaponeurotic tissues. There is now a new technique to face the musculoaponeurotic flaccidity and in this way achieve acceptable abdominal contour. The major oblique muscle is sutured to the rectus fasciae.

Somalo and Gonzalez-Ulloa extended the transverse abdominal incision circumferentially and introduced the belt lipectomy. This concept would provide the stepping stone for many subsequent "radical" lifting procedures [13, 14].

3. History of upper body contouring procedures

Similarly as with the improvements in abdominal contour surgery, procedures to ameliorate redundant skin on other parts of the body were being devised. The arms of a weight loss patient often manifest sagging deflated skin, downward descent of the posterior axillary fold, and redundant axillary skin. Initial attempts to correct these anomalies were performed in the 1920s by Thorek and his contemporaries and involved primarily elliptical excisions of skin [15]. The procedure did not change significantly and was pretty exotic until 1973. Here, Lewis carried the resection into the patients' axilla and performed a Z-plasty to reduce the effects of scar contracture. Soon after, Pitanguy again developed alternative solution for patients with excessive lateral axillary skin tissue, in which he continued the arm scar into the inframammary fold. Afterward, he developed a method of a so-called bat-wing torsoplasty in the 1970s. This technique combined brachioplasty with vertical axilloplasty in a single scar bilaterally [16]. Another big contribution was made by Regnault, who created a fishtail version of the arm reduction that is still used with small modifications by many surgeons [17].

4. History of lower body contouring procedures

The lower extremities have also suffered the unwanted effects of massive weight loss as well as effects of gravitational forces. In the beginning of the twentieth century, Dr. Kelly and Dr. Noel realized the aesthetic impact of thigh morphologic abnormalities and performed local excisions of the thigh tissue in combination with abdominal lipectomy [18, 19]. They managed to achieve success with elliptical excisions of skin and fat. This method was brought to life at the moment when Lewis created the notion of a thigh lift in 1957, using a circular resection with vertical components, in order to minimize overall circumference; thus thigh contour was altered greatly in a most positive way [20]. Pitanguy's contribution to trochanteric lipodystrophy in the 1960s [21] has inspired Farina to devise "riding trousers" resection type [22]. It differs from obesity because, according to Pasqualini [23] the latter is a state in which an excess of fat accumulate, predominantly in subcutaneous cellular tissues, and a remarkable change in the shaping of the body occurs as a consequence. From a clinical standpoint, trochanteric lipomatosis is like a real lipoma, since, according to Bergmann and his coworkers [24], it remains unaltered even when the patient loses significant weight. The incision must be fusiform and deep to the aponeurotic layer, from the iliac crest up to the mediocrural level. The upper end of this incision has to be lengthened backward, following the iliac crest to about 15 or 10 cm from the posterior midline [32]. Fusiform excision of the dermofat together with undermining of the crural flaps is carried out after that. Large undermining of the incision's lower end is carried out in parallel to the iliac crest in a way to expose the aponeurosis of the gluteus maximus. By pulling upward and forward, the angle of this large pelvicrural flap, a right-angled triangular part is achieved for the excision. Next, a cutaneous suture is carried out with simple interrupted stitches, and a few Donati's stitches are tied upon rollers of gauze. A pressure dressing of gauze that has been impregnated with Vaseline petroleum jelly is applied and fixed with adhesive tape [22].

The fusiform excision, which continues from the iliac crest, up to a quite high point on the lateral face of the thigh, needs to be done towards the posterior side, in order to be hidden from the front side [22]. Schrocher advised to leave one or two centimeters of fat on the aponeurosis because, in his opinion, when the aponeurosis is exposed there is excess exudation [25]. In Farina's opinion this is caused by lipolysis, a natural phenomenon when fat tissues are handled, so we must not hesitate to undermine at the fascial plane.

Abundant lipolysis can modify the aesthetics by changing the general volume of the limbs. The upper end of the abovementioned incision, when it gets near the iliac crest, needs to follow the line in an anteroposterior direction until the middle to the posterior midline. Farina not only removed the disfigurement but also succeeded in improving the aesthetic aspect of the buttocks by making them look higher using this method. The patient must stay absolutely stable for a week, when we start to remove alternate stitches [22].

This method eventually ended up with scars in a position which was neither desired nor expected.

This method has been further improved by Pitanguy using a semicircular excision technique, which at once took care of trochanteric adiposity and medial and lateral thigh laxity. Baroudi, Regnault, and Grazer came up with further modifications in this method. In the end, the semicircular thigh reduction has been completely revised by Regnault and we got the circular thigh reduction [26]. One of the unwanted side effects of these methods was known as gluteal depression. It is a contour shape loss between the iliac crest and femoral trochanter. Agris, Aston, and many others rectified this by filling up this area with excess deepithelized skin [27]. Agris J. Use of dermal-fat suspension flaps for thigh and buttock lifts..

In the early 1990s, Dr. Lockwood would further revolutionize the rejuvenation of the lower extremity and move onto entire thigh-abdomen-trunk aesthetic unit by describing the anatomic features and making use of the superficial fascial system (SFS) to anchor tissues after excisional lifting procedures [28, 29]. His precise description of the medial thigh anchoring technique in 1988 allowed a more durable lift of the inner thigh with less scar migration [30]. The introduction of the high-lateral-tension abdominoplasty and the lower body lift expanded upon the earlier belt lipectomy concept of Somalo and Gonzalez-Ulloa to fix and perfect the entire thigh-trunk-abdomen aesthetic unit [13, 14].

5. History of breast reduction

Male and female breast tissue would also experience unpleasant and significant conformational changes as a result of massive weight loss. The female breast is one of the most attractive aesthetic areas in female anatomy. There are numerous testimonies to the crucial and often devastating role that feminine beauty and figure of breasts had in many different cultures. Depending on the cultures and the era, vision of what makes beautiful and sensuous breasts have more or less stayed the same for the past 2500 years. First of all their size, but also shape, and maybe the breasts' symmetry can have a greater effect on the women's self-esteem and/or confidence. Reduction mammaplasty is certainly one of the frequently asked surgeries—plastic surgeons can make a crucial effect to a woman's quality of both physical and social life. Plastic surgery has seen quite high satisfaction rate of the patients constantly, although there are not always success stories to be told [33].

Majority of women with extremely large breasts might suffer from poor self-esteem, altered self-image, and other psychological effects. Women, whose breasts are abnormally large relative to their body built, are often limited in their choice of clothing and even lifestyle. Exercise, sports, and participation in other daily activities might be very difficult for them. Breast sizes are a powerful factor in woman's attitudes, career choices, as well as personal life in so many ways.

Urgent medical conditions, such as skin lacerations and intertrigo, chest tightness, or for example, chronic headaches as well as pains in the breast, neck, back, or shoulder are well known complaints of women with breasts larger than usual. These symptoms are either eliminated or significantly improved by reduction mammaplasty. After surgery, majority of these women enjoy a positive new outlook, cured from their medical complaints and engage in activities that were previously impossible for them.

Breast reduction surgery continues to develop, improve and is being refined constantly with a large number of procedures. Each procedure presents particular advantages in terms of symptoms, vascular preservation, technique design, ease of realization, minimum scarring, maintenance of innervation, and long-term results.

Usually seen anomalies are asymmetric volume loss, or for instance loose inelastic and redundant skin, or medialized nipple-areola complex (NAC) position in women. There is also lateral outward migration of tissue, which results with axillary skin excess. Rejuvenation of chest is still one of the most challenging areas in body contouring surgery.

Long time ago, in the 6th ct. AD, Paulus Aegineta described a technique of reduction mammaplasty in order to correct the gynecomastia. Furthermore, in 1561 Hans Schaller has successfully performed a reduction mammaplasty by breast amputation [31]. Dieffenbach [32] was the first surgeon to make a reduction mammaplasty in a female patient, leaving the scar in the inframammary fold. Thomas [33] and Guinard [34] underlined the inframammary fold as an entrance site for the operative treatment of surplus breast tissue.

Most of the surgical treatments made during the 1800s and the early 1900s were aiming at correcting ptosis. Different skin types, as well as glandular excisions were involved, attaching or sometimes suspending the breasts on a higher position at the chest wall, however, without the true nipple-areola complex (NAC) transposition. The whole idea of nipple-areola complex transposition has been improved in between 1909 and 1925. Morestin in 1909 [35] was the first surgeon who transposed the nipple-areola. He was followed by Villandre, cited in 1925. He referred to a surgery that he performed in 1911 [36]; and later Lexer continued the work [37].

The following phase in the evolution of breast reduction surgery was mainly focused on the knowledge of the blood supply of the skin, mammary glands, and nipple-areola itself. The subdermal blood supply to the breast skin and glands was object of many detailed considerations.

In 1937, Schwarzmann [38] proposed to leave a periareolar dermal ring in order to improve arterial and venous blood supply directly to the nipple-areola. This has improved viability of the nipple-areola complex and improved its transfer. It is a beginning of methods involving deepithelized nipple pedicle flaps.

The extreme significance of incisions' marking beforehand the operation was well presented by Bames in 1948 [39]. The following year, Aufricht [40] remarked that ultimate breast form is determined by the postsurgical "skin brassiere". Wise in 1956 [41] described a pattern for preoperative marking of the breast that resulted an aided in accurate and reproducible resection of parenchymal tissue while minimizing complications and resulting in satisfactory breast shape.

Resulting and following refinements in breast reduction surgery evolved around pedicle designs to preserve vascularity and place the scars in more aesthetic area. Different orientations of the breast dermal and parenchymal pedicles were described. Strombeck [42] described a horizontal dermal bipedicle flap that helped maintain innervation to the nipple-areola complex. McKissock [43] described a vertical bipedicle flap; Weiner et al. [44] a superiorly based flap; finally, Courtiss and Goldwyn [45] along with Georgiade et al. [46] used inferiorly based flaps.

A few authors described substantial innervation of the breasts. Marchac and de Olarte [47], Góes [48], Lejour [49], and Lassus [50] implemented vertical as well as short-scar reduction methods. Most of the methods developed during the 1960s and 1970s. However, during the last decade or more, they achieved common popularity, acceptance, as well as regular utilization.

However, Beisenberger's dermoglandular separation [51] as well as nipple transposition at the unilateral vascular pedicle which Skoog did in 1963 [52], Regnault's B type reduction [53], Lassus's vertical mammaplasty [54], or Benelli's periareolar reduction [55] have helped discovering new methods and techniques to recreate satisfactory breast shape in both women and men. Various authors described in detail glandular reshaping and dermal suspension.

6. History of liposuction

Removing excess fat from localized body sites is not a new idea [56]. In 1921, in France, Charles Dujarrier tried to remove subcutaneous fat using a uterine curette on a dancer's calves and knees [57]. Unfortunately, he damaged the femoral artery, and the patient has lost her leg as a result. One of the original and creative initiatives came from Schrudde in 1964, when he extracted fat from lower areas of the limb, through a visibly small incision, utilizing a curette. The unfortunate results from this surgical initiative were unpleasant hematomas and seromas [34, 58]. Pitanguy, on the other hand, was in favor of a removal of both fat and skin in a block, in order to remove excess thigh adiposities in one act. However, significant visible incisions made this method quite unpopular [20].

The field of modern liposuction began with the technique and new instruments developed by Arpad and Fischer [59, 60]. During their work in Rome, Italy, they managed to develop a blunt hollow cannula, with additional function of suction. Some of the previous cannula designs contained a cutting blade also. They made their results public in 1976 [61]. Fischers also started the crisscross tunnel formation method, from several incision sites. The new instruments have brought very promising results. The abovementioned complications were avoided using these instruments. Kesselring and Meyer [62] published their surgery results of sharp curettage aided by a suction device in 1978, but their method did not receive a wide acceptance.

Fournier, in Paris, showed an early interest in the Fischer's liposculpture technique [63]. He was an initial enthusiasts of the "dry technique" in which no fluids were infiltrated into the patient prior to liposuction. Fournier would become a world leader in liposuction and fat transplantation, eventually insisting on the benefits of tumescent anesthesia and making a great contribution in opening new horizons and ideas to surgeons from different parts of the world.

Illouz, a Parisienne, was quite attracted by the Fishers' work. His preferred method was a *"wet* technique", where they implemented a solution of hypotonic saline together with hyaluronidase inserted into the adipose tissue before the aspiration. lllouz thought that the solution itself was a "dissecting hydrotomy" which would catalyze the removal of fat and thus reduce trauma, as there was smaller amount of bleeding. lllouz received worldwide publicity and promoted this method.

The first US surgeon to visit France to learn the new area of liposuction was Lawrence Field in 1977, a Californian dermatology surgeon [64]. Other surgeons from the States, coming to conferences and educating themselves about new methods in the literature, also showed an interest in the area. One of them was Norman Martin, an otolaryngologist. He visited to Illouz in 1980 and quickly started with liposuction surgeries in Los Angeles in 1981 [65].

It was 1982 when a group of physicians from various specialty disciplines received lectures from Illouz and Fournier. Among them, dermatologists Claude Caver and Arthur Sumrall attended these classes. Rhoda Narins, a dermatologist from New York, also visited France in 1982 to learn the techniques. At the same time, a task group formed by the American Society of Plastic and Reconstructive Surgeons visit to Europe to learn and form opinions about this new procedure. Recognizing its potential, the abovementioned attempted to monopolize the whole field by having lllouz sign a contract with them to exclusively teach plastic surgeons worldwide. Fournier in turn refused to sign that kind of contract, and in spite continued to teach physicians from various fields [65]. Julius Newman, otolaryngologist and cosmetic surgeon, together with his associate Richard Dolsky, who was a plastic surgeon, together taught the first American course on liposuction, held in Philadelphia in 1982. The five live surgery workshops were held in Hollywood, California, in June 1983, under the authority of the American Society of Cosmetic Surgeons and the American Society of Liposuction Surgery. There were altogether 10 dermatologists in attendance.

Interest in liposuction has been on the upward spiral since and continued to expand in the United States. In 1983 and 1984, several interspecialty courses were sponsored by the American Academy of Cosmetic Surgery. "Lipo Suction" term was coined by Newman and soon he eventually established the ASLS—American Society of Liposuction Surgery. Some of the first publications about liposuction were noted in the dermatological literature, back in July 1984 [66, 67].

Already in 1984, liposuction training was ongoing in some residency programs. For instance, the dermatology section at the Tulane University School of Medicine was one of the first ones to teach residents about liposuction on a regular basis. Liposuction was soon a part of the "Core Surgical Curriculum in Dermatology" in 1987. Dermatologic surgeons also had a greater role in postgraduate education in liposuction, and established special training courses. Doctors Patrick Lillis, Rhoda Narins, and Jeffery Klein organized many workshops that gained much interest.

The dermatological literature of the 1980s is filled with numerous interesting and important articles describing liposuction methods [67–71]. Klein designed the tumescent technique, showcasing almost entirely bloodless session of liposuction with application of just local anesthesia [72]. This creative innovation was a turning point and dramatically altered the future of liposuction. The first dermatological textbook to contain a chapter on liposuction was *Cosmetic Dermatologic Surgery,* published by Year Book in 1984, authored by Samuel Stegman and Theodore Tromovitch.

In 1987, Klein's description of the tumescent technique and subsequent demonstration of its safety and efficacy revolutionized the art and practice of suction lipectomy [31].

The American Academy of Dermatology (AAD), the American Society for DermatoJogic Surgery (ASDS), and the International Society of Dermatologic Surgery (ISDS), all practiced extensive educational program on liposuction subject at their annual gatherings starting in 1984. Coleman and Fournier were guest editors of a special liposuction issue in *Journal of Dermatologic Surgery and Oncology* in 1988. Lillis and Coleman were guest editors for a special issue of *Dermatology Clinics* on liposuction in 1990 and again in 1999. William Coleman and Naomi Lawrence were guest editors for a special issue of *Dermatologic Surgery* in 1997.

The first detailed instructions on care [73] for liposuction procedures have been approved by the American Academy of Dermatology in 1989 and published in 1991. The Tumescent Liposuction Council has been formed in 1992, with the aim of increasing level of awareness about the advancing tumescent method for liposuction treatment. Their newsletter was first published in 1993. Many postgraduate courses were organized to help teaching dermatologists how to master this method.

During the 1980s, dermatologists were major contributors to this field. Some of the contributions were the use of liposuction for the face alone or in combination with microlipoinjection, face-lifting [74, 75], and liposuction for axillary hyperhidrosis, lipomas, gynecomastia, and reconstructive surgery [76, 77].

In the beginning, large cannulas were employed for liposuction, some up to 1 cm in diameter. These large instruments may have caused damage to neurovascular bundles and occasionally may have led to uneven contours and seromas or hematomas in some patients. Gentle touch was needed for use of local anesthesia, which was favored by dermatological surgeons. Different, smaller-diameter cannulas have been developed by dermatological surgeons [78–80]. The cannulas that are normally used at the present time are extremely small in diameter, some with an inner diameter of less than 0.6 mm. Blunt-tipped cannulas are IJOW standard, due to significantly decreased injury to blood vessels. The use of several side entry points opens the possibility for removal of adipocytes. Hand-operating instruments, combinations of syringes and cannula tips were also invented [81–84]. Many surgeons chose the usage of these quiet, disposable instruments, so they became quite popular as backup items. The aspiration units that manufacturers designed in cooperation with dermatological surgeons gradually became more powerful but more quiet as well, making surgical environment pleasant and positive experience.

In 1987, dermatologist Jeffery Klein, MD, presented his development in the field tumescent anesthesia [85]. His innovation consisted of infiltration of a dilute solution of lidocaine with epinephrine to allow for more extensive liposuction using only local anesthesia, significantly minimizing bleeding [72]. This revolutionized the field of liposuction for all specialties [86, 87]. Klein [88] and Lillis [89, 90] showed in presentation that the hematocrit of the aspirate fat was minimal. The expected complications of hematoma and seroma formation became rare. Complex calculations of fluid and blood loss or autologous transfusion were no longer needed. Peri- and postoperative monitoring was all of a sudden made much more simple.

Klein showed that diluted combinations of lidocaine together with epinephrine are really not absorbed in the same way as normally used commercial lidocaine. Klein [91] proved that when tumescent liposuction is performed in combination with previous application of 0.05% lidocaine and 1:1,000,000 epinephrine, maximal doses of 35 mg of lidocaine per kilogram of body weight were very safe and quite effective. This pharmacological discovery made possible for large volumes of fat to be removed. This development of tumescent anesthesia eventually encouraged some surgeons to progressively explore the different options and limitation of lidocaine. Lillis reported no complications what so ever in tumescent lidocaine doses of more than 70 mg/kg. Ostad et al. [92] suggested the max tumescent safe lidocaine dosage to be 55 mg/kg of the body weight. The rate of application of the tumescent anesthesia was found not to be dependent of lidocaine levels in plasma [93]. The tumescent procedure has been of utmost importance in the field and experts around the world recognize its importance.

Nowadays, some specialties still perform liposuction in the hospitals, but dermatological surgeons have clearly shown that tumescent liposuction is harmless, just as an office-based outpatient surgical treatment [94]. There were quite a low number of cases with complications, however with no fatalities, when the tumescent anesthesia method was implemented as a local anesthetic with no excess intravenous fluids or for instance general anesthesia [95, 96]. Complications and even fatalities in some cases have been reported when liposuction was performed under total anesthesia and deep intravenous sedation, after implementation of tumescent fluids. The mentioned variations of the tumescent technique have been strongly criticized by most dermatological surgeons all over the world [97]. Dermatological surgeons have also proven without any doubt that limiting the amount of fat aspirated contributes in general to the safety of the procedure [94].

Documentation of safety in liposuction procedures that are performed by dermatological surgeons has been impeccable [95, 96]. The number of lawsuits has been shown to be significantly decreased when liposuction is performed applying the tumescent technique, in an outpatient setting by a dermatological surgeon. Hospital-based liposuction, which more often than not involves general anesthesia, have resulted in 3.5 times as many malpractice claims [94].

Liposuction, as a procedure, is practiced by several specialties, and interspecialty rivalries have formed and exist to this day. Competing personal economic interests by different branches have led to attempts to restrict who should be allowed to perform liposuction and in what setting [56, 57]. Several states have accomplished introducing negative impact legislation in order to limit the physical location in which liposuction can be carried out. Without a doubt liposuction is safest as an outpatient procedure. Demanding by law the performance of liposuction in a hospital setting may increase the risks and complications and endanger patients. These politically and economically-based restrictions on such activities will continue due to influence of wealthy medical lobbies.

At first, ultrasonic liposuction has been developed in Europe in the beginning of 1990s by Zocchi [98]. The procedure exposes fat cells to ultrasound, which acts as a fat-aspiration catalyst. Ultrasonic techniques may be cannula based (internal) and by external application. Although the American Society of Plastic and Reconstructive Surgeons promoted ultrasonic liposuction in the past, dermatological surgeons generally gave up on this technique. Use of internal ultrasound increases the risk for cutaneous burns and seroma formation, and has almost no benefits over regular liposuction. Several studies by dermatologists who were studying external ultrasonic liposuction have found almost no benefit to it, when used before, during, or after a procedure. Moreover, complications have occurred from both forms of ultrasound, and it gives the right to the above-mentioned dermatological surgeons [99–103].

It has been the case that shaving instrument with suction to remove fat has been used in submental resection [104, 105]. Furthermore, a full-body version of this technology as well as new more powerful liposuction cannulas has been developed and used by dermatologic surgeons [106]. These devices use a rotary internal blade built into the cannula and are designed to facilitate tunneling through fibrous adipose tissue. Newer powered liposuction devices make use of a reciprocating cannula that facilitates fat removal and may decrease the physical work of the surgeon, which is in those interventions substantial [106].

Noncosmetic applications of procedures such as liposuction have been introduced or even invented by creative dermatological surgeons from all around the world [77]. They clearly showed that liposuction could be used to remove lipomas [107–109] angiolipomas [110], and improve hyperhidrosis [76, 111, 112]. Liposuction techniques can greatly assist in hematoma situations, with successful evacuation of hematoma [113]. Klein demonstrated and performed liposuction techniques for breast reduction. The field pioneered liposuction method in order to achieve flap movement in cutaneous reconstruction [114–117]. Gynecomastia [118, 119] benign symmetrical lipomatosis (Madelung's disease) [120], Dercum's disease [121], Cushing's disease [122], and insulin-induced lipohypertrophy [123, 124] have been treated with liposuction as well. Lymphedema, most often following breast cancer treatment, has benefited from liposuction and controlled compression therapy [125, 126]. Liposuction has become a valuable technique in situations where a surgeon intends to improve stomal dysfunction [127, 128].

Liposculpture has become a proven modality that can avoid unseemly scars in patients with good skin tone and provide a significant adjunct to excisional lifting procedures. Ultrasonic liposuction techniques have the potential to improve aesthetic results.

7. Body contouring after massive weight loss

Massive weight loss (MWL) is normally defined as an excess weight loss (EWL) of 50% or more in an effort to combat morbid obesity [129]. A comprehensive and detailed preoperative evaluation is mandatory as the body-contouring procedures following MWL are often extensive with potential morbidity and even mortality [130]. Although this amount of weight loss is most commonly found in bariatric surgery settings, plastic surgeons should separate between patients who have undergone bariatric/metabolic surgery and those who have lost weight only through diet and exercise, because malabsorptive procedures produce a number of nutritional deficiencies not otherwise seen. Furthermore, they need to understand the differences between various bariatric surgical techniques and take their basic working mechanism into consideration as patients having purely restrictive procedures are less likely to suffer from many of the metabolic complications and deficiencies that may be seen after malabsorptive weight loss operations [131]. The terms, body contouring or post-MWL body contouring, can be applied to any surgical procedure used to modify the skin envelope, subcutaneous layer, and/or investing fascia, and include a wide range of operations performed to treat the MWL patient. After a rapid and massive weight loss, there is a sudden change in BMI which leads to skin and soft tissue becoming excessive and redundant with a poor tone. Surplus skin and malpositioned adipose deposits can contribute to medical conditions such as irritation, fungal infections, poor hygiene, skin breakdown, physical function impairments, and low self-esteem [131]. Therefore, excisional surgery may relieve these symptoms and, for all these reasons, it must be considered to be reconstructive rather than cosmetic [132]. However, MWL patients are also seeking an aesthetic outcome to improve their body image and self-esteem.

All of the advances made in body contouring, from the original work of Dr. Kelly and his contemporaries to the modifications seen every once in a while since, have contributed to a dynamic and evolving specialty. Currently, there is no field within the realm of plastic surgery which is growing with the same rapidity, and with worldwide obesity continually on the rise, the growth of this field is unlikely to abate in the near future. The contributions of Thorek, Passot, Pitanguy, Baroudi, Grazer, Wise, Regnault, Lassus, Illouz, Klein, Lockwood, and others have provided the necessary armamentarium to approach the post-weight loss patient knowledgably, thoughtfully, and adequately equipped to restore pleasing contour to the patients we as surgeons care for. The combination of regional dermolipectomies, lifts, and suction lipoplasty has the potential to restore the elegant human form, to recreate gesture, and to restore appropriate structure.

Author details

Balkovic Marija[1*] and Jankovic Irena[2]

*Address all correspondence to: m.balkovic@yahoo.com

1 Clinic for Plastic and Aesthetic Surgery, Medical Beauty Center, Belgrade, Serbia

2 Clinic for Plastic and Reconstructive Surgery, Clinical Center Nis, Nis, Serbia

References

[1] Persichetti P, Simone P, Tambone V. About beauty. Plast Reconstr Surg. 2004;114(1): 270–271.

[2] Saldanha OR. Lipoabdominoplasty. 1st edition. Rio de Janeiro (Brazil): Di-Livros, 2006;1.

[3] Kelly HA. Report of gynecological cases (excessive growth of fat). Johns Hopkins Med J. 1899;10:197–201.

[4] Peters L. Resection of Pendulous fat abdominal wall in cases of extreme obesity. Ann Surg. 1901;33:299–304.

[5] Babcock W. The correction of the obese and relaxed abdominal wall with special reference to the use of the buried silver chain. Am J Obst. 1916;1:596–611.

[6] Regnault P, Daniel R. Aesthetic Plastic Surgery: Abdominoplasty. Boston: Little Brown; 1984. p. 618.

[7] Thorek M. Plastic Reconstruction of the Female Breast and Abdomen Wall. Springfield, IL: Thomas; 1924.

[8] Passot R. Chirurgie Esthetique Pure. Paris: Doin; 1931. pp. 260–267.

[9] Grazer FM. Abdominoplasty. Plast Reconstr Surg. 1973;51:617–623.

[10] Pitanguy I. Abdominal lipectomy: An approach to it through an analysis of 300 consecutive cases. Plast Reconstr Surg. 1967;40:384–391.

[11] Regnault P. Abdominoplasty by the W technique. Plast Reconstr Surg. 1975;55:265–266.

[12] Psillakis JM. Abdominoplasty: some ideas to improve results. Aesthetic Plast Surg. 1978;2:205–215.

[13] Somalo M. Dermolipectomia circular del trunco. Cir Clin Exper. 1942;6:540–543.

[14] Somalo M. Dermolipectomia circular del trunco. Cir Clin Exper. 1942;6:540–543.

[15] Thorek M. Esthetic surgery of the pendulous breast, abdomen and arms in females. Illinois Med J. 1930;3:48–57.

[16] Pitanguy I. Dermolipectomy of the abdominal wall, thigh, buttocks and upper extremity. In: Converse JM, editor. Reconstructive Plastic Surgery. 2nd ed. Philadelphia, PA: WB Saunders; 1977. pp. 190–198.

[17] Regnault P. Brachioplasty, axilloplasty and preaxilloplasty. In: Ely JF, editor. Transactions of the Seventh International Congress of Plastic and Reconstructive Surgery. Sao Paulo, Brazil: Cartgraf; 1980.

[18] Kelly HA. Excision of the fat of the abdominal wall lipectomy. Surg Gynecol Obstet. 1910;10:229–231.

[19] Noel A. La Cirurgie Esthetique: Son Role Social. Paris: Mason; 1926.

[20] Lewis JR. The thigh lift. J Int Coll Surg. 1957;27:330–334.

[21] Pitanguy I. Trochanteric lipodystrophy. Plast Reconstr Surg. 1964;34:280–286.

[22] Farina R, Baroudi R, Goleman B, Decastro O. Riding trousers-like pelvicrural lipodystrophy. Br J Plast Surg. 1961;13:174–178.

[23] Pasqualini RG. Endocrinologia. 2nd ed. Buenos Aires: E1 Ateneo; 1951.

[24] Von Bergmann G, et al. Tratado de Patologia Medica. Vol. 2. Rio de Janeiro: Labor SA. 1936.

[25] Schrőcher F. Kosmetische Operationen. Munich: J. F. Lehmanns; 1955.

[26] Regnault P, Baroudi R, Carvalho C. Correction of lower limb lipodystrophy. Aesthetic Plast Surg. 1979;3:233–249.

[27] Aston SJ. Buttocks and thighs. In: Regnault P, editor. Aesthetic Plastic Surgery. Philadelphia, PA: WB Saunders; 1980. pp. 1038–1039.

[28] Lockwood T. Superficial fascial system (SFS) of the trunk and extremities: a new concept. Plast Reconstr Surg. 1991;87:1009–1018.

[29] Lockwood T. Lower body lift with superficial fascial system suspension. Plast Reconstr Surg. 1993;92:1112–1125.

[30] Lockwood T. Fascial anchoring technique in medial thigh lifts. Plast Reconstr Surg. 1988;82:299–304.

[31] Schaller H. Cited in Grimm K, Fritche E. Reduction of breasts. Hans Schaller and the first mammaplasty in 1561. Contribution to history of medicine. Handchir Mikrochir Plast Chir. 2000;32(5):316–320.

[32] Dieffenbach JF. The extirpation of bruestdruese. In: Dieffenbach JF, editor. The operative surgery, vol. 2. Leipzig: Blockhouse; 1848. pp. 359–373.

[33] Thomas TG. On the removal of benign tumors of the mamma without mutilation of the organ. NY Med J Oster Rev. 1882;35:337.

[34] Guinard M. Comment on Aesthetic ablation of breast tumors, by M.H. Morestin. Bull Mem Soc Chir Paris. 1903;29:568.

[35] Morestin H, Guinard A. Mammary hypertrophy treated by discoid resection. Bull Soc Chir (Paris). 1907;33:649–651.

[36] Villandre C. Cited in Dartigues L. Surgical treatment of breast prolapse. Arch Franco-Belg Chir. 1925;28:325.

[37] Lexer E. Hypertrophy of both mammea. Munch Med Wochenschr. 1912;59:1702.

[38] Schwarzmann E. Avoidance of nipple necrosis by preservation of corium in one-stage plastic surgery of breast. Rev Chir Struct. 1937;7:206–209.

[39] Bames HO. Reduction of massive breast hypertrophy. Plast Reconstr Surg. 1948;3(5): 560–569.

[40] Aufricht G. Mammaplasty for pendulous breasts. Empiric and geometric planning. Plast Reconstr Surg. 1949;4:13–29.

[41] Wise RJ. A preliminary report on a method of planning the mammaplasty. Plast Reconstr Surg. 1956;17(59):367–375.

[42] Strombeck JO. Mammaplasty: report of a new technique based on the two pedicle procedure. Br J Plast Surg. 1960;13:79–90.

[43] McKissock PK. Reduction mammaplasty with a vertical dermal flap. Plast Reconstr Surg. 1972;49(3):245–252.

[44] Weiner DL, Aiache AE, Silver L, Tittiranonda T. A single dermal pedicle for nipple transposition in subcutaneous mastectomy, reduction mammaplasty, or mastopexy. Plast Reconstr Surg. 1973;51(2):115–120.

[45] Courtiss E, Goldwyn RM. Reduction mammaplasty by the inferior pedicle technique. Plast Reconstr Surg. 1977;59(1):500–507.

[46] Georgiade NG, Serafin D, Morris R, Georgiade G. Reduction mammaplasty utilizing an inferior pedicle nipple-areolar flap. Ann Plast Surg. 1979;3(3):211–218.

[47] Marchac D, de Olarte G. Reduction mammaplasty and correction of ptosis with a short inframammary scar. Plast Reconstr Surg. 1982;69(1):45–55.

[48] Góes JS. Periareoral mammaplasty: double skin technique with application of polyglactine or mixed mesh. Plast Reconstr Surg. 1996;97(5):959–968.

[49] Lejour M. Vertical mammaplasty: early complications after 250 personal consecutive cases. Plast Reconstr Surg. 1999;104(3):764–770.

[50] Lassus C. Update on vertical mammaplasty. Plast Reconstr Surg. 1999;104(7):2289–2298.

[51] Beisenberger H. Eine neue methode der mammaplastik. Zentrabl Chir. 1928;55:2382–2387.

[52] Skoog T. A technique of breast reduction: transposition of the nipple areolar complex on a cutaneous vascular pedicle. Acta Chir Scand. 1963;126:453–465.

[53] Regnault P. Reduction mammaplasty by the "B" technique. Plast Reconstr Surg. 1974;53:19–24.

[54] Lassus C. A technique for breast reduction. Int Surg. 1970;53:69–72.

[55] Benelli L. A new periareolar mammaplasty: the "round block" technique. Aesthetic Plast Surg. 1990;14:93–100.

[56] Coleman WP III. The history of liposculpture. J Dermatol Surg Oncol. 1990;16:1086.

[57] Dolsky RL, Newman J, Ferzek JR, Anderson RW. Liposuction: history techniques, and complications. Dermatol Clin. 1987;5:313–333.

[58] Schrudde J. Lipexheresis (liposuction) for body contouring. Clin Plast Surg. 1982;11:445–456.

[59] Coleman WP III. The history of Dermatologic liposuction. Dermatol Clin. 1990;8:381–383.

[60] Fischer G. Liposculpture: the correct history of liposuction: part 1. J Dermatol Surg Oncol. 1990;16:1087–1089.

[61] Fischer A, Fischer G. First surgical treatment for molding body's cellulite with three 5 mm incisions, Bull lnt Acad Cosmet Surg. 1976;3:35.

[62] Kesselring UK, Meyer RA. Suction curette for removal of excess local deposits of subcutaneous fur. Plast Reconstr Surg. 1978:62:305–306.

[63] Coleman WP III. The history of liposuction and fat transplantation in America. Dermatol Clin. 1999;7:723–727.

[64] Field LM. The dermatologist and liposuction – a history. J Dermatol Surg Oncol. 1987;13:1040–1041.

[65] Herter CP. The history of LSNA. Lipoplasty. 1999;16:9.

[66] Field LM. Liposuction surgery: a review. Dermatol Surg Oncol. 1984;10:530–538.

[67] Chrisman BB, Field LM. Facelift surgery update: suction-assisted rhytidectomy and other improvements. J Dermatol Surg Oncol. 1984;10:544–548.

[68] Stegman SJ, Tromovitch TA. Cosmetic dermatologic surgery. Chicago: Yearbook, 1984.

[69] Stegman SJ. The application of lipo-suction surgery in dermatology. Adv Dermatol. 1986;1(21):l–9.

[70] Coleman WP III. Liposuction and anesthesia. J Dermatol Surg Oncol. 1987;13:1295–1296.

[71] Coleman WP III. Complicated surgical techniques. II. Liposuction. Clin Dermatol. 1987;5:110–119.

[72] Klein JA. Anesthesia for liposuction in dermatologic surgery. J Dermatol Surg Oncol. 1988;14:1124–1132.

[73] Air TH, Coleman WP III, Skouge JV, Stegman SJ, Torok HM. Guidelines of care for liposuction. Committee on Guidelines of Care. J Am Acad Dermatol. 1991;24:489–494.

[74] Asken S. facial liposuction and microlipoinjection. J Dermatol Surg Oncol. 1988;14:297–305.

[75] Chrisman BB. Liposuction with facelift surgery. Dermatol Clin. 1990;8:501–522.

[76] Lillis PJ, Coleman WP III. Liposuction for treatment of axillary hyperhidrosis. Dermatol Clin. 1990;8:479–482.

[77] Coleman WP III. Non-cosmetic applications of liposuction. J Dermatol Surg Oncol. 1988;14:1085–1090.

[78] Weber PJ, Wulc AE, Jaworsky C, Dzubow LM. Warning: traditional liposuction cannulas may be dangerous to your patient's health. J Dermatol Surg Oncol. 1988;14:J 136–138.

[79] Collins PS. Selection and utilization of liposuction cannulas. J Dermatol Surg Oncol. 1988;14:1139–1143.

[80] Klein JA. Tumescent technique: tumescent anesthesia and microcannular liposuction. St. Louis: Mosby; 2000.

[81] Weber PJ, Dzubow LM. A new, more flexible mechanism and method of liposuction. J Dermatol Surg Oncol. 1988;14:715–717.

[82] Fournier PF. Who should do syringe liposculpturing? J Dermatol Surg Oncol. 1988;14:1955–1956.

[83] Fournier PF. Reduction syringe liposculpturing. Dermatol Clin. 1990;8:539–551.

[84] Bisaccia E, Scarborough DA, Swensen RD. Syringe-assisted liposuction: a cosmetic surgeon's office technique. J Dermatol Surg Oncol. 1988;14:982–989.

[85] Klein JA. The tumescent technique for liposuction surgery. Am J Cosmet Surg. 1987;4:263–267.

[86] Klein JA. Tumescent technique for local anesthesia improves safety in large-volume liposuction. Plast Reconstr Surg. 1993;92:1085–1098.

[87] Klein JA. The history of tumescent liposuction. In: Klein J. Tumescent technique: tumescent anesthesia and microcannular liposuction. Sr. Louis: Mosby; 2000.

[88] Klein JA. The tumescent technique. Anesthesia and modified liposuction technique. Dermatol Clin. 1990;8:425–437.

[89] Lillis PJ. The tumescent technique for liposuction surgery. Dermatol Clin. 1990;8:439–450.

[90] Lillis PJ. Liposuction surgery under local anesthesia: limited blood loss and minimal lidocaine absorption. J Dermatol Surg Oncol. 1988;14:1145–1148.

[91] Klein JA. Tumescent technique for regional anesthesia permits lidocaine doses of 35 mg/kg for liposuction. J Dermatol Surg Oncol. 1990;16:248–263.

[92] Ostad A, Kageyama N, Moy Rl. Tumescent anesthesia with a lidocaine dose of 55 mg/kg is safe for liposuction. Dermatol Surg. 1996;22:921–927.

[93] Butterwick KJ, Goldman MP, Sriprachya-Anunt S. Lidocaine levels during the first two hours of infiltration of dilute anesthetic solution for tumescent liposuction: rapid versus slow delivery. Dermatol Surg. 1999;25:681–685.

[94] Coleman WP III, Hanke CW, Lillis P, Bernstein G, Narins R. Does the location of the surgery or the specialty of the physician affect malpractice claims in liposuction? Dermatol Surg. 1999;25:343–347.

[95] Bernstein G, Hanke CW. Safety of liposuction: a review of 9478 cases performed by dermatologists. J Dermatol Surg Oncol. 1988;14:1112–1114.

[96] Hanke CW, Lee MV, Bernstein G. The safety of dermatologic liposuction surgery. Dermatol Clin. 1990;8:563–568.

[97] Klein JA. Risks of systemic anesthesia. In: Klein J. Tumescent technique: tumescent anesthesia and microcannular liposuction. St. Louis: Mosby; 2000.

[98] Zocchi M. Ultrasonic liposculpting. Aesthetic Plast Surg. 1992;16:287-98.

[99] Igra H, Satur NM. Tumescent liposuction versus internal ultrasonic assisted tumescent liposuction. A side to side comparison. Dermatol Surg. 1997;23:1213–1218.

[100] Lawrence N, Coleman WP III. Ultrasonic assisted liposuction. Internal and external. Dermatol Clin. 1999;17:761–771.

[101] Lawrence N, Coleman WP III. The biologic basis of ultrasonic liposuction. Dermatol Surg. 1997;23:1197–1200.

[102] Maxwell GP, Gingrass MK. Ultrasound assisted lipoplasty: a clinical study of 250 consecutive patients. Plast Reconstr Surg. 1998;101:189–204.

[103] Scheflau M, Tazi H. Ultrasound assisted body contouring. Aesthetic Surg Q. 1996;16:117–122.

[104] Gross CW, Becker DG, Lindsey WH, Park SS, Marshall DD. The soft-tissue shaving procedure for removal of adipose tissue. A new less traumatic approach than liposuction. Arch Otolaryngol Head Neck Surg. 1995;121:1117–1120.

[105] Becker DG, Weinberger MS, Miller PJ, et al. Liposhaver in facial plastic surgery. A multi-institutional experience. Arch Otolaryngol Head Neck Surg. 1996;122(116):l–7.

[106] Coleman WP III. Powered liposuction. Dermatol Surg. 2000;26:315–318.

[107] Carlin MC, Racz JL. Multiple symmetric lipomatosis: treatment with liposuction. J Am Acad Dermatol. 1988;18:359–362.

[108] Field LM. Liposuction surgery (suction-assisted lipectomy) for symmetric lipomatosis. J Am Acad Dermatol. 1988;18:1370.

[109] Pinski KS, Roenigk HH Jr. Liposuction of lipomas. Dermatol Clin. 1990;8:483–492.

[110] Kaneko T, Tokushige H, Kimura N, Moriya S, Toda K. The treatment of multiple angiolipomas by liposuction surgery. Dermatol Surg Oncol. 1994;20:690–692.

[111] Hasche E, Hagedorn M, Sattler G. Subcutaneous sweat gland suction curettage in tumescent local anesthesia in hyperhidrosis axillaris. Hautarzt. 1997;48:817–819.

[112] Payne CM, Doe PT. Liposuction for axillary hyperhidrosis. Clin Exp Dermatol. 1998;23:9–10.

[113] Goldberg LH, Humphreys TR. Surgical pearl: using the liposuction cannula/syringe apparatus for conservative evacuation of postoperative hematomas. J Am Acad Dermatol. 1996;34:1061–1062.

[114] Field LM. Adjunctive liposurgical debulking and flap dissection in neck reconstruction. J Dermatol Surg Oncol. 1986;12:917–920.

[115] Field LM, Novy FG III. Flap evaluation and mobilization by blunt liposuction cannula dissection to repair temple defect. J Dermatol Surg Oncol. 1987;13:1302–1305.

[116] Field LM, Spinowirz AL Flap elevation and mobilization by blunt liposuction cannula dissection in reconstructive surgery. Dermatol Clin. 1990;8:493–499.

[117] Field LM, Skouge J, Anhalt TS, Recht B, Okimoto J. Blum liposuction cannula dissection with and without suction-assisted lipectomy in reconstructive surgery. J Dermatol Surg Oncol. 1988;14:1116–1122.

[118] Samdal F, Kleppe G, Amland PF, et al. Surgical treatment of gynecomastia. Five years experience with liposuction. Scand J Plast Reconstr Surg; Hand Surg. 1994;28:123–130.

[119] Dolsky RL. Gynecomastia: treatment by liposuction subcutaneous mastectomy. Dermatol Clin. 1990;8:469–478.

[120] Amicucci G, Sozio ML, Rizzo RM, Sozio A. Madelung's disease. Clinical case and review of the literature. Minerva Chir. 1998;53:655–657.

[121] Berntorp E, Berntorp K, Brorson H, Frick K. Liposuction in Dercum's disease: impact on haemostatic factors associated with cardiovascular disease and insulin sensitivity. J Intern Med. 1998;243:197–201.

[122] Narins RS. Liposuction surgery for a buffalo hump caused by Cushing's disease. J Am Acad Dermatol. 1989;21:307.

[123] Hanner H, Olbrisch RR. The treatment of type-1 diabetics with insulin-induced lipohypertrophy by liposuction. Dtsch Med Wochenschr. 1994;119:414–417.

[124] Samdal F, Amland PF, Sandsmark M, Birkeland KI. Diabetic lipohypertrophy treated with suction-assisted lipectomy. J Intern Med. 1993;234:489–492.

[125] Brorson H, Svensson H. Complete reduction of lymphoedema of the arm by liposuction after breast cancer. Scand J Plast Reconstr Surg Hand Surg. 1997;31:137–143.

[126] Brorson H, Svensson H, Norrgren K, Thorsson O. Liposuction reduces arm lymphedema without significantly altering the already impaired lymph transport. Lymphology 1998;31:156–172.

[127] Sharma S, Bryson JR. liposuction for retracted urostomy. Br J Urol. 1996;78:472–473.

[128] Margulies AG, Klein FA, Taylor V. Suction-assisted lipectomy for the correction of stomal dysfunction. Ann Surg. 1998;64:178–181.

[129] Shermak MA, Chang D, Magnuson TH, Schweitzer MA. An outcomes analysis of patients undergoing body contouring surgery after massive weight loss. Plast Reconstr Surg. 2006;118:1026–1031.

[130] Michaels J 5th, Coon D, Rubin JP. Complications in postbariatric body contouring: postoperative management and treatment. Plast Reconstr Surg. 2011;127:1693–1700.

[131] Bossert RP, Rubin JP. Evaluation of the weight loss patient presenting for plastic surgery consultation. Plast Reconstr Surg. 2012;130(6):1361–1369.

[132] Bruschi S, Datta G, Bocchiotti MA, Boriani F, Obbialero FD, Fraccalvieri M. Limb contouring after massive weight loss: functional rather than aesthetic improvement. Obes Surg. 2009;19:407–411.

6

New Concepts on Safer Abdominoplasty

Guillermo Blugerman, Diego Schavelzon,
Boris Martínez , Gabriel Wexler,
Andrea Markowsky and Marcelo Lotoki

Abstract

Abdominoplasty was one of the first techniques described in literatura, and in some of his writings, Hippocrates mentioned the resection of skin and the apron-like abdominal flaps. The first standardization of this procedure was carried out by H.A. Kelly, who was a gynecologist, in 1890, but the procedure gained some popularity when Pitanguy published his report in 1967. With the advent of liposuction, they tried to replace abdominoplasty; however, in many cases, they yielded unreliable results. It was in the year 2000, with the advent of the pull down abdominal flap technique proposed by Avelar and then spread by Saldanha, surgeons significantly increased the indications for abdominoplasty. This was reflected in international statistics since abdominoplasty climbed from the 15th place in the 1990s to the 4th place in 2012. According to some publications, traditional abdominoplasty generally includes extensive dissection of upper abdominal flap all the way to the costal margin with a consequent decrease of blood flow of 50–70%. We present a technique with no flap undermining, including in-bloc resection of premarked área from the umbillicus scar to the suprapubic area, dissecting the tissue with an instrument called Iconoclast, thus preserving blood flow, after hydrodissection with tumescent solution, which varies if the patient is under general anesthesia or sedation. It has been shown that simultaneous liposuction of flap and flanks in the conventional abdominoplasty technique increases the risk of necrosis and seromas, so in many cases it is contraindicated. Therefore, our technique allows us to perform the liposuction of the upper abdominal flanks and waistline without running any risks. In this technique umbilicus scar its recreated with the use of skin graft. Unlike conventional abdominoplasty techniques, the presence of previous abdominal wall scars is not a limitation. In the case of smokers patients, risks are reduced by keeping the blood flow of the upper flap constant. We do not recommend this technique for very thin patients, with multiple pregnancies and regularly an important rectus muscles diastasis where we indicate the abdominal wall.vertical plicature.

Keywords: TULUA, conventional abdominoplasty, laser lipolysis, hydrodissection, neoumbilicus

1. Introduction

Abdominoplasty was one of the first techniques described in medical-surgical literature. In some of his writings, Hippocrates mentioned the resection of skin and the apron-like abdominal flaps. The first standardization of the procedure was carried out by H.A. Kelly, who was a gynecologist, in 1890 [1] but only gain some popularity when Pitanguy published his report in 1967 [2].

Although the abdomen is the part of the body that undergoes most changes during pregnancy due to changes in body weight, these techniques did not gain in popularity because of the high rate of complications that this surgery had regardless of the surgeon's experience.

With the advent of liposuction, in many cases it attempted to replace abdominoplasty, obtaining dissimilar and unreliable results.

It was in the year 2000, with the advent of the pull down abdominal flap technique proposed by Avelar [3] and then spread by Saldanha [4], when surgeons significantly increased the indications for abdominoplasty. This was reflected in international statistics since abdominoplasty climbed in popularity from the 15th place in the 1990s to the 4th place in 2012. This increase is linked to a higher number of bariatric surgeries, resulting in a greater number of patients interested in skin rehabilitation procedures, but it is also linked to the fact that surgeons felt more confident to obtain acceptable results with less risk to the patient and to the surgeon himself.

Since 1999 in our practice, we have been performing Juarez Avelar's technique—albeit modified by us—to work with tumescent anesthesia. Despite a significant reduction in the rate of serious complications, we continue to see a few cases of dehiscence of the flap, and infections by the presence of subcutaneous devitalized tissues likely to be colonized by skin flora bacteria. In February 2013 we attended the lecture delivered by Dr. Francisco Villegas about his personal technique called with the acronimTULUA (Transverse plication, no Undermining, full Liposuction, neoUmbilicoplasty, Abdominoplasty) in the ISAPS Congress in Santiago de Chile

We found very interesting concepts in this presentation, and that is why after our return we implemented a modified protocol in order to perform this technique with the assistance of tumescent anesthesia. For 18 months we performed 188 tucks with this new technique with a very low complication rate.

2. History

In 1890, Demars and Marx reported the first limited tummy tuck in France. H.A. Kelly, a surgeon gynecologist, was the first to report this procedure in the US, which took place at Johns Hopkins hospital in Baltimore in 1899. Kelly called this procedure "transverse abdominal lipectomy". In Germany in 1909 S. Weinhold [5] reported the cloverleaf incision, a combination of vertical and oblique incisions.

In 1916, W. Babcock [6] was the first to report the vertical elliptical resection with wide undermining of the abdominal wall. In 1918, E. Schepelmann [7] modified the Babcock elliptical incision into transverse teardrop incision extending from the xiphoid appendix to the pubis. This resulted in a better contouring of the lower abdomen.

In 1924, M. Thorek [8] described the technique of placing the incision below the umbilicus in a transverse fashion and removing excess skin and fat down to the fascia in a wedge-shaped form. He called this technique plastic "adipectomy". This researcher described the removal of the umbilicus if required in a crescent incision and transplanting it to the new place as a composite graft. In 1931, M. Flesh-Thebesius and K. Wheisheimer [9] modified Thorek's incision and included the umbilicus. In 1949, I.F. Pick [10] reported his technique, followed by A.J. Barsky [11] in 1950, which was a modification of the Thorek transverse incision with the addition of the vertical incision at its ends.

In 1955, M. Galtier [12] reported the four quadrants resection technique. Vernon in 1957 reported his low transverse abdominal incision procedure with wide undermining and transposition of the umbilicus. This was followed by C. Dufourmentel [13] and R. Mouly [14] in 1959, which included Vernon's technique [14] with the addition of a small vertical incision at the midline.

M. Gonzalez-Ulloa [15] in 1960 and Dubouset J.R. Vilain [16] in 1964 reported a similar technique to I.F. Pick and A.J. Barsky's circular abdominoplasty. In 1965, Spadafora [17] described a similar technique to Vernon's, but he lowered the incision to a less conspicuous site. His incision started at the center, curving around the mons pubis, and then at the inguinal crease the incision curved upward toward the anterior superior iliac spine.

When reviewing the literature up to 1967, researchers divided the tummy tuck procedure into three main categories:

(1) Surgeons who favored transverse incision, (2) those who favored the vertical incision, and (3) those who described a combination of transverse and vertical incisions.

In 1967, Pitanguy published his technique, which was considered to produce successful results. From 1967 to 1975 he reported more than 500 cases of abdominoplasty and mammoplasty performed simultaneously.

In 1972, P. Regnault [18] reported "W" shaped incision technique which was later modified in 1975. In 1978, J. Planas [19] advocated the "vest over pants" technique. The belt lipectomy was replaced by suction-assisted lipectomy and abdominoplasty in 1980, which was popularized by Y. Illouz. Between 2000 and 2004, Avelar together with Saldanha published the concept of Lipoabdominoplsty.

3. Anatomy

The anterolateral abdomen is divided into nine regions by four imaginary planes: two vertical (medioclavicular/midinguinal) and two horizontal (transpyloric/intertubercular) planes. The transpyloric plane corresponds to the midpoint between the umbilicus and the xiphoid appendix, crossing the pylorus at the lower border of the first lumbar vertebra. The subcostal plane that passes across the costal margins and the upper border of the third lumbar vertebra can be used instead of transpyloric plane. The lower horizontal plane, designated as the intertubercular line, crosses the anterior abdomen at the level of the fifth lumbar vertebra, and connects the anterior superior iliac spines on both sides. Thanks to these planes, these 9 regions are formed (epigastric region, hypochondriac region, flanks, mesogastric region, umbilicus and iliac fossa) [20].

The anterolateral abdominal wall consists, from the outside in, of the skin, superficial fascia, deep fascia, external and internal abdominal oblique, transverse abdominis, rectus abdominis and pyramidalis, as well as the transversalis fascia.

3.1. Blood supply

The abdominal wall receives blood supply through branches of the femoral, external iliac, subclavian and intercostal arteries as well as from the abdominal aorta. These branches include the superficial epigastric, superficial circumflex iliac, superficial external pudendal, deep circumflex iliac, superior and inferior epigastric, posterior intercostal, subcostal, musculo-phrenic, and lumbar arteries.

3.2. Venous drainage

It is drained via the superficial epigastric, thoracoepigastric, paraumbilical and the superficial circumflex iliac veins [21].

3.3. Innervation

The skin of the anterior abdominal wall is innervated by the ventral rami of the lower five or six thoracic (thoracoabdominal) spinal nerves that continue from the intercostal spaces into the abdominal wall. The anterolateral abdominal also receives nerve fibers from the anterior roots of the twelfth thoracic pair (subcostal) and from the iliohypogastric, and ilioinguinal nerves. Each intercostal nerve is connected to a sympathetic ganglion by a connecting adjacent white branch that carries presynaptic sympathetic fibers, and a communicating branch gray transmitting postsynaptic sympathetic fibers [22].

4. Research methods

Scientific basis of traditional abdominoplasty.

According to some publications, traditional abdominoplasty generally includes extensive dissection of the upper abdominal flap all the way to the costal margin with a consequent decrease of blood flow of 50–70%. Furthermore, this technique involves the vertical plication of the fascia of the rectus abdominis muscles and certain techniques of the oblique muscles, demanding traumatic separation maneuvers of the flap which results in trauma on adipose tissue that is also exposed to surgical environment for a long time. It has been shown that simultaneous liposuction of flap and flanks in conventional abdominoplasty increases the risk of seroma and necrosis, so it is contraindicated in many cases.

In most conventional techniques, reinsertion of the umbilicus is performed by exteriorization through an incision in the flap and suturing techniques of different designs [23].

4.1. Patient selection

Unlike other conventional abdominoplasty techniques, the presence of previous abdominal wall scars is not a limitation for this procedure. In the case of patients who smoke, risks are reduced by keeping the blood flow of the upper flap constant. We do not recommend this technique for very thin patients, with multiple pregnancies and regularly an important rectus muscles diastasis where we indicate the abdominal wall.vertical plicature in combination with the transverse one.

4.2. Surgical technique

Preoperative photographs are taken with the patient in a standing position. For marking surgeons can use laser levels as those used in architecture which allow us to draw lines and reference points in a symmetric fashion.

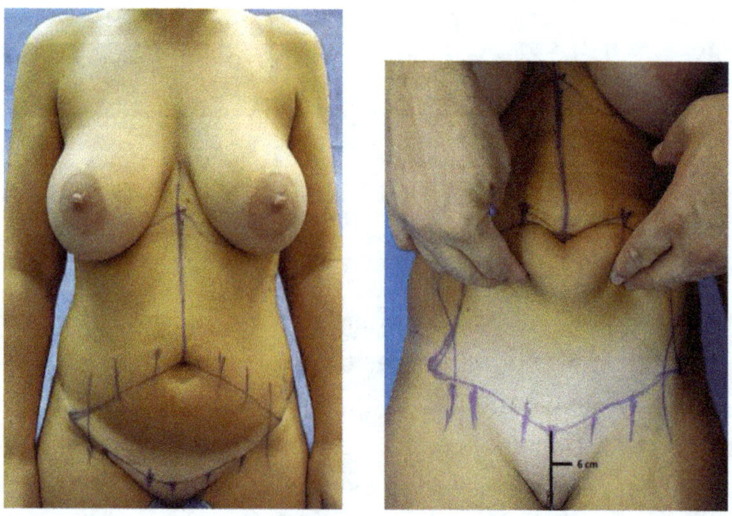

Figure 1. Surgical resection design on the anterior abdominal Wall.

It is very important to use a good quality, long lasting surgical skin marker so that the lines are not erased during liposuction with tumescent anesthesia and glove rubbing on the skin.

The first line to mark is the vertical line that goes from xiphoid to anterior vulvar commissure. This is very important because the umbilicus will be located on this line. The lower edge of the lozenge, indicating the place of the scar, is usually planned 6 cm above the superior vulvar commissure to ensure an anatomically regular pubis. The lozenge marked, must be mented by vertical lines that guide us when closing the wound **(Figure 1)**.

This surgery can be performed under general, regional, or local tumescent anesthesia. In all cases we use local tumescent infiltration, but the concentration of lidocaine varies. If the patient is under general or regional anesthesia we use solutions that contain 300 mg of lidocaine per liter; however, when we don't work with benerl anesthesia we use 600 mg per liter of saline solution.

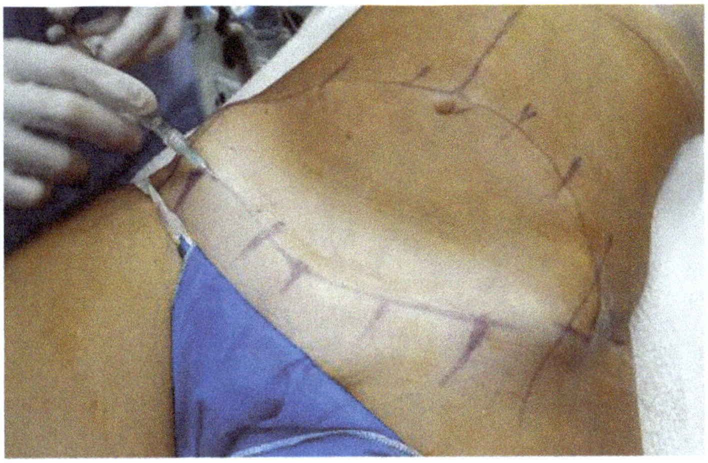

Figure 2. Superficial tumescent local anesthesia infiltration with a 50/8 needle and peristaltic pump.

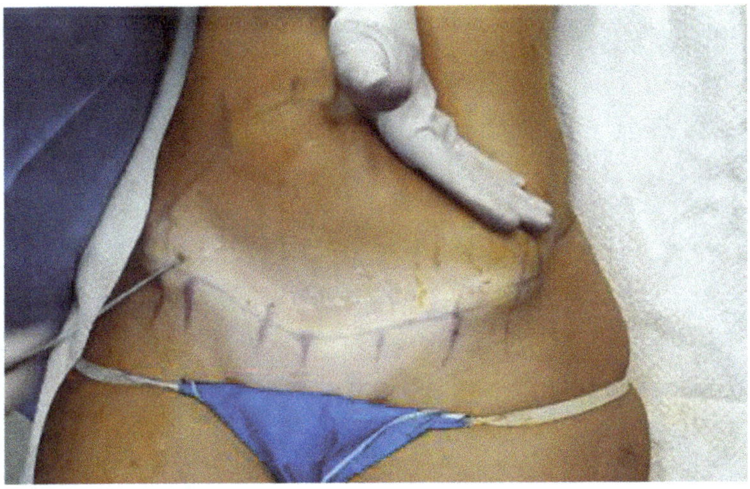

Figure 3. Suprafascial tumescent hidrodisection.

Two different types of anesthetic infiltration are performed. In the areas where liposuction is performed, all planes of subcutaneous tissue are infiltrated, starting by the deepest layer until reaching more superficial subcutaneous layers. The area to be resected is hydrodissected with 500 cc of anesthetic solution just above the aponeurotic fascia using a 2.5-mm blunt tip cannula. In addition, it is infiltrated with a 50/8 needle below the lines on which the incision will be made, **Figures 2** and **3**.

After finishing the local anesthesia infiltration, laser assisted liposuction of previously marked and infiltrated areas is performed, making sure to preserve the fat in the area where the new umbilicus will be placed so that it has the correct depth.

Once liposuction, which usually covers the superior abdomen and flanks, is finished, we disinfect the surgical field by changing the surgical gloves of the surgical team to reduce the risk of contamination.

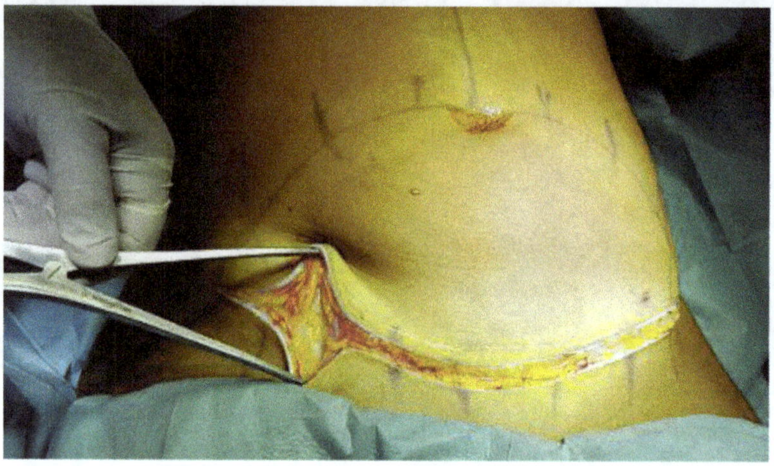

Figure 4. Dissection of adipose tissue with an instrument called Iconoclast.

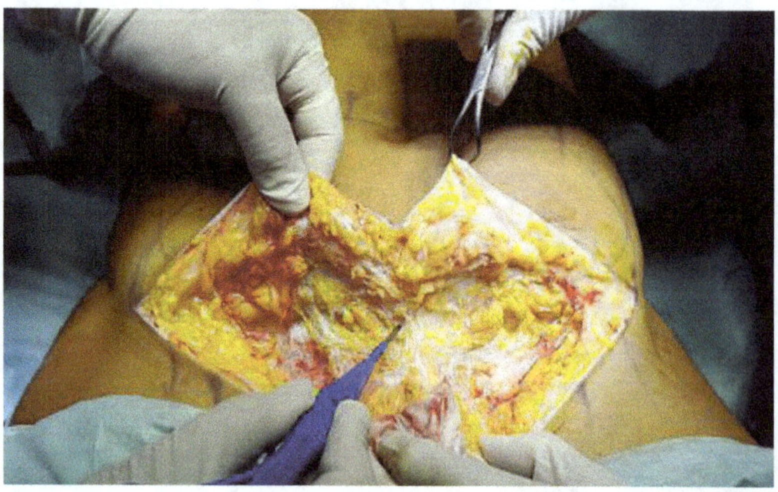

Figure 5. Redundant block integument disection between the fat and the anterior fascia.

The skin is incised superficially to expose adipose tissue and dissection is performed with an instrument known as Iconoclast [4] that facilitates the identification of blood vessels running under the skin, which are cauterized by the assistant doctor as they become visible. The Iconoclast allows, if necessary, the preservation of scarpa fascia as shown in **Figures 4**, **5** and **6**.

Once the lower border of the cutaneous adipose island/tissue is dissected, we advance over the aponeurosis, cauterizing perforating vessels in its emergence from the fascia.

All these dissection maneuvers can be performed with minimal bleeding thanks to the combination of hydrodissection and the use of the Iconoclast together with the simultaneous cauterization of vessel.

After complete dissection of the premarked area, the following step is the deatachment of umbilical scar. We palpate the cylinder that connects the fascia with the skin to determine the presence or absence of hernias. If some degree of hernia is observed, it is mobilized to the abdominal cavity by squizing movements. The bottom of the umbilical scar is exposed as a "bun" of hard, elastic consistency. This bun is then cut from beneath with a scalpel, making sure to remove all the skin to avoid future complications. The remaning deffect on the abdominal wall after aumbilicus deatachment is closed by means of a cross-shaped suture of braided, nonabsorbable material (nylon or polyester).

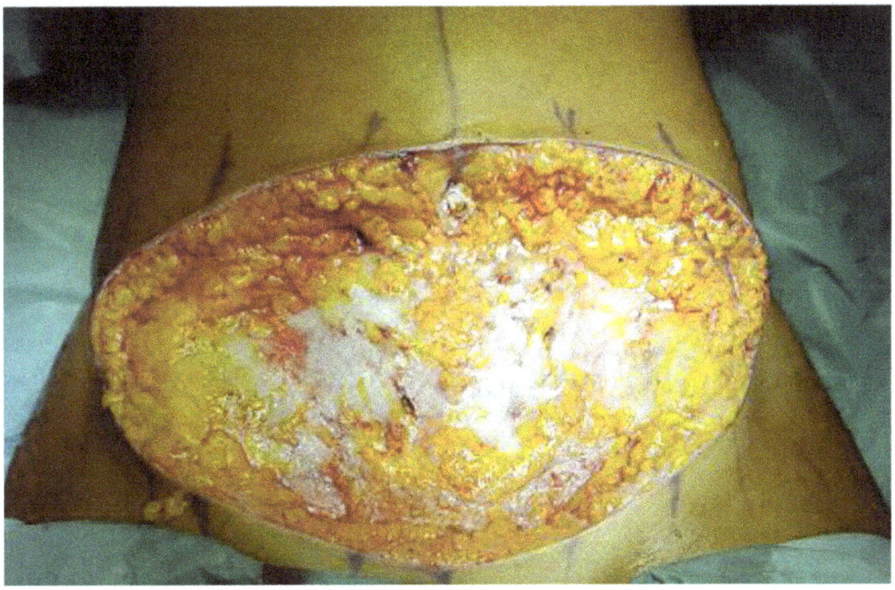

Figure 6. After In-Block redundant tissues resection including the umbilical scar.

At this point the patient should be placed in a semi-upright sitting position (45°) (bayonet position) **Figure 7**, to facilitate transverse plication of the aponeurotic fascia of the abdomen.

The first stitch we place is the central one that goes from the old umbilical scar to the nearest point of the suprapubic incision. Generally this distance is 5–10 cm depending on the degree of abdominal wall laxness, **Figure 8**.

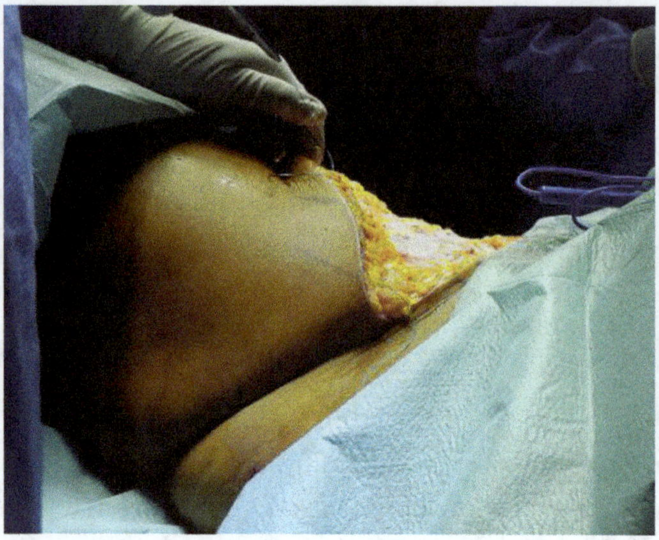

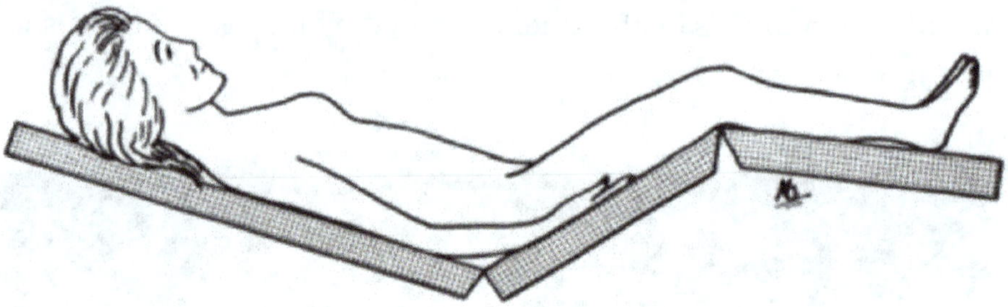

Figure 7. Patient it's placed in a Jacknife position

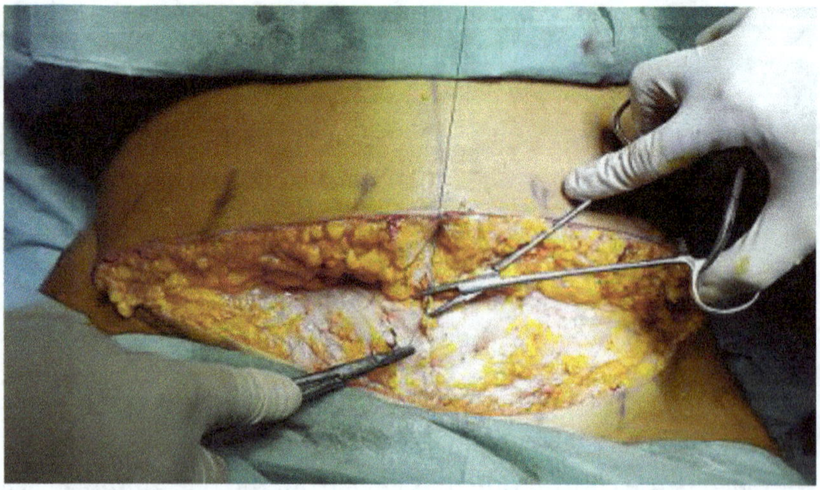

Figure 8. Closure of old umbilical defect and first stitch of thansverse plicature.

Then with the same nonabsorbable material we perform a simple interrupted suture placing stitches on each side of the first one, every 3 cm, until we cover all the width of the anterior abdominal wall.

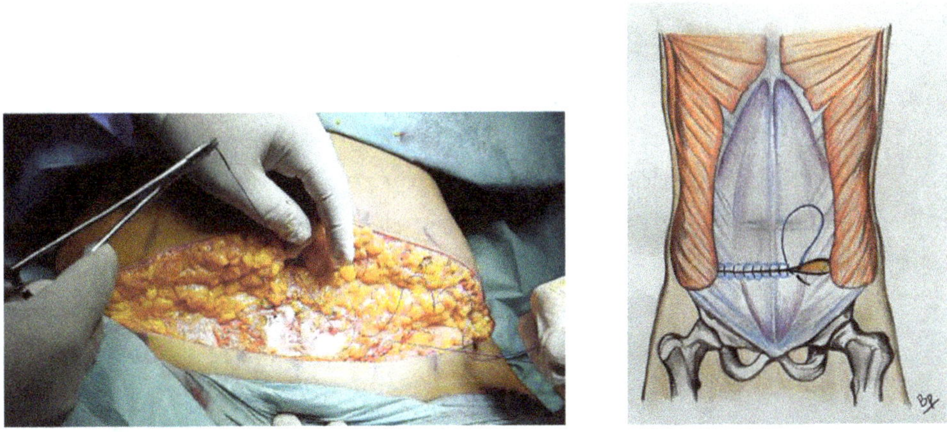

Figure 9. Transverse plicature final aspect.

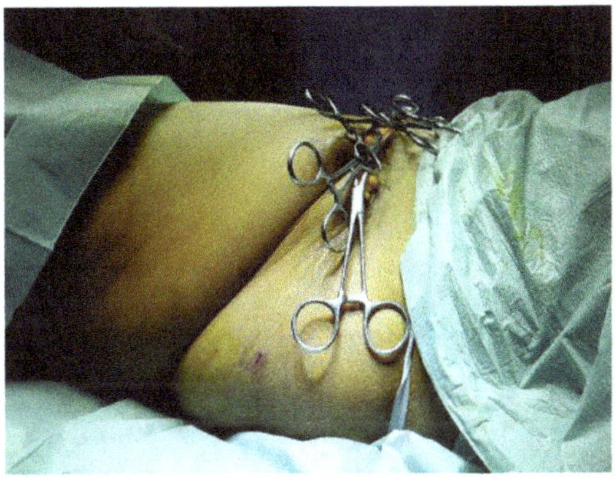

Figure 10. Transitory wound closure with the help of towll clamps.

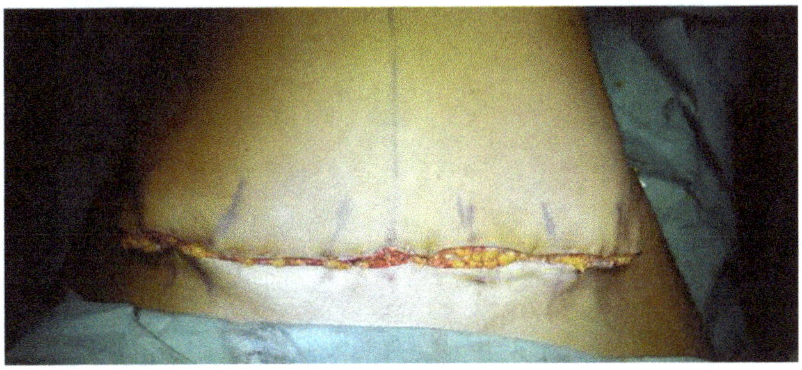

Figure 11. Closure of subcutanous layer.

The suture takes an oblique direction so that the plicature takes a vector from out to inside, thus improving the shape of the waist and avoiding a dog-ear formation. We perform a suture from scarpa fascia to mons pubis in order to stabilize the final scar position and then continius running suture with nonabsorbable monofilament number 0. Before subcutanous closure a careful control of hemostasis with electrocautery its done, **Figure 9**.

Bupivacaine 1% 10 cc solution its infiltrated at the subfascial plane on the inferior abdomen in order to control postoperative pain during the first 12 hours. The Scarpa fascia plane its closed using 2–0 vicryl sutures, for the subcutaneous cellular tissue, with 2-0 monocryl mattress suture and 3–0 monocryl for the dermis and skin using an intradermal continuous pattern, The surgical table return to the original position in order to stablish the position of the new umbilical scar **Figures 10** and **11**.

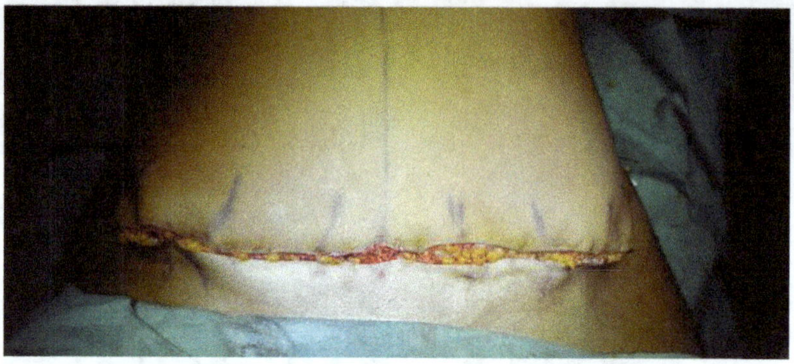

Figure 12. Skin and subcutaneous layer closure.

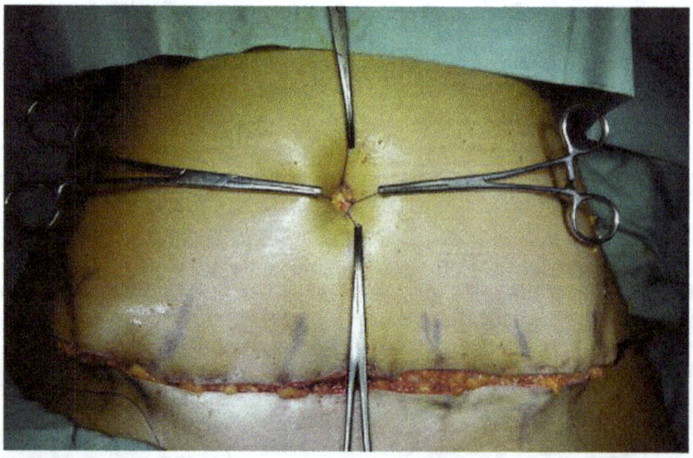

Figure 13. Umbilical reconstruction.

Through an oval-shaped incision in the midline, 3 cm cephalic direction from the iliac crests, the neoumbilicus is recreated by resecting skin, then the borders of the aponeurosis are folded with 3–0 monocryl and a full thickness skin graft is placed at the bottom fixed with 3–0 monocryl, careful control of hemostasis with electrocautery, **Figures 12** and **13**.

5. Results

From 2013 to 2015, 188 patients were operated on, of which 178 were women and 10 were men; the age range was 24–74 years. Likewise, other combined surgeries were performed such as mastopexy, breast inclusion, face-lifting, rhinoplasty, and blepharoplasty, among others. The most common combined surgery was TULUA with laser lipolysis 4 regions 123 cases, then mastopexy with implants 18 cases, mastopexy without implants 13 cases, gluteoplasty increase by lipotransference 9 cases, TULUA 7 cases, breast inclusion 4, upper blepharoplasty 3, gynecomastia 3, facelift 2, breast lipotransference 2, bichat 2, rhinoplasty 1, and vaginoplasty 1 (see **Figure 14**).

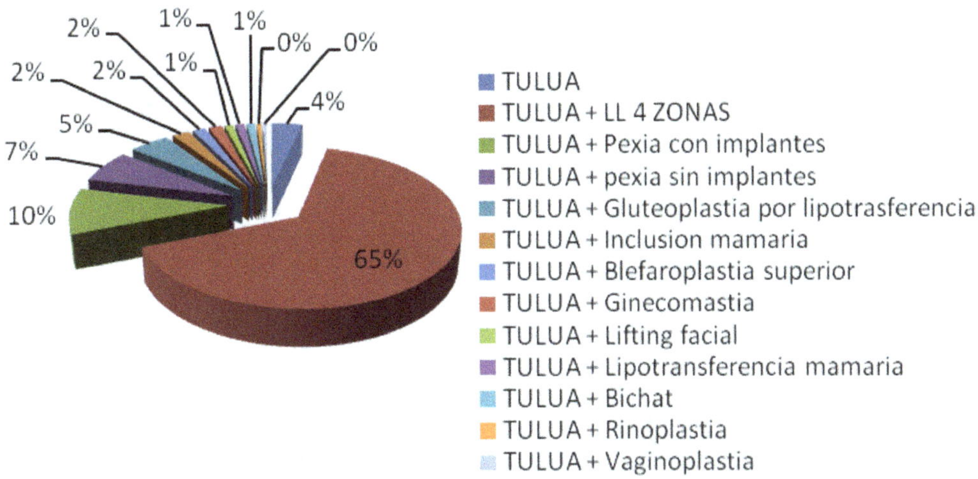

Figure 14. The summary of all the results of the technique combined procedures and complications.

Combined surgeries and TULUA	
TULUA	7
TULUA + LL 4 regions	123
TULUA + mastopexy with implants	18
TULUA + mastopexy without implants	13
TULUA + gluteoplasty by fat graft	9
TULUA + breast inclusion	4
TULUA + superior blepharoplasty	3
TULUA + gynecomastia	3
TULUA + facelife	2
TULUA + breast lipotransference	2
TULUA + bichat	2
TULUA + rhinoplasty	1
TULUA + vaginoplastia	1

Complications	
Seroma	17
Dehiscence	11
Umbilical flap loss	7
Hypertrophic scar	3
Dog-ear formation	2
Infected wound	1
Umbilical granuloma	1
Seroma + dehiscence	1

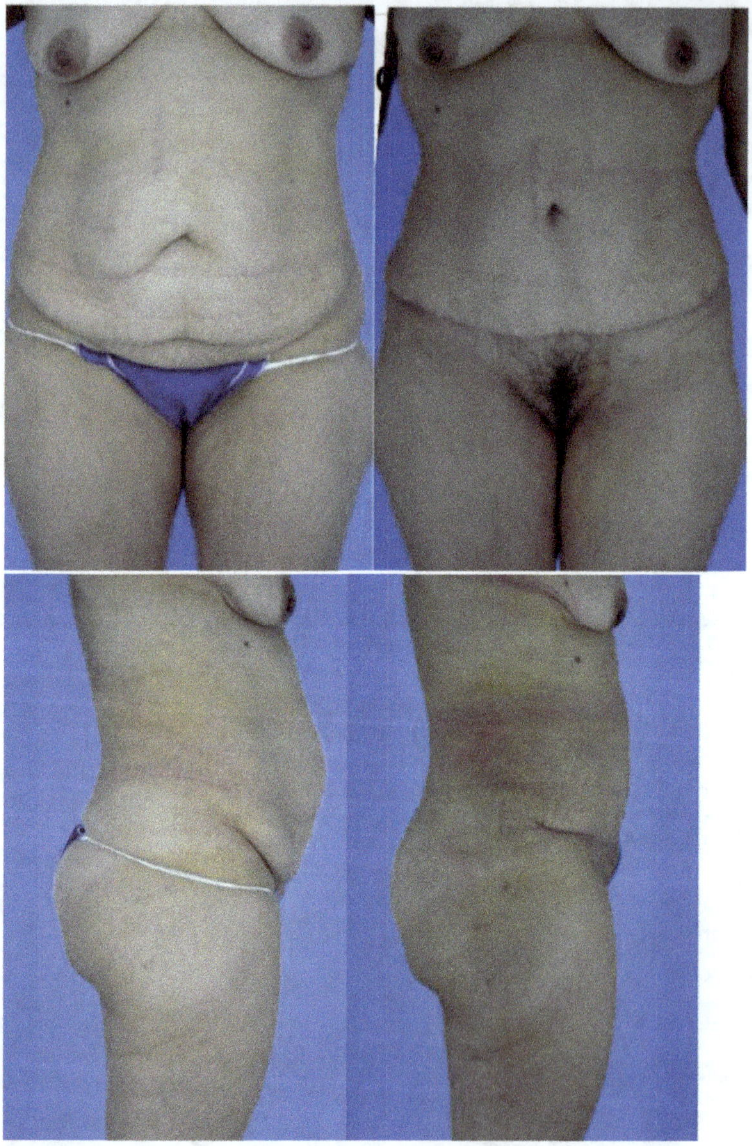

Figure 15. Before and after result in patient with a previous surgical scar.

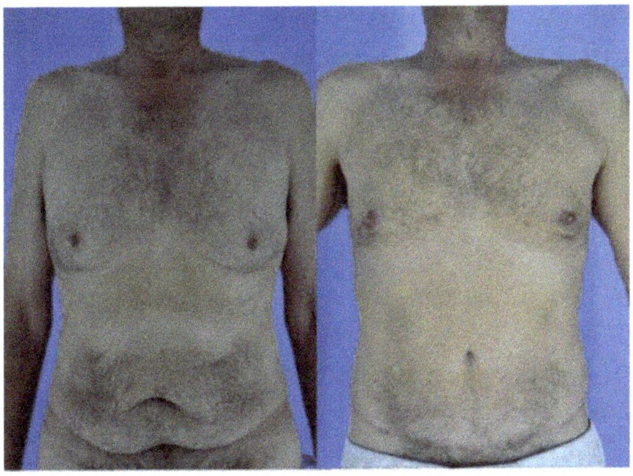

Figure 16. Before and after result in a male patient after massive weight loss.

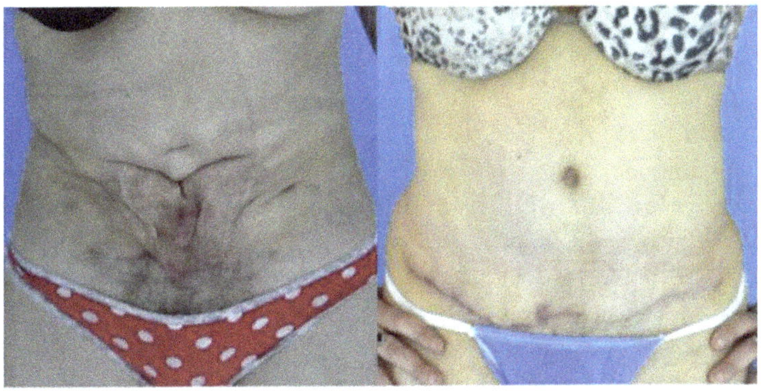

Figure 17. Before and after result in a patient that present fibrotic séquelas after liposuction.

The most common complications were seroma after liposuction, 17 cases; partial dehiscence —no more than 1 cm—, 11 cases; umbilical flap loss, seven cases; hypertrophic scar, three cases; dog-ear formation, two cases; infected wound, one case; umbilical granuloma, one case; seroma combined with dehiscence, one case.

Postoperative recovery—to resume activities—takes 15 days; the drain is not left, and manual lymphatic drain is prescribed 1 week after surgery for 1 month **Figures 15**, **16** and **17**.

6. Conclusion

This paper attempts to show that the TULUA (transverse plication, no undermining, full liposuction, neoumbilicoplasty, and low transverse abdominal scar) technique offers abdominoplasty patients greater safety because no dissection of the upper flap is performed, preserving the major vessels of the integument in the anterior wall, they can be corrected hernias of the abdominal wall, low-rate infections, etc. Indicated for patients with multiple comorbidities; hypertension, diabetes, autoimmune diseases, along with tumescence. In our hands, patients are discharged the same day, without relying on strong painkillers. This technique could be consdered a modified lipoabdominoplasty focused in diminish the complications rate of this tyoe of procedures and the one observed in the classic abdominoplasty.

Author details

Guillermo Blugerman, Diego Schavelzon, Boris Martínez*, Gabriel Wexler, Andrea Markowsky and Marcelo Lotoki

*Address all correspondence to: drblugerman@gmail.com

B & S Center of Excellence in Plastic Surgery, Buenos Aires, Argentina

References

[1] Kelly HA, Excision of the fat of the abdominal wall. Surg Gynec Obstet 1910; 10: 229.

[2] Pitanguy I, Abdominal lipectomy: an approach to it through an analysis of 300 consecutive cases. Plast Reconstr Surg 1967; 40: 384.

[3] Avelar J, Fat suction versus abdominoplasty. Aesth Plastic Surg 1985; 9: 265.

[4] Saldanha OR. Lipoabdominoplasty without undermining. Aesth Surg J 2001; 21: 518.

[5] Weinhold S, Bauchdeckenplastik. Zentralbl F Gynak 1909; 38: 1332.

[6] Babcock W, The correction of the obese and relaxed abdominal wall with special reference to the use of buried silver chain. Phila Obstet Soc May 14, 1916.

[7] Schepelmann E, Bauchdeckenplastik mit besonderer Berucksichtigung des Hangebauches. Beitr Klm Chir 1918; 3: 372.

[8] Thorek M, Plastic surgery of the breast and abdominal wall, Charles C. Thomas, Springfield, II, 1924.

[9] Flesh-Thebesius M, Wheisheimer K, Operation des hangebauches. Chirug 1931; 3: 841.

[10] Pick IF, Surgery of repair: principles, problems, procedures. Abdomen (abdereplasty), vol 2. Lippmncott, Philadelphia, 1949, p. 435.

[11] Barsky AJ, Principles and practice of plastic surgery, Williams & Wilkins, Baltimore, 1950.

[12] Galtier M, Surgical therapy of obesity of the abdominal wall with ptosis. Mcm Acad Chir 1955; 81: 341.

[13] Dufourmentel C, Mouly R, Chirurgie plastique. Flammarion, Paris, 1959, pp. 381–389.

[14] Vernon S, Umbilical transplantation upward and abdominal contouring in lipectomie. Am J Surg 1957; 94: 490–492.

[15] Gonzalez-Ulloa M, Belt lipectomy. Br J Plast Surg 1960; 13: 179.

[16] Vilain R, Dubousset J, Technique et indications de la lipectomie circulaire. 1250 observations. Ann Chir 1964; 18: 289.

[17] Spadafora A, Abdomen adiposa y péndulo-dermolipectomia iliaco-inguino-pubiana. Prensa Universitaria (Buenos Aires) 1965; 114: 1839.

[18] Regnault P, Abdominoplasty by the W technique. Plast Reconstr Surg 1975; 55: 265.

[19] Planas J, The vest over pants abdominoplasty. Plast Reconstr Surg 1978; 61: 694.

[20] Shiffman MA, Cosmetic surgery of the abdominal wall, 2007, ISBN: 978-958-8328-10-2.

[21] Hester TR Jr. Nahai F, Beegle PE, Bostwick J, Blood supply of the abdomen revisited, with emphasis on the superficial inferior epigastric artery. Plast Reconstr Surg 1984; 74: 657–670.

[22] Linszka TG, Dellon AL, Manson PN. Iliohypogastric nerve entrapment following abdominoplasty. Plast Reconstr Surg 1994; 93: 181–184.

[23] Neaman KC, Armstrong SD, Baca ME, et al., Outcomes of traditional cosmetic abdominoplasty in a community setting: a retrospective analysis of 1008 patients. Plast Reconstr Surg 2013; 131: 403e–410e.

7

High-Definition Liposculpture

Carlos Oaxaca

Abstract

In this chapter, we describe the author's experience with the technique, the characteristics of the ideal patients and the postoperative management of these patients to obtain positive outcomes. It is of clinical importance to underline that a good skin quality is mandatory to get the best results.

We operated on various patients between 20 and 30 years of age.

Several authors have described different techniques using different devices, but skin quality, the volume of fat to be suctioned and the surgeon's skill are critical to achieving good results.

Keywords: Liposculpture, High-definition body contour, Liposculpture small volume, minimal liposculpture

1. History "Who does not know the history is condemned to repeat it"

Charles H. Willi (1926) was the first surgeon to inject small quiantity of fat for aesthetic purposes. Giorgio Fischer (1975) was the first to describe the removal of fat through small incisions (5 mm) using a cannula, with an internal mechanism to cut and was called the "planotome" that was attached to a suction machine. Syringe-assisted, ultrasound-assisted, laser-assisted-, water jet-assisted, power-assisted, and percussion massage-assisted liposuction techniques have evolved since. Bircoll (1982) described the use of autologous fat from liposuction and then use it for contouring and filling defects.

Morever, the addition of stem cells to fat that has been transferred to improve fat survival is considered the newest method. We also know that cosmetic surgery is changing and improving through new instruments (machines, cannulas), as well as through new ideas as noted by several authors, and modifications of old techniques. We believe that more advances and development in the field will continue in the years to come.

2. Introduction

No sculpture can carve an aesthecially and shapely body without the knowledge of its anatomy, and this is where this surgery (high-definition liposculpture) is quite amazing. Therefore, as surgeons, we must know exactly and almost in a perfect fashion, the tendons, muscles, valleys and zenith (cancavities and convexities) of every single muscle in the abdomen for it to be recreated.

Over the years, the concepts of liposculpture have changed and we know about the different techniques such as super wet and wet and dry that are used to beautify body countouring.

3. What is High-Definition Liposculpture?

This is an advanced body sculpting technique for the rectus abdominis and oblique muscles that can give a properly selected patient excellent results, specifically a highly sculpted, athletic body shape. Alfredo Hoyos from Colombia [1, 2] was among the first surgeons who has describedthis technique with VASER, with excellent results. Generally, patient selection or eligibility to undergo this procedure to créate a highly defined body contour is critical. Thus, talking to the patients about the clinical requirements, and overall, being objective with the results, are essential.

Note that there are different body forms: mesomorph, ectomorph, and endomorph. Depending on the body type identified, we must find the body proportion.

However, these body types will be different between women and men, and so we must have these in mind before planning the surgery.

In the abdomen, specificall for the men, there isa tendency to gain more intra-abdominal fat in the whole abdomen, including the epigastric, mesogastryc and hipogastric areas, compared to the women because men accumulate more fat in the hipogastric area but more extra-abdominal.

The anatomical form of women (**Figure 1**) is rounded and different from men that is an inverted trapezoid (**Figure 2**. Male abdomcn).

Optimal male body contouring should consider the entire torso and skin draping tightly over well-developed muscles through abdominoplasty and multiple oblique ellipses [5]. Nowadays, not just the men, but also women are seeking this kind of surgery, more to impress, especially when they are In swimsuit clothes.

Thus, to recreate this kind of abdomen, several descriptions on the techniques: VASER, laser, and standard Liposuction have been published.

When there is skin excess, this will have to be removed horizontally to have the skin tightly bound to the muscle. In this case, the surgery must be done in two stages.

How will the best results be obtained? Is it true that expensive devices are needed to perform it?

The answer is "not always," as has been described and experienced by some surgeons from the USA.

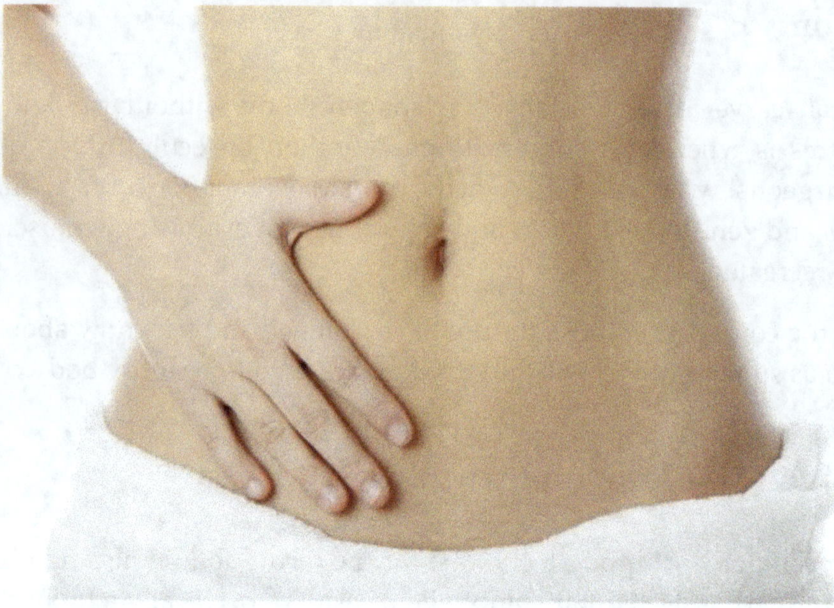

Figure 1. Female Abdomen.

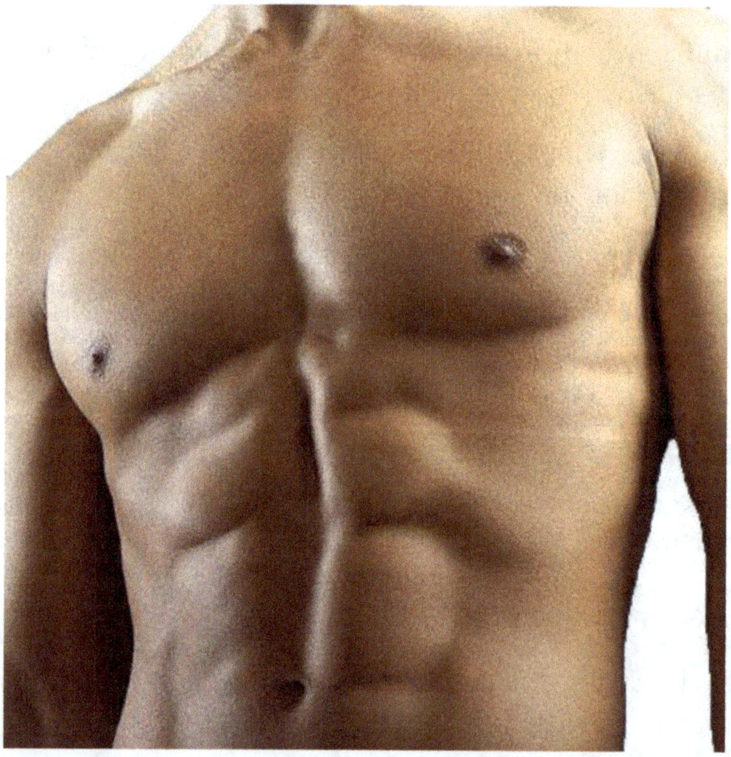

Figure 2. Male Abdomen.

It is important to mention that for best results, a good skin quality is mandatory because flaccidity will not give us high definition. In consultations with the patient, male or female, their expatatives are asked.

4. Anatomy

We must know about the ideal anatomy of the abdomen:

4.1. Rectus Abdominis

This muscle arises from the symphysis, crest, and pecten of the pubis and runs upward to insert into the xiphoid process and costal cartilages of the fifth to seventh ribs. Its main action is to flex the trunk (**Figure 3**).

4.2. External Oblique

This muscle forms the lateral abdomen. It originates from the external and inferior surfaces of the lower seventh to eighth ribs. The external oblique has two parts: an upper thoracic portion and a lower flank portion.

4.3. Serratus Anterior

This quadrilateral muscle originates anteriorly as fingerlike bundles from the external surfaces of the upper eighth to ninth ribs and wraps around the rib cage to insert into the vertical, medial edge of the scapula. It acts to draw the scapula laterally and around the rib cage, as in punching.

The below parts are not in the abdomen but form part of the aesthetic anatomy of the anterior chest:

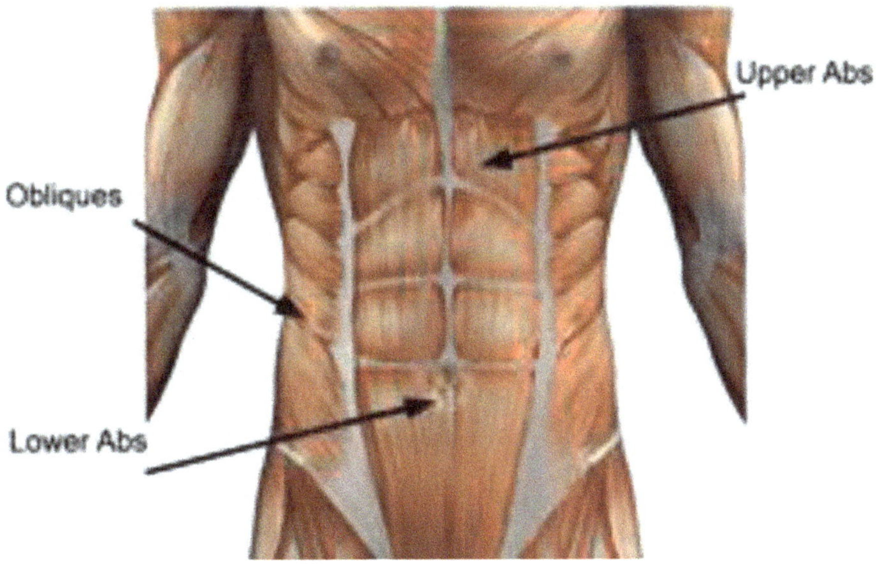

Figure 3. Anatomy of the Abdomen.

4.4. Pectoralis Major

The pectoralis major forms most of the muscle bulk of the chest and gives the chest a smooth, convex form, particularly when the muscle is well developed and defined. It originates from the medial half of the clavicle, anterior surface of the sternum, costal cartilages of the first 6th–7th ribs, and inferiorly, the superior part of the external oblique aponeurosis of the abdomen.

4.5. Latissimus Dorsi

The latissimus dorsi is a triangular muscle that passes from the midline to the arm like a cape, covering the deeper muscles of the mid and lower back. It originates from the spinous processes of the seventh to twelfth thoracic vertebrae, those of all of the lumbar and sacral vertebrae, the posterior one-third of the iliac crest, and the external surfaces of the lower three ribs.

5. Fat Metabolism

Fatty tissue represents at birth, about 17 % of bodyweight;and in adolescence, around 20% in women and 10 % in men with some phenotypic variations. In normal adults, fat approaches 15–20%in men and 25–30% in women. Two types of fat are described in the human body: white adipose tissue and brown adipose tissue.Fatty tissue also plays an important role as an energy source during exercise. Fat, the major energy stored in the body, is mobilized from adipose tissue as free fatty acids to provide metabolicfuel. At lower exercise intensities, fats may provide 50–60% of the energy for muscle contraction, but this process cannot keep pace withthe high demands for energy that occurs during heavy exercise. Energy liberation from fat is slower than the liberation of glucose from glycogen.Moderate activity, in fact, favors the consumption of fat as muscle fuel. The depletion of body fat reserves is almost never a limiting factorin muscle activity. In the absence of other fuels, proteins can serve as an energy source for contraction, particularly as it occurs during heavy,prolonged, or intense exercise.

6. Anatomy of the Fatty Tissue

We must consider anatomy before liposculpture can be done. We have the skin, the superficial and deep fat layer, divided by the superficial fascia (Scarpa) and the deep fascia (Camper).

Additionally, the fat thickness in the body varies. The superficial adipose tissue in the abdomen is thicker and in the gluteal and thigh, it is thinner. In the leg, there is only superficial and no deep adipose tissue.

It is extremely important to consider the fat percentage between women and men, and for the purpose of this chapter, note always that the less the fat percentage, the better the result will be (**Figure 4**).

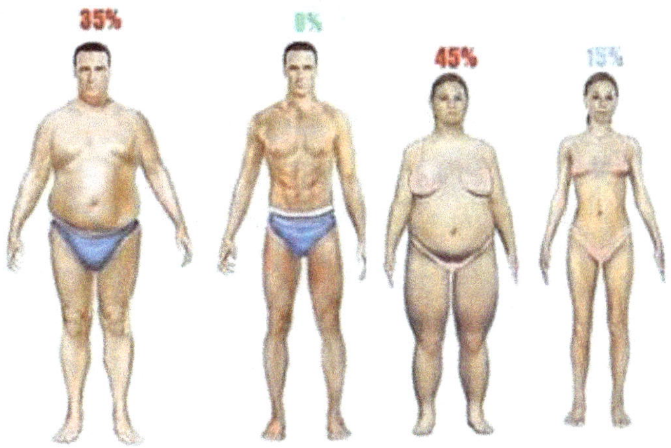

Body Fat Percentages

Description	Men	Women
Essential fat	2-5%	10-13%
Athletes	6-13%	14–20%
Fitness	14–17%	21–24%
Acceptable	18–24%	25–31%
Obese	25%+	32%+

* American Council on Exercise Guidelines

Figure. 4. Body differences between women and men.

7. Who is the Ideal Patient?

The medical history of each patient is essential. Inquiring about patient intake of salicilates or other medicines is also important. Most importantly, regardless if laboratory test results are normal, we need to ask and verify if they are taking dietary complements, such as vitamin E, vitamin A, or artichoke, green tea, ginko and other similar complements that extend coagulation time.

7.1. Indications

The most critical factors in selecting patients are the following:

1. Skin elasticity.

2. Work up in the gym (for better results).

3. Age variability.

Patients with poor skin quality and strias are not ideal candidates for this procedure because their skin will not shrink appropriately.

Patients whose work up on gym or regularly exercising on daily basis, are preferred, because are expected that there will be less amount of fat to be suctioned, so after surgery will result in high definition muscle.

7.2. Contraindications

Age is an important factor with older age, there is more flaccidity. Patients who are obese are also not good candidates for this procedure.

Ahigh tendency to gain weight is also a factor.

Patients have to be analyzed in standing and sitting positions to check if muscle diastasis of the rectus abdominis muscle exists.

Grasping the skin to look for flaccidity that could be an important factor to get the best results is also important.

Having photographs of the patient are likewise essential. First, these will help in supporting comments and observations during consultation.

Second, this could help to protect us, because many times, patients will appreciate better the result, when they see their former physical body.

That is why we always take photos pre and postoperatively and dispaly them on a big screen, after every consultation. This will avoid any claim.

8. Preparation of the Patient

In consultation, the availability and analysis of the patients' lab tests incluiding Haematic counts, protein levels, partial thromboplastin time and prothrombin time, and glucose, urea and creatinin levels are necessary.

The protein level is a prognostic factor to determine if there is alowriskoflung thromboembolism.

It is equally important that the patient read and sign an informed consent form where details including the type of anesthesia, the kind of the surgical procedure, and even possible complications, such as allergy, bleeding, infection, pain, pulmonary embolism, scarring, and seroma, are explained.

9. Anesthesia

Although there are two options for anesthesia, general anesthesia is preferred. For this type of surgery, this is not a problem because the amount of aspiration is about 600 ml on average, but the operative time is long. Intraoperative tumescent anesthesia, using the Klein solution is as follows:

- Saline solution, 1 lt
- Sodium bicarbonate, 10 ml
- Lidocaine 2%, 50 ml
- Epinephrine, 1 ml

As the total aspirated volume is less than 600 to 800 ml, then we use the same amount of volume. This will decrease the bleeding.

Remember that lidocaine has two effects: create vasoconstricticon to lessen the bleeding and slow the systemic absorption of lidocaine.

It is crucial that the surgeon always verifies the prepared solution, to avoid, in some occasions, potential mistakes from nursing staff when they prepare the solution.

10. Markings

The markings are the most important factor because we delineate the belly of the rectus abdominis muscle and the oblique muscles to be tailored (**Figure 5**).

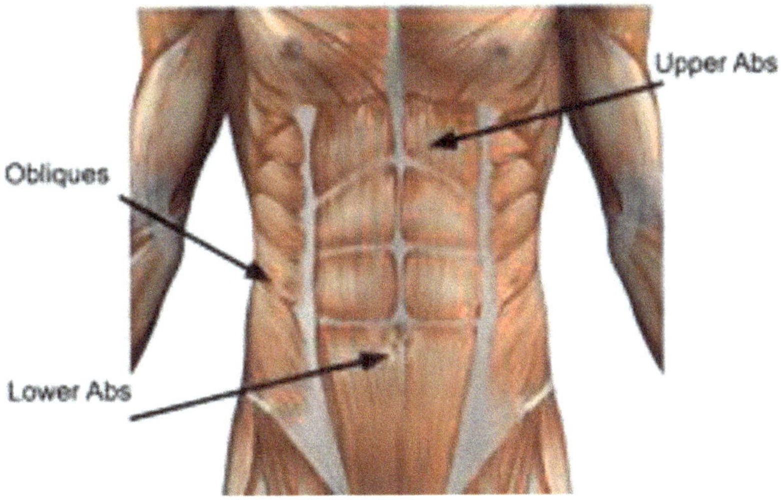

Fig. 5. Valleys and peaks to be mimicked during the liposculpture.

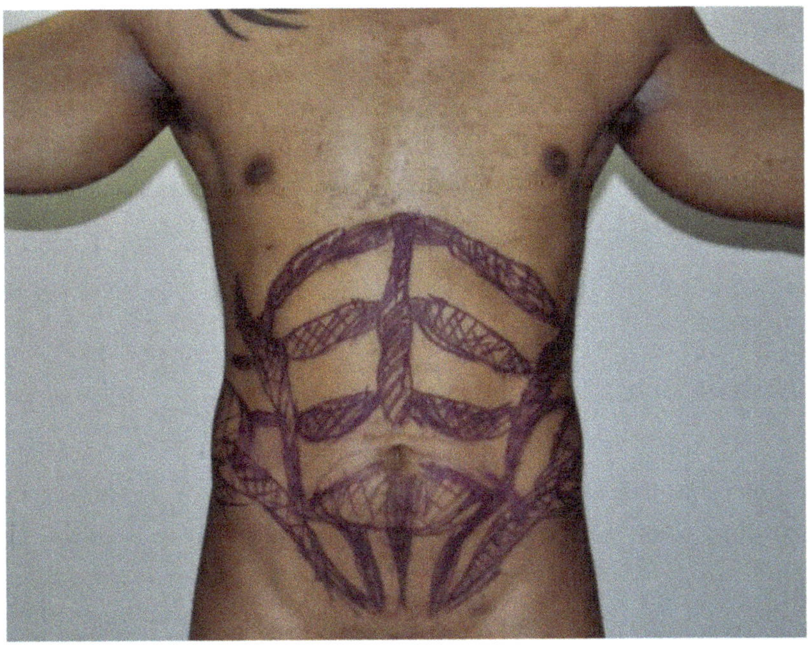

Fig. 6. Marking the patient.

The patient must be marked in a standing position and this will take several minutes, but this is one of the most crucial parts of the procedure (**Figure 6**). The muscular anatomy must be recreated with the surgery and here, the valleys and peaks must be done with the cannula. This procedure takes more tan 30 minutes. An artistic drawing on the patient's body is done before the surgery in standing position.

11. Technique

The patient is always operated on under general anhestesia. In a standing position, the area is cleaned with betadyne and the surgical table is covered with sterilized clothing.

Saline solution (one liter), epinephrine (one ampule) and sodium bicarbonate (one) are added to infiltrate the area to be suctioned. We won't need more than 600 ml of this solution.

Small incisions are placed as marked in **Figure 6**.

The male patients are completely marked because they request for a "six-pack" abdomen. Sometimes we have to define the pectoral area and this can be done by high-definition liposculpture or adding pectoral implants [4].

The treatment for women is different because they want the medial depression of the alba line to be recreated and that the demarcation between the oblique and rectus muscle (semilunar line) be defined. These are important points to be remembered or considered [4].

Another point is thinking about the intra-abdominal and extra-abdominal fat, with the former being more challenging.

Liposculpture is done with a 20-ml syringe and a 2- or 3-mm cannula. It takes about 4 hours on average and the tip of the cannula is turning up to the skin to create fibrosis from the underside of the skin to the fascia. An aggressive cannula is used like a chisel in the subcutaneous tissue for superficial liposuction, removing the fat at the level of the tendinous inscriptions, the anatomic lines, and the muscular borders, toemphasize the muscle bulk, which means recreating muscle valleys and peaks as mentioned previously.

Patients who used to be obese could be required to undergo two stages of surgery, one to excise the abdominal skin excess and then do liposuction, and the second to sculpt the abdominal muscles [4].

The critical point in attaining high definition is to highlight adherence in the tendinuous area.

The incisions are placed in the suprapubic area, generally two of 2-mm in length, another one in the umbilicus and epigastric area. Sometimes it may be required in the lateral area of the abdomen to recreate the tendinous inscriptions of the muscles. The cannulas used are 6 hole with 2- to 4-mm diameter, generally with a 20-ml syringe. If an area has more fat deposit, then a 5 mm diameter cannula is used, with 50 ml siringe. Then the final touch is done with 2 mm cannula.

The infiltration is done by areas, because it is time-consuming procedure, that takes more tan 4 hours, on average. Normally, infiltration is started from the hypogastric area and flanks, going superiorly, and then going from the epigastric incision and lateral incisions to create the oblique and six-pack abdomen desired by the patient. Sometimes micro-fat grafting may be required to get the best results.

Note that it is important not to simply think about creating a symmetrical "six-pack abdomen, as doing it so symmetrical, may lead to an unnatural result.

The incisions are sutured with nylon 6-0 or subcutaneous monocryl 5-0. Then a special garment is used, but in the area where surgery was performed, a foam tapped with a 1- inch wide micropore will be added and left there for at least 1 week. The garment will be retained for one month all day long and for the second month, it will be just be during the day, and then resting by night. Care must be taken not to use tied garment if micro-fat grafting has been used, otherwise it will reduce the viability of the grafted fat.

Moisturizing the skin at this moment is mandatory.

Drains are never used for these patients because the amount suctioned

12. Postoperative Care

The author used levofloxacine 500 mg daily for 1 week and ibuprofen 400 mg twice daily for 1 week. For a small amount of fat suctioned, enoxaparine is prescribed, due to the length of time of surgery.

The goal in the postoperative period is to reduce bruising, avoid hypertrophic scars and allow adhesions where there must be retraction in the tendinuous areas of the muscles, therefore, postoperative ultrasound must be avoided.

Arnica is used one tablet twice a day for 2 weeks to reduce bruising.

Manual lymphatic drainage (MLD) [3] pioneered by Emil Vodder in 1930's is done after the first postoperative week, and this will reduce postoperative edema. The strategically induced change in pressure in the subcutaneous tissues enhances filling and emptying of initial lymphatics, increases the rate of contraction of lymphatics, and increases lymphatic transport capacity. Firmer, deeper movements may be employed in localized areas to soften hardened tissue due to fibrosis or fibrosclerosis, but excessively deep, diffuse pressure is avoided to minimize capillary filtration. The benefits of manual lymphatic drainage are stimulation of the lymphatic flow and circulation; stimulation of the immune system, parasympathetic nervous system with relaxation and anti-spastic effects, and as perineural edema is lessened, pain is also reduced; fibrosis reduction, improvement of cellular nutrition; and tissue recovery. The frequency of each session must be 2 days each for at least 2 weeks. The duration of each session must be anywhere from 40 to 60 minutes. Care must be taken to ensure that MLD is carried out gently and without pain to the patient.

The stitches are taken out on the at 7th day, postoperatively, but if the suture material used is monocryl, then this will no longer be necessary.

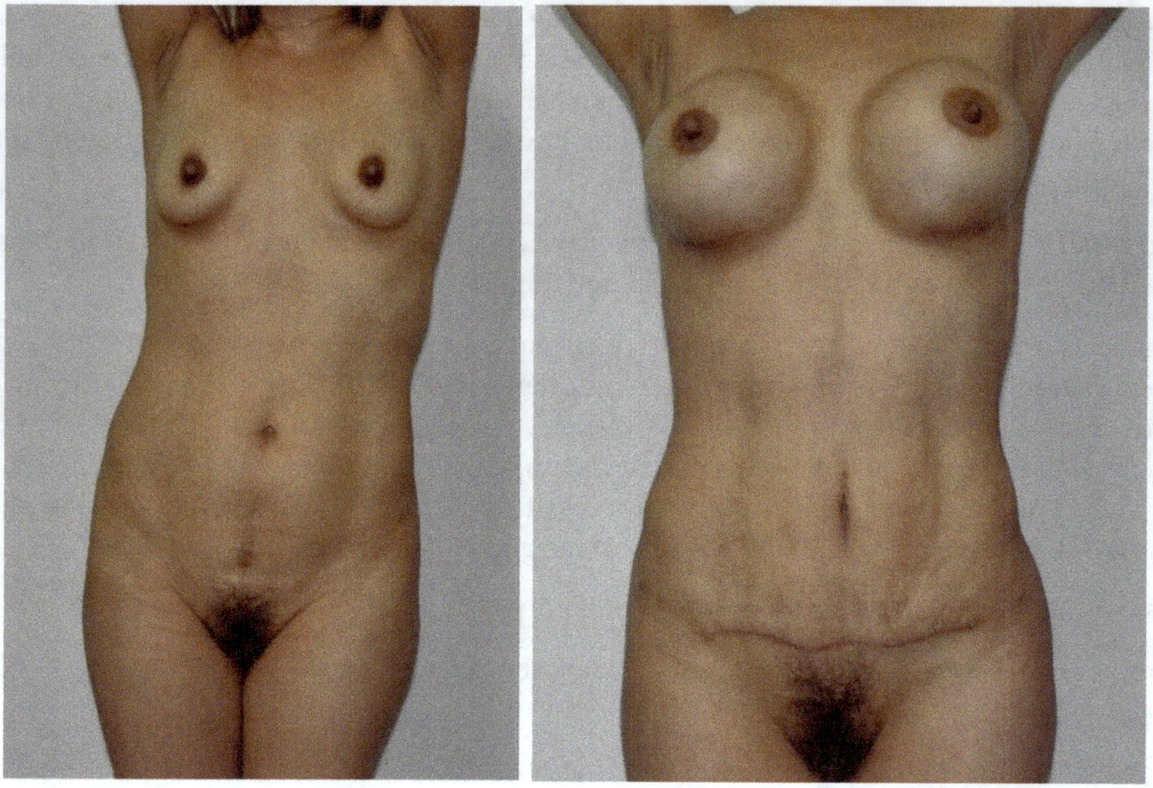

Figure 7. Frontal pre and postoperative photos: female patient with miniabdominoplasty.

Garments are used day and night for the first month postoperatively, and taken out only for cleansing. For the second month, garments are used just during the day, and taken out by night. Epifoam is used in the areas where depressions have been created in the tendinuous areas, for 3 weeks and over the garments.

13. Starting activities

The patients are asked to walk the next postoperative day using anti-thromboembolism socks for 1 week.

14. Results

The best results are obtained between 3 and 6 months postoperatively. This is always mentioned to the patients because they ask in the first postoperative consultations about the results, and they are eager to see the final result in the first month. The appointments are made in the office at Day 7 and then 1, 3, 6 and 12 months postoperatively. At 3rd month, (before and after) photos are taken and shown to the patient on a big screen, this way, they will see the results and feel more comfortable about the outcome. Results for the female patients are shown in **Figures. 7**, **8**, and **9**. Results for the male patients are shown in **Figures 10**, and **11**.

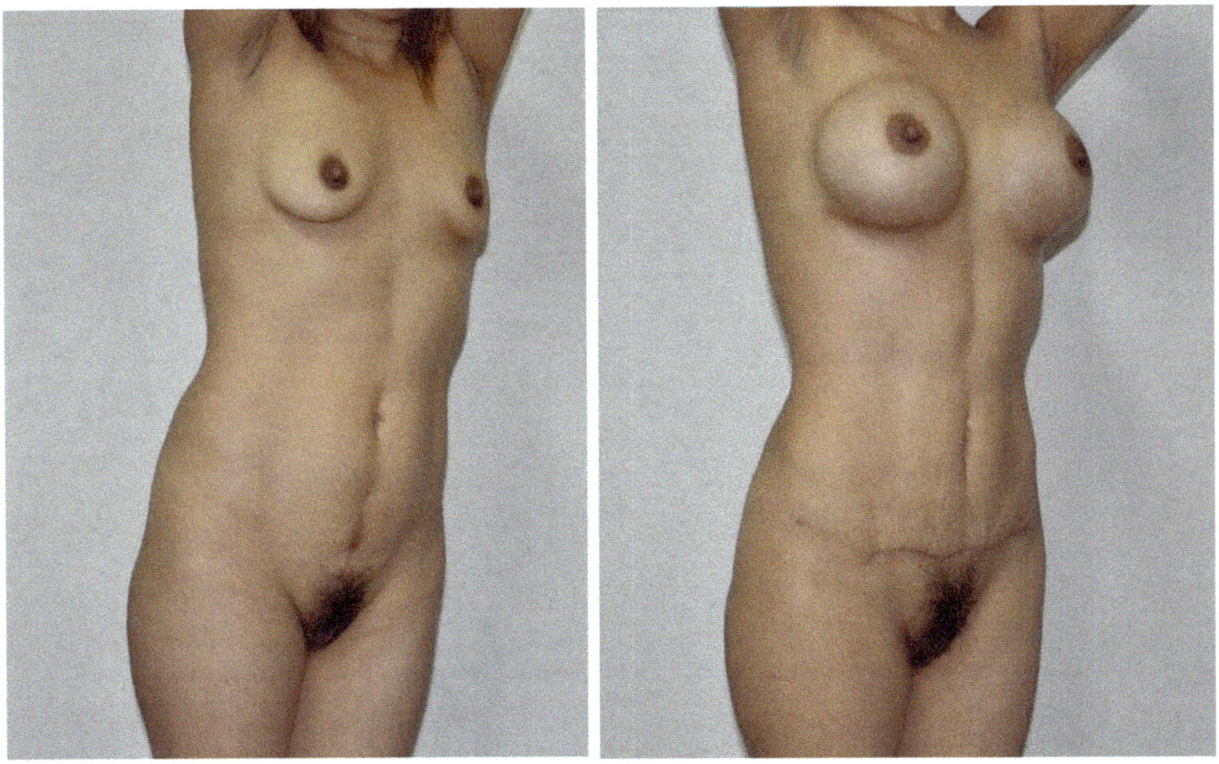

Figure 8. Pre and postoperative photos, right oblique on a female patient.

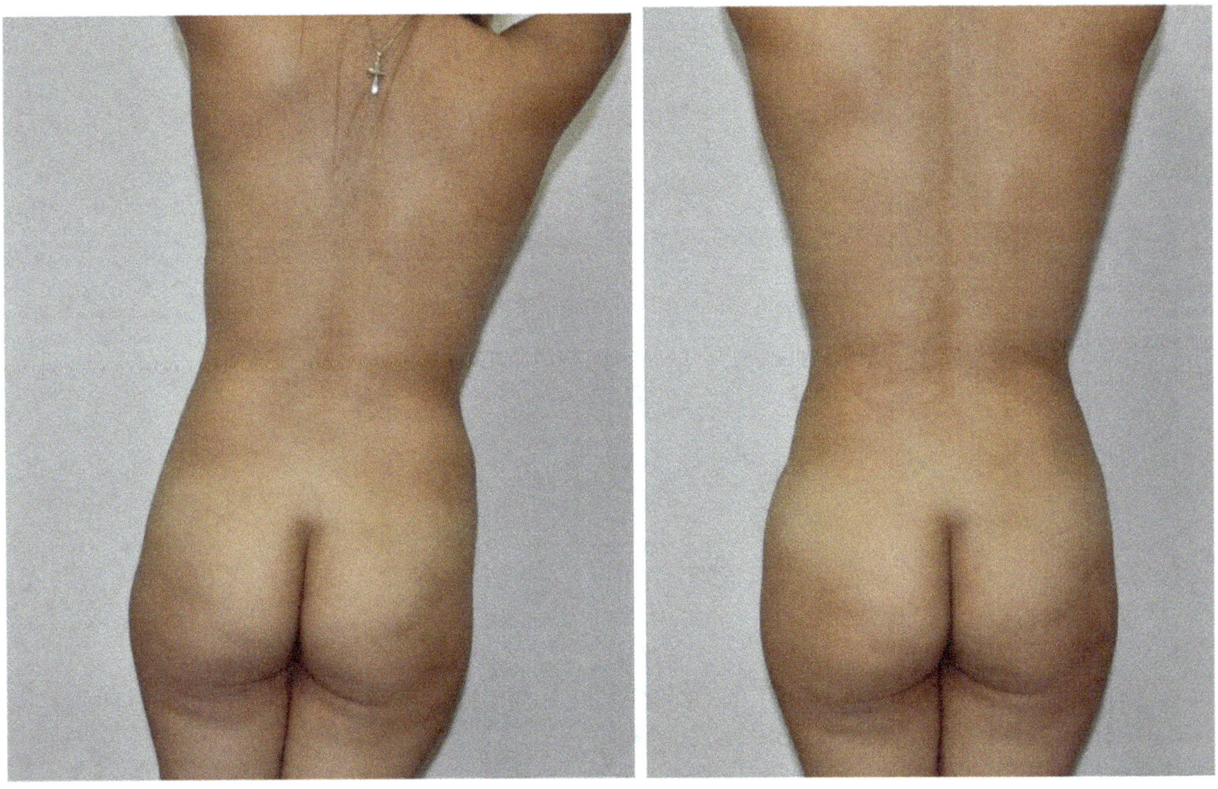

Figure 9. Pre and postoperative photos: female patient.

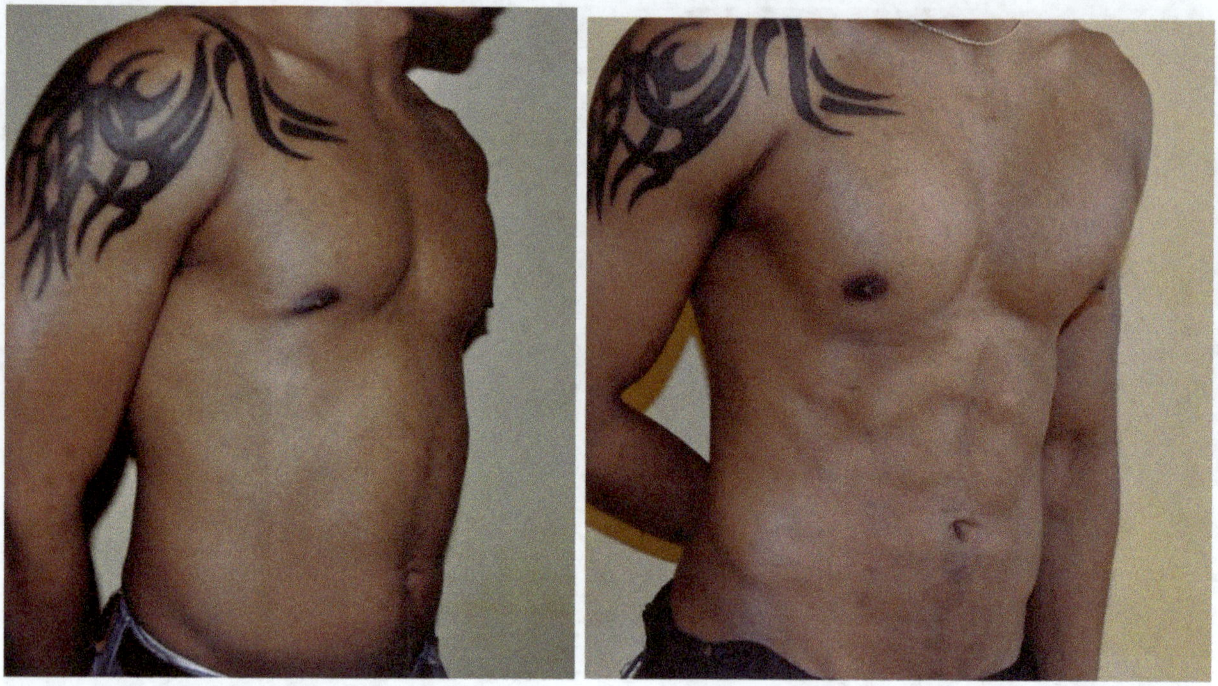

Figure 10. Right oblique pre and postoperative on a male patient.

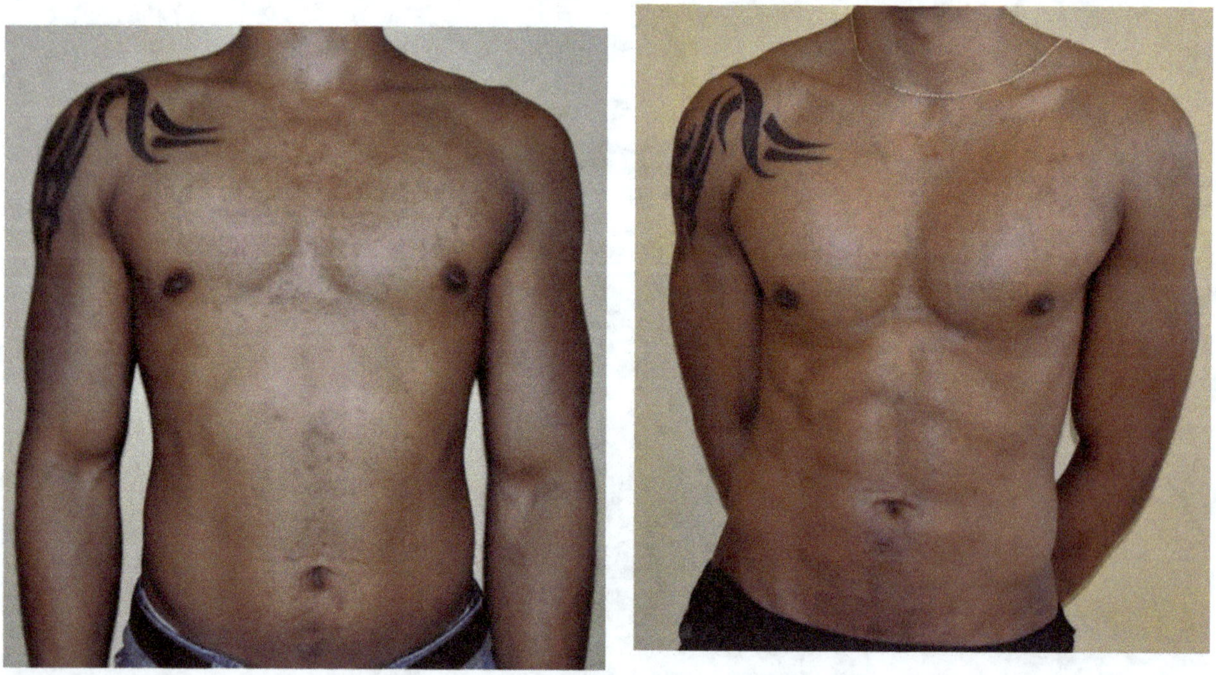

Figure 11. Frontal pre and postoperative photos on a male patient: mild assymetry on the abdomen that looks more natural.

15. Complications

It is very seldom to have complications for this surgery,given that patients are well-evaluated during preoperative stage. Bleeding is also rare as per the author's experience.

Infection may be a possibility, and so antibiotics should be started 30 minutes prior to surgery and continuing for 7 days in the postoperative period.

Skin necrosis is a high possibility with aggressive suction with the cannula when it is turned against the skin.

Seroma, pulmonary edema, thromboembolism and perforation are another complications reported, but these may be reduced, if not eliminated, with careful administration of the technique, given that it is superficial; Pinching the skin all the time, with the other hand, while cannula is passing under the skin, is necessary and helpful.

Lidocaine toxicity is rare because the amount of fluid infiltrated in the areas to be treated is very small. On large liposuctions, this complication can occur, but now, the author, has abandon its use, because the patient is under general anesthesia, then lidocaine is no longer required and this will reduce chances of toxicity.

Burns on the skin incisions because of friction caused by cannulas going in and out of the skin is a high possibility. Instiling water over the entrance of the incisions is recommended.

The absence of depressions in the sculpted areas after the surgery could be considered as a complication, but well-selected patients do not develop it. Skin retractions on sites that are not planned could happen sometimes when the cannula shifts during suctioning.

Skin flaccidity is a more common complication when patients are not selected properly.

Another potential and critical complication that must be shared to the patients is that if they gain weight and become fat in the future, the appearance of their abdomen may be likened to that of a turtle, but with a "six pack". Therefore, it is important to highlight to patients the need to always be in check of their weight.

16. Discussion

High-definition liposculpture is a highly demanding surgical procedure that needs the expertise of plastic surgeons who perform this procedure regularly. As always, the expertise is mandatory to get the best results.

Having experienced plastic surgeons and the accurate analysis as well as adequate selection of patients are crucial because these will impact having satisfied patients.

Always remember that the final result will be seen after 3 months, generally, and this must be mentioned to the patiens.

17. Conclusion

We have presented the critical points in this chapter, beginning with the anatomy, preoperative markings, standardized photos, and how the procedure must be done, apart from the ideal cannulas to be used. The purpose of this chapter is to establish the critical points to ensure a successful surgery.

Author details

Carlos Oaxaca

Address all correspondence to:droaxaca@hotmail.com

Plastic Surgeon, Torre Medica Santé, Leon, Guanajuato, México

References

[1] Hoyos E. Alfredo, Millard John. VASER assisted High Definition Liposculpture. Scientific Forum, 2007, Nov 27 (6) 594-604.

[2] Hoyos E. Alfredo, Perez Mauricio. Arm Dynamic Definition by Liposculpture and Fat Grafting. Aesthetic Surg J. 2012 32(8) 974-987.

[3] Hoyos Alfredo, Prendergast Peter. High Definition Body Sculpting. Springer Editorial, 2014.

[4] Yi Xin Zhang, David Lazzer, et al. Three-Dimensional Superficial Liposculpture of the Hips, Flanks and Thighs. Plast Reconstr Surg Global Open, 2015; 3: e291.

[5] C. Monarca, M. I. Rizzo. New Body Contouring Technique in Male: The Muscular Sculpture Aesth Plast Surg (2015) 39: 199–202.

8

Body Contour Surgery in Massive Weight Loss Patients

Redefining Body Lift Surgery and Other Contour Deformities

Marcelo A. Cuadrado, Gabriel Moina and Daniel Moina

Abstract

Background: Massive weight loss population presents different body deformities due to deflation and poor skin tone. Deformities in the lower trunk, upper torso, arms, and thighs are based on age, degree of skin laxity, and adipose tissue. Traditional plastic surgery techniques like abdominoplasty will not work in this kind of patients. Surgeon's major challenge is how to restore the skin and overlaying fat in patients that do not have the same deformities. Identifying the vectors of dropping tissue will lead to classifying this kind of deformities and planning the best surgical procedure.

Methods: Different operative techniques are described in this article to safely manage the main areas of the body. The use of combined liposuction to improve lipodystrophy areas is well indicated to avoid any complication of the main surgical treatment. A step-by-step description on postoperative indications and management is included.

Results: Plastic surgery office consultation has increased in massive weight loss patients, so it is very important to understand new body contouring techniques. It is critical that overall patient satisfaction is (mostly) achieved.

Conclusions: With a comprehensive diagnosis, patient classification, dynamic marking, and postoperative patient management, body contouring techniques have evolved from a traditional abdominoplasty, brachioplasty, thighplasty to a multiple vector correction. Results are consistent over time.

Keywords: body contouring, massive weight loss, body shaping, body lift, arm lifts, thigh reduction

1. Introduction

Today, massive weight loss patients are a big population in terms of plastic surgery office consultation. Since bariatric surgery evolution, many of the severe obese patients have become improved their health and life quality and the results of this change usually impacts their body. Skin tone and adipose tissue have their first impact revealing lax and lipodystrophy leading to hanging skin and fat all over the body.

One of the biggest problems is the correct diagnosis of patient's contour deformities.

It is our duty to exam all areas that we must treat as sections to have the contour as accurate as possible.

There are (**Figures 1** and **2**):

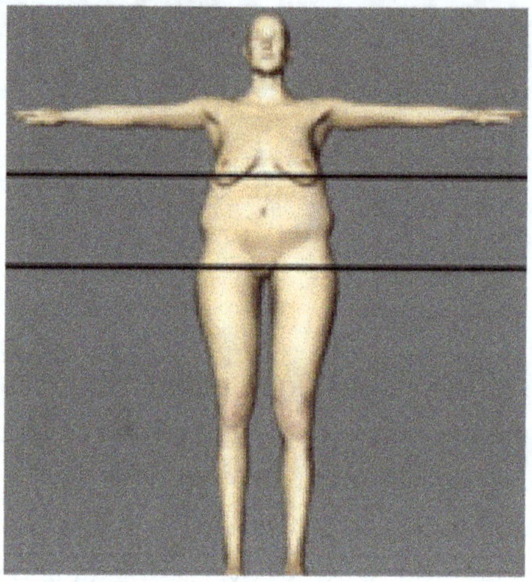

Figure 1. Front upper, middle, and lower section.

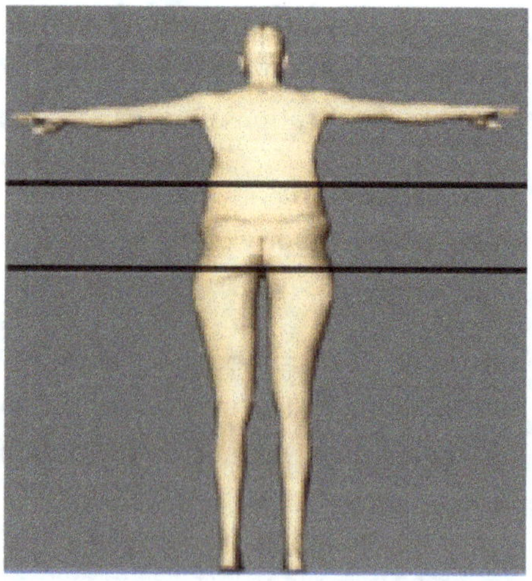

Figure 2. Back upper, middle, and lower section.

- Upper section (arms, thorax, and upper back).
- Middle section (central part of abdominal wall, lateral wall, buttocks, and back).
- Lower section (medial and lateral thighs and legs).

2. Body lift surgery

In the middle section, there are many surgical treatments and we must identify the best one for every patient.

So for a better classification, we must address patients' variability patterns (**Figures 3** and **4**):

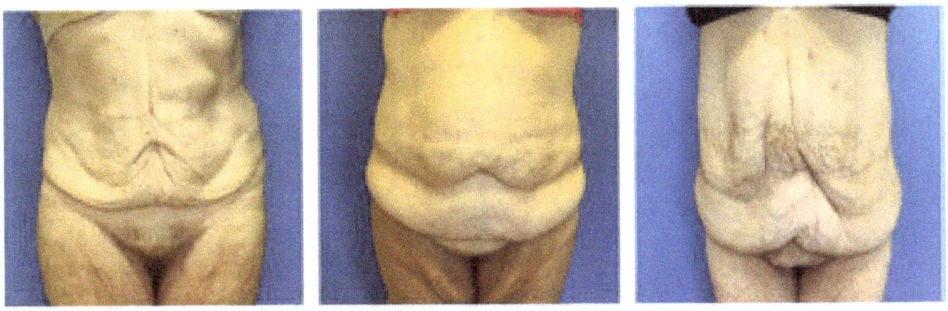

Figure 3. Variability patterns at front.

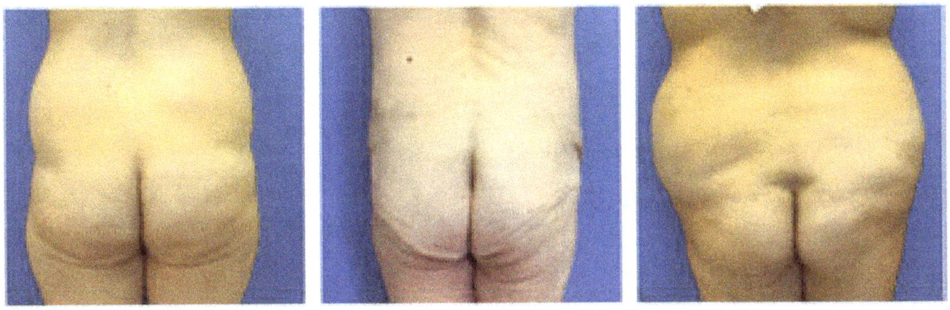

Figure 4. Variability patterns at back.

- In lax skin and rolls at the front and back in every patient.
- Previous scars (Special attention in anatomical blood supply).
- Structural body shape (android or gynecoid).
- Intra-abdominal excess.

Knowing the anatomical shape, we could see which one will have a better contour:

- Severe skin laxity, low adipose tissue, and medium size skeletal muscle will be the best body contouring patients, only need to re-drape skin to the continent underneath.
- Large and oblique scars are a big problem due to vascularization. If so, discuss with patient about necrosis and complications.
- Women mostly have a pear shape or gynecoid and are narrow from torso and wider at the hips, so stretching skin laxity contour improves. Men and some women have an android or pear shape so circumferential procedures are a standard treatment avoiding denting or heavy dog ears.

Why are body lifts the best procedures in the massive weight loss patients?

A common example is to watch the anterior abdominal wall and discard lateral and back or pretend to treat the anterior part and improve contour on lateral and back.

As shown in **Figure 5**, classic abdominoplasty has an ellipse pattern with a wider medial resection that have a 100% of skin tension, reaching the most lateral resection with no tension at the end of the closure is achieved and final dog ear or bulky tissue is revealed.

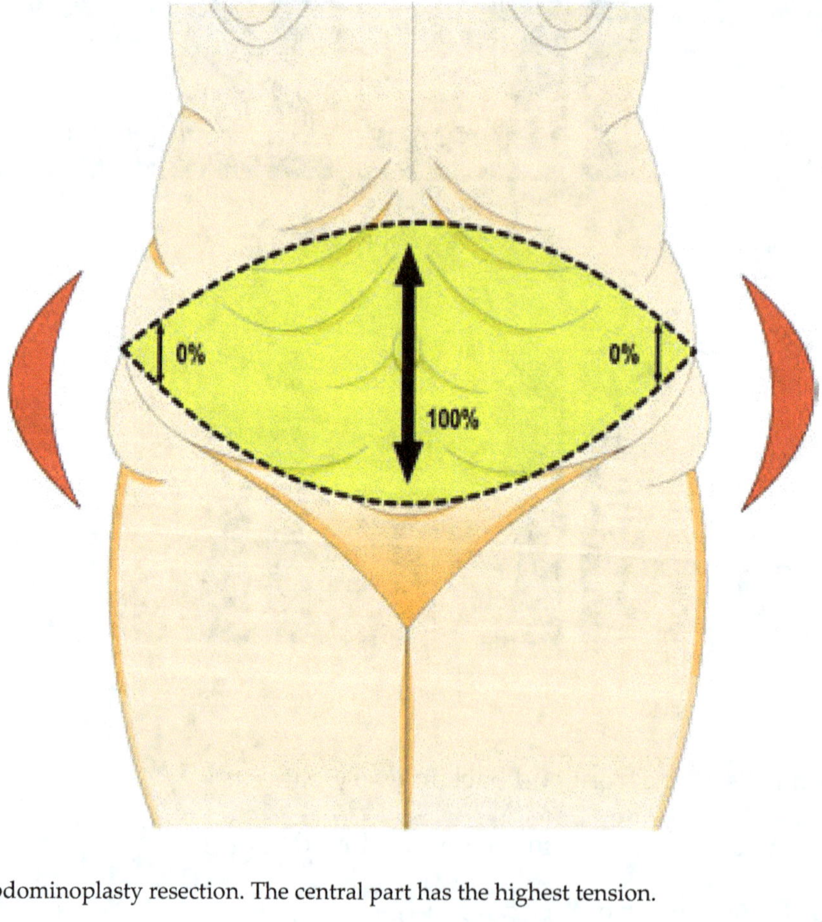

Figure 5. Classic abdominoplasty resection. The central part has the highest tension.

With a circumferential procedure, skin is resected over the front and back and a 100 percent of high tension applied to the skin ends with the best improvement in contour [1] (**Figures 6** and 7).

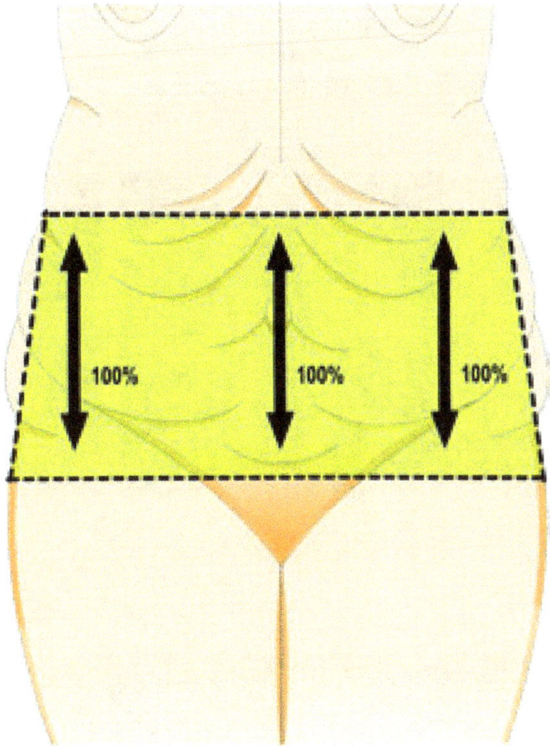

Figure 6. Highest tension in a circumferential procedure is applied at front and back.

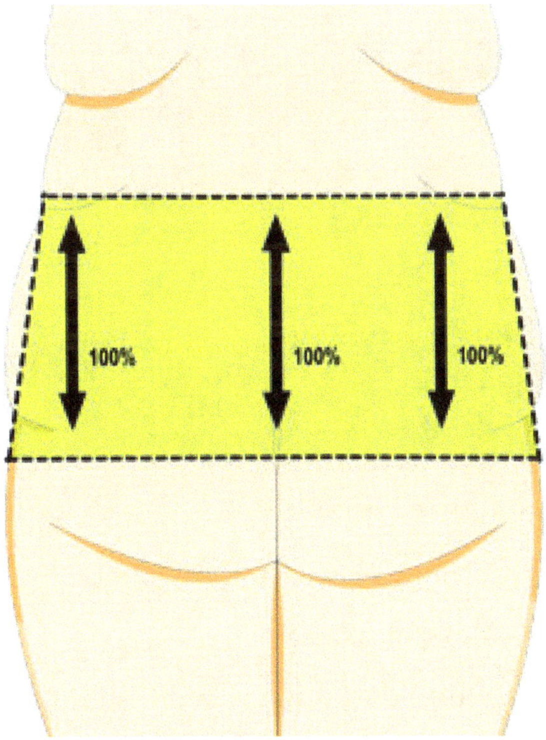

Figure 7. Higher tension at the back makes a better gluteal shape.

2.1. Markings

Start with the patient in a standing position (**Figures 8** and **9**).

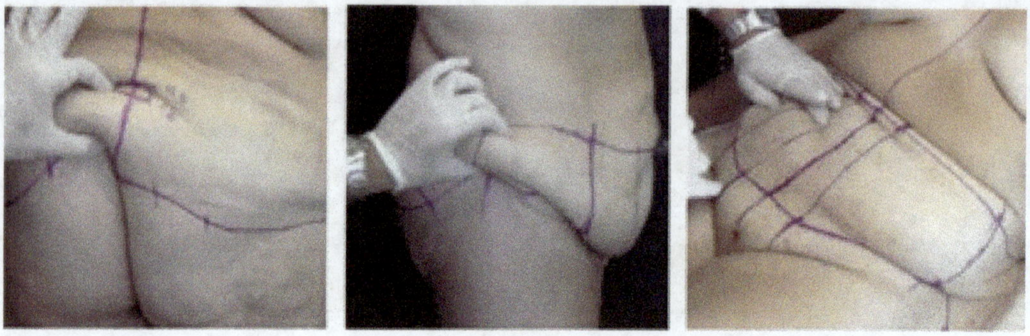

Figure 8. Dynamic pinch.

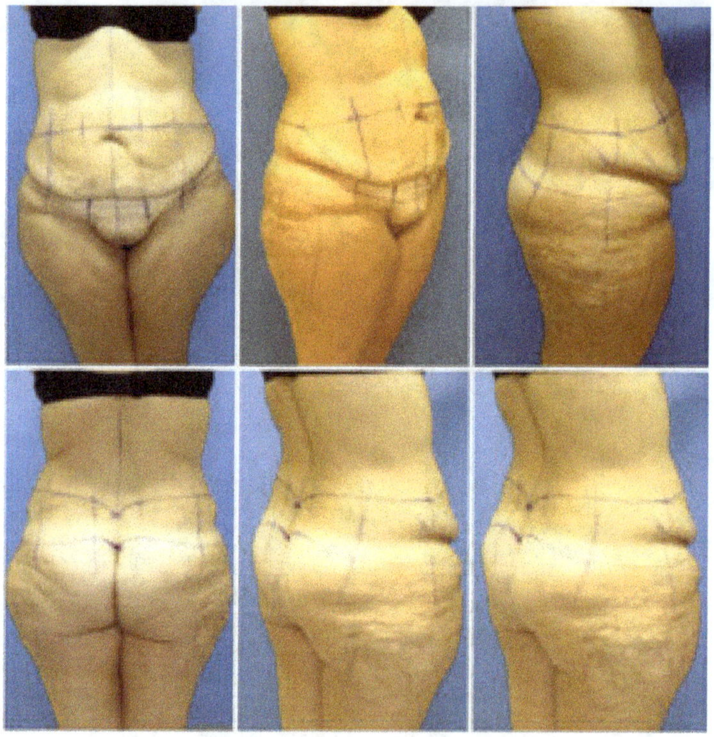

Figure 9. V-S pattern at the back and trapezoidal at front.

- Midline marking reaches xiphoid process to midline pubis.
- Midline marking of the back to gluteal crease.
- Dynamic pinch in the back lifting gluteal and lateral tissue in a V-S fashion

  V (superior) and Italic S (inferior) improve buttocks shape.
- Dynamic pinch in the anterior part lifting pubis and inguinal area in a trapezoidal fashion.

- Always in the midline back decrease tension about 2 cm than pinch avoiding over resection.

  Marking tips: Always use landmarks to keep anatomical references.

  If not sure about resection, do not do it. It is better to decrease the amount of resection to keep surgery safe.

2.2. Operative technique

- The patient in prone position, incision, and dissection from upper marking down (**Figures 10** and **11**).
- Subfascial dissect avoiding lymphatic injury.
- Lift the flap and tailor tacking avoiding over resection.
- Fascial closure with absorbable sutures and subdermal [2].
- Drains placed under closure.
- Lateral ending with a dog ear to continue in the anterior part.
- In supine position, pubic marking incision as classic abdominoplasty.
- Subfascial dissection towards xiphoid, umbilical transposition.
- If needed, muscle plication will improve contour.
- Abdominal flap is descended and fascial and dermal closure is made.

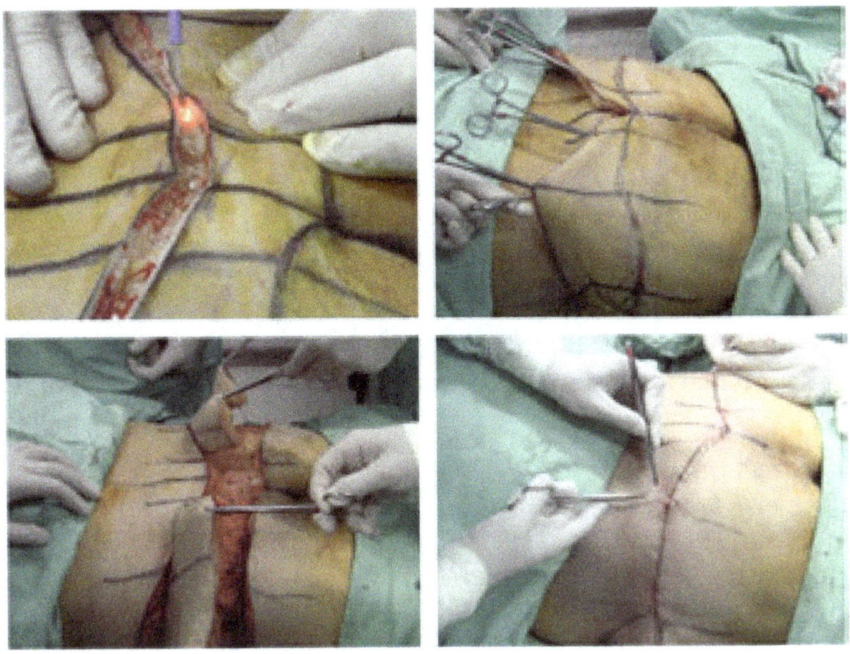

Figure 10. Body lift surgery pictures, starting in prone position. At the upper right, lifting the buttocks.

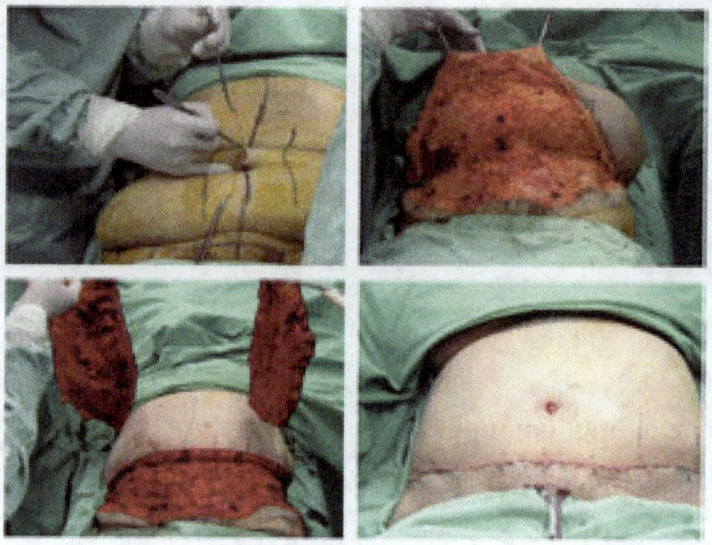

Figure 11. Body lift at the abdominal time, subfascial undermining.

Tips: Keep the subfascial tissue intact, decrease postoperative seromas.

Reaching the umbilicus area, look for any little hernia, and if so, repair it.

Safe liposuction area: Only at the lateral thighs with mild-to-severe lipodystrophy.

Patients who underwent a previous abdominoplasty have a different approach:

- The back is marking as usual.
- The lateral and anterior area is treated as an inverted ellipse fashion keeping most of the tension at lateral aspects than in the midline

Marking tips: Always look at the umbilicus position. A higher position improves in contour.

Try to lower the previous abdominoplasty scar. This is the most visible area.

Surgery tips: Umbilicus is the danger zone. Dissect the flap near the insertion and descend the new flap in a block.

If infra umbilical skin redundancy requires a higher resection, umbilical transposition is mandatory.

In lower position, umbilicus sometimes is better to repositioning a little bit higher and leaving a minimal vertical scar.

2.2.1. Postoperative care

- Do not fully extend for 1 week. It is a high-tension technique and dehiscence may occur.
- Drains will be kept until 20 ml serohematic/day.
- Compression garments for 1 month.

2.2.2. Pre- and post-op results

See **Figures 12** and **13**.

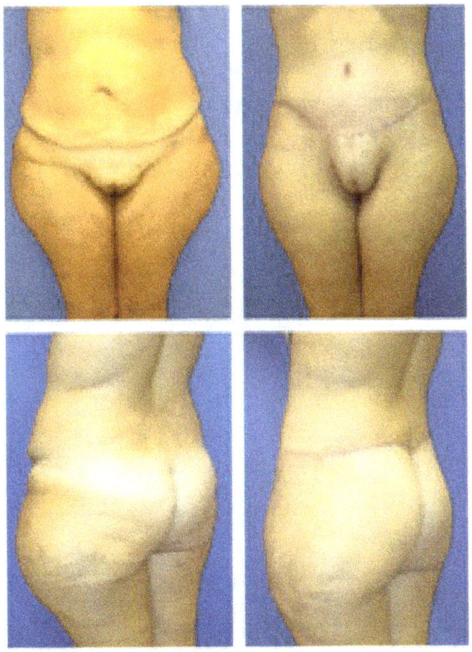

Figure 12. Left side, pre-op; right side, post-op. Improving contour and gluteal shape.

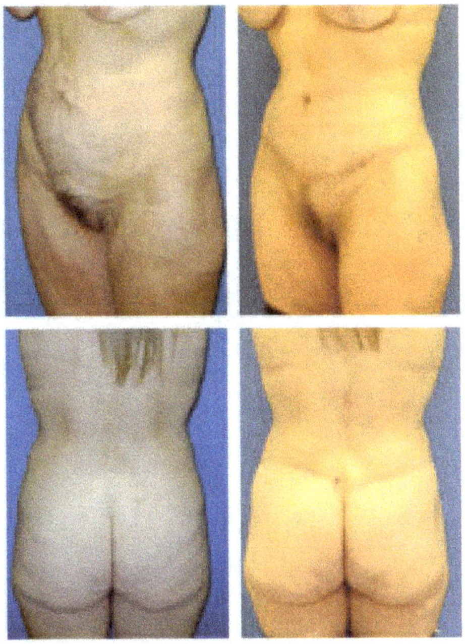

Figure 13. Left side pre-op, right side post-op, 2 years.

3. Arm lift and surrounding areas

After weight loss arms and axilla area often deflated and gravity vectors lead to a typical tent-like deformity from elbow to medial axillary line.

Patients feel uncomfortable about their upper extremities due to their visual movement of hanging tissue. This is usually patients' first consultation.

This hanging tissue reveals the drop vector due to gravity [1].

With the upper arm, horizontal extent (15°) and palms up the deformities show up.

Our goal is to reshape the arms to their natural looking.

Extension to medial axilla line is often needed due to tissue excess and not to falling in a dog ear final scar.

This is the natural extension line from the arm to the lateral chest area.

Arm deformities types and treatment classification (**Figure 14**)

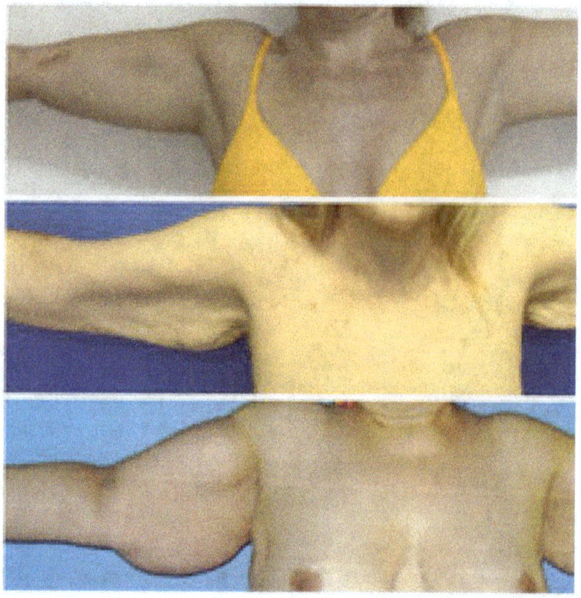

Figure 14. Different types of deformities.

Type 1: Mild adipose pinch—Good skin tension

Type 2: Severe adipose pinch—Severe skin laxity

Type 3: Low adipose pinch—Mild skin laxity

Type 1: Treatment: Liposuction (classic liposuction or ultrasound assisted)

Type 2: Treatment: Sequential ellipse skin resection

Type 3: Treatment: Skin resection with surrounding areas liposuction. Contour results may vary among patients

3.1. Scar placement

There is a controversial issue about placing the scar in a more medial fashion than a posterior place.

It is obvious that a scar placed in the bicipital crease will be in a more natural and anatomical area. But the truth is that after a long postoperative time, the scar will expand or migrate because of the gravity.

A scar placed at the lowest point of the posterior axillary fold is better because it extends to axilla defects and maintains the arm reduction over time without migration (**Figure 15**).

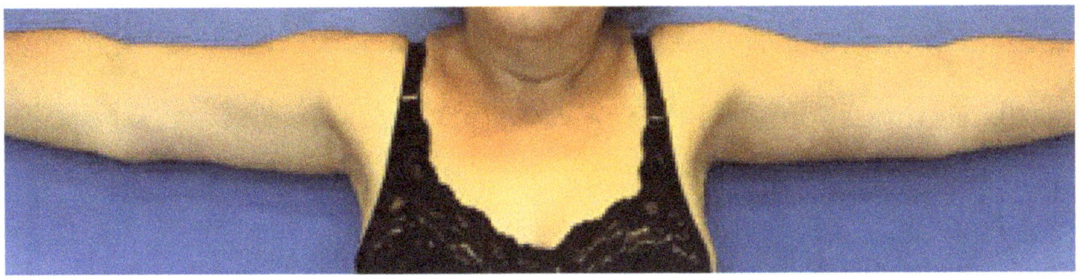

Figure 15. With arms open, scar is nonvisible.

At this time, you can combine arm lift with breast and upper back roll surgery and improve contour in the arms, lateral torso, back, and breast.

3.2. Markings

In standing position (**Figure 16**)

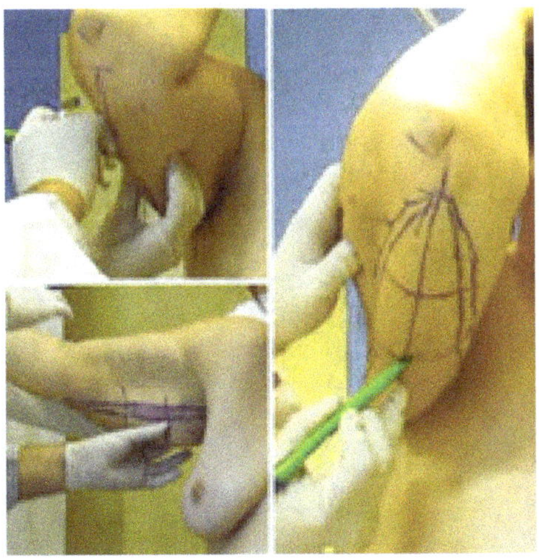

Figure 16. Pinch and hatch marks. Resection always is less than marked.

- Dynamic pinch at the posterior axillary fold towards axilla.
- This pinch will be about 1.5–2 cm less avoiding high tension in closure.
- Crossing axilla pinch will reclute lateral torso tissue.
- No marking Z-plasty is needed in the axilla.

3.3. Operative technique

- Patient positioned with arms open and movable to a position higher than the head (**Figure 16**).
- Partial Incision made from the elbow towards axilla maintaining superficial fascia.
- Sequential to the hatch marks to avoid over resection.
- Each hatch mark is accessed closure made from fascia and subdermal.
- Reaching axilla continue more subdermal to avoid lymph injury.
- Cross-axilla and resect until the last markings.
- Final closure made, skin glue.
- Drains under closure.

Tips: Arms are not collapsible, and compartmental syndrome could occur so less resection (**Figures 17–19**).

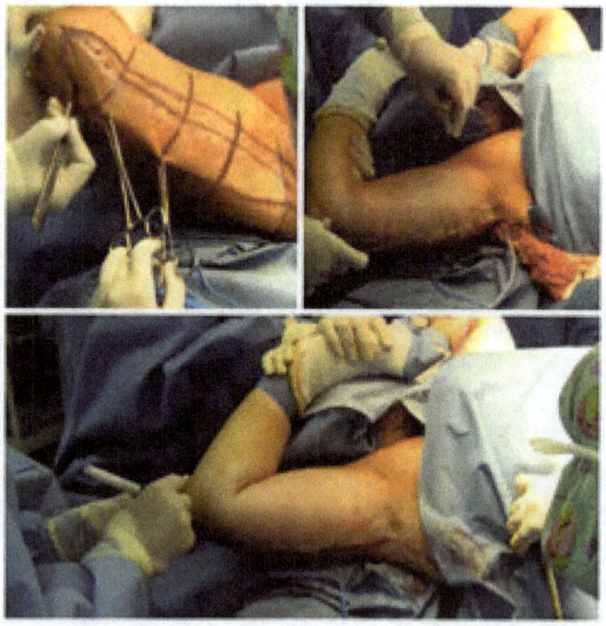

Figure 17. Upper left hatch marks are relevant in this surgery.

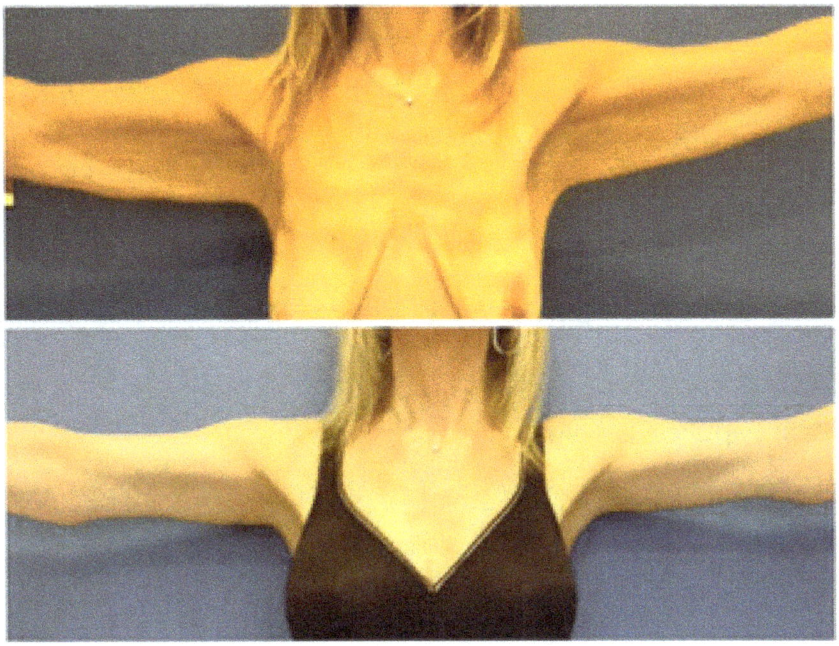

Figure 18. Deflated arm reaching axilla and lateral thorax. Pre- and post-op.

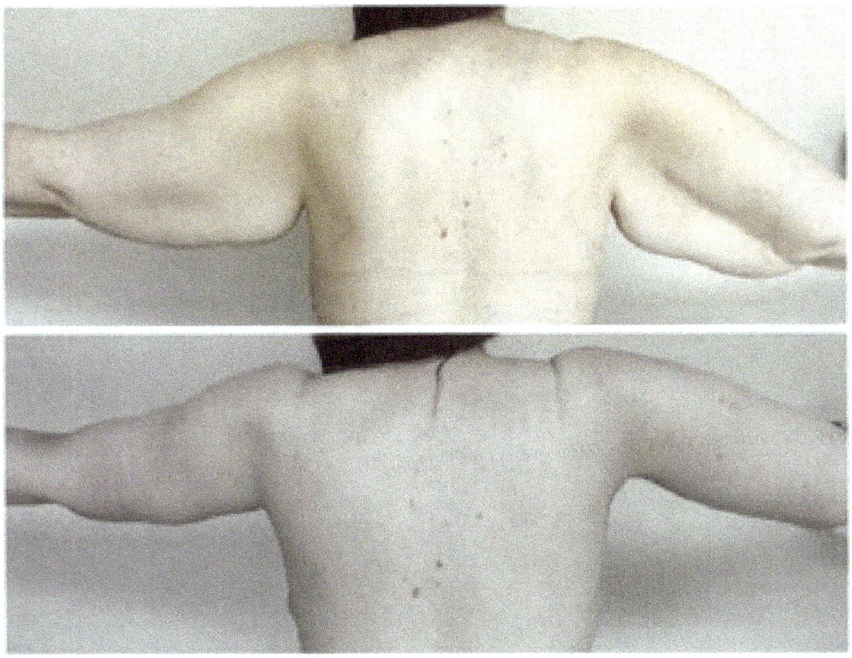

Figure 19. Aesthetic problem with adipose excess and scar due to trauma. Pre- and post-op.

Be gentle when moving, nerve compression or injury may happen.

Lateral torso resection shapes under the axilla and the lateral aspect of the breast and sometimes could lateralize the nipple, so if you are planning to combine surgery, be aware at this point.

3.4. Postoperative care

- Compression garments after surgery are mandatory from the hand to the axilla.
- The same day after surgery the surgeon must see patients hand for swelling and blood supply. Sometimes compression is too high and must free some pressure of the garment.
- Patient must elevate arms above the chest to avoid excessive swelling.
- Smooth movements and no lifting heavy objects.
- Drains kept a few days until 20 ml/day.
- Silicone sheets are applied 4–6 months.

Some male patients could benefit the chest wall with the lateral torso resection with marking extension and variation.

This selection is made in patients with (**Figure 20**).

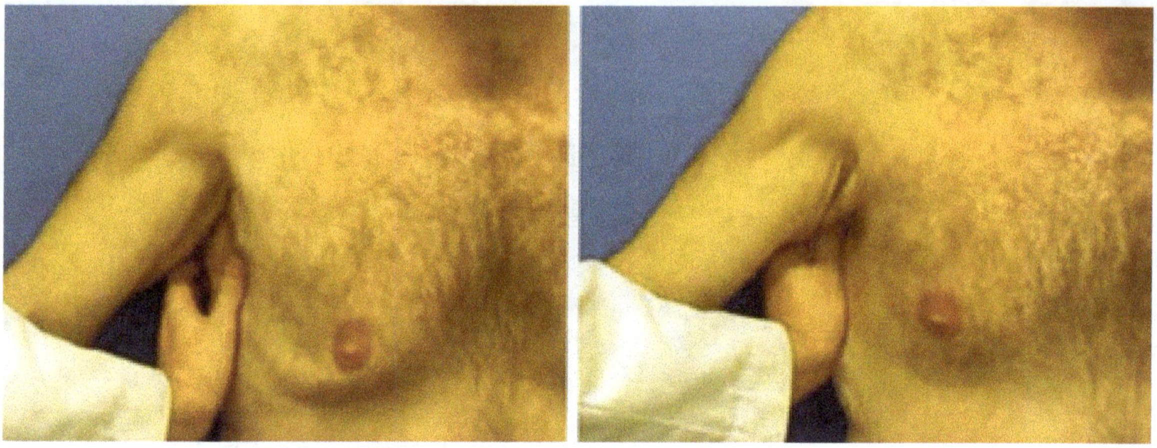

Figure 20. Notice the lateral traction improve NAC position.

- Deflation of the breast and position of NAC higher than inframammary fold.
- Lateral torso skin laxity.

Marking tips:

- Arm lift as described, crossing axilla and reaching lateral torso vertical dynamic high pinch is made.
- Evaluate NAC position as pinch.
- Sand clock shape is made with wider part at the NAC position.
- Extension will vary between patients (**Figure 21**).

With selected patients, we could perform upper body lift surgery resecting back rolls and leaving a final scar that cross from back to submammary fold.

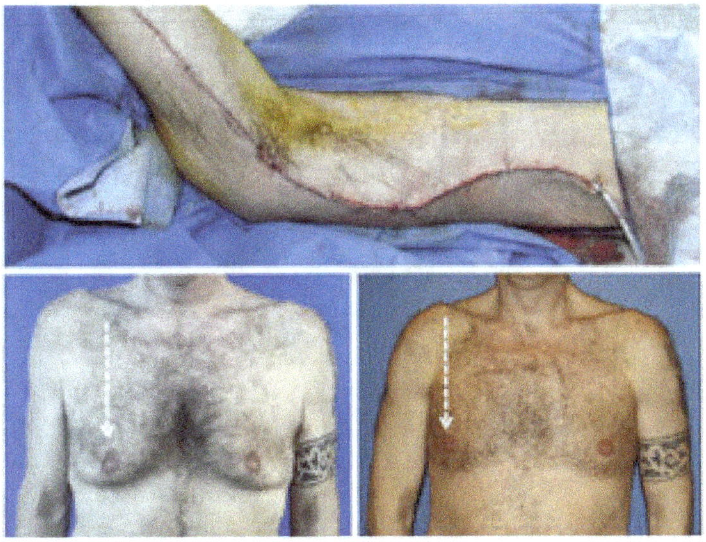

Figure 21. Long extension in lateral aspect. Pre- and post-op results.

This type of procedure requires changing position at the surgery table like the lower body lifts.

Markings:

- Standing position at the back elevate the excess in upward fashion.
- Dynamic pinch keeping the upper line just above the bra line.
- Continue to lateral hatch marks addressing submammary fold.

3.5. Operative technique

- Excise over the upper line and dissect downwards.
- Elevate the flap and tailor tack.
- Continue to the lateral aspect ending at the middle axillary line.
- Then rotate patient and continue in supine position.

Tips: Always keep the superficial fascia it will help you to anchor the flap in an upward position.

It is better to do lower body lift first as major skin tension body procedure it will tight some upper part excess leading to scar predictable positioning.

If breast or upper chest surgery will not be performed at this time, extend to the inframammary fold, dog ears at the lateral torso are too visible.

3.6. Results

See **Figures 22** and **23**.

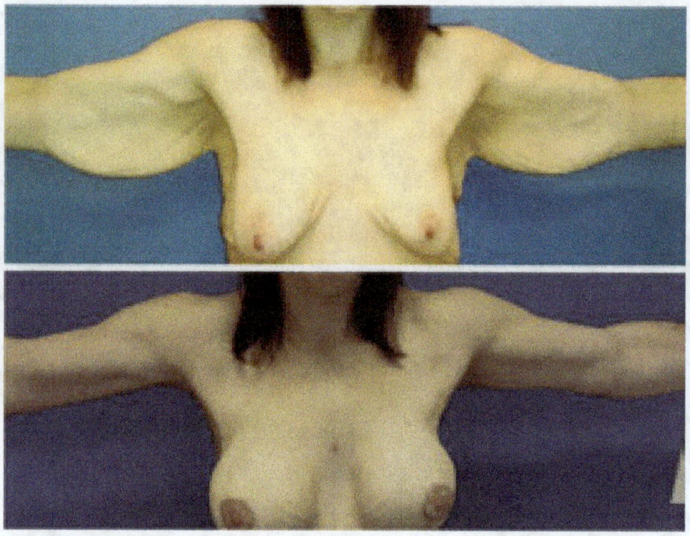

Figure 22. Brachioplasty, augmentation mastopexy, and back rolls surgery. Front view.

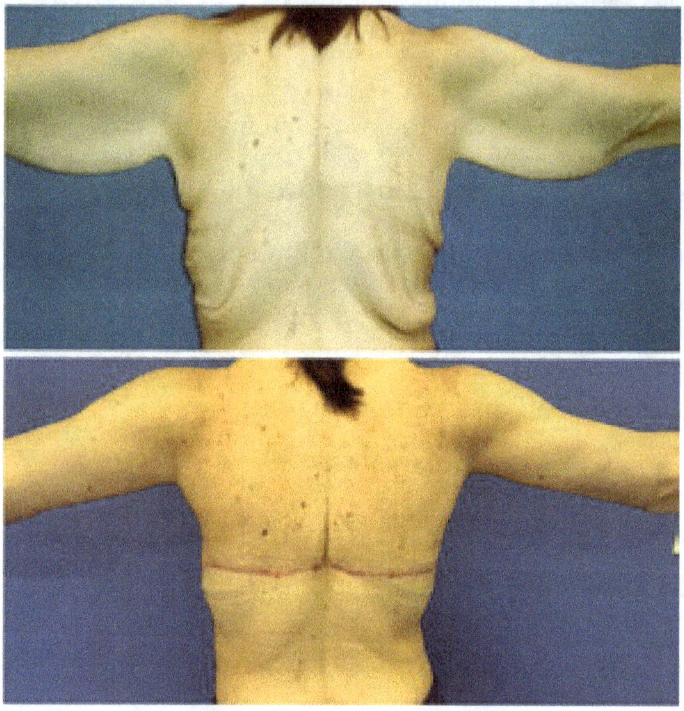

Figure 23. Back view.

4. Thigh lifting and reduction

The inner thighs are one of the areas that many plastic surgeons try to avoid mainly because the complication rate is higher than other surgical procedures [3].

Skin laxity and lipodystrophy vary according to patients so the thighs are divided into three zones (**Figure 24**):

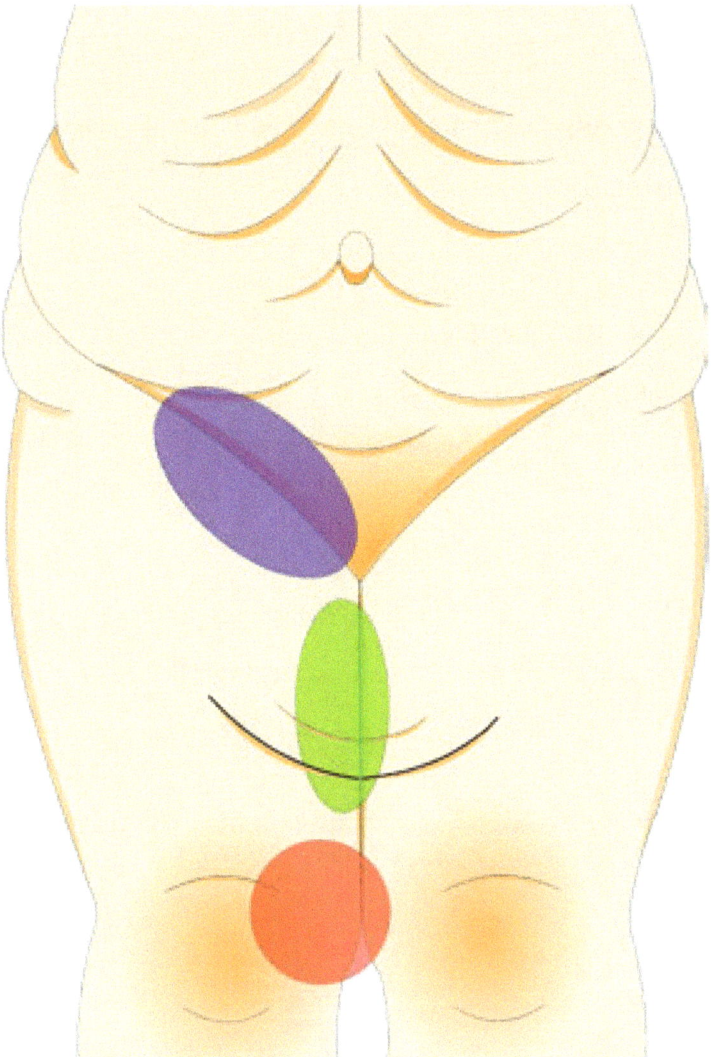

Figure 24. Thigh zones inguinal (purple), medial (green), upper knee (red).

- The inguinal zone.
- The medial inner thigh.
- The upper knee section.

The inner thigh as we describe it has two negative vectors due to gravity, skin laxity, and amount of fat in the area. The retaining skin ligaments in the inguinal and throcanther area are responsible for the vectors.

For reshaping the area, we propose to reinvert these critical vectors by anchoring the superficial fascia to the Colles ligament in the horizontal vector and resect the amount of skin and fat in the vertical one.

4.1. Planning inner thigh reduction

Which is the extension of the deformity?

- Pinch diagnosis in stand-up position.
- Elevation of the horizontal (subinguinal) vector.
- Careful examination of inner thigh and extension of vertical vector.
- Evaluate if deformity reaches or passes the knee.

4.2. Scar placement

- Inguinal scar should be placed in the inguinal crease.
- Vertical incision should not be too anterior or posterior.
- In stand-up position not visible scars.
- Evaluate patients with previous thigh incision.

4.3. Use of liposuction

- Only in areas that should not be excised (e.g., knee, lateral thigh).

4.4. Marking and tips

Pinch dynamic markings are used and marks are less than the original 1 or 1.5 cm to avoid over resection (**Figure 25**).

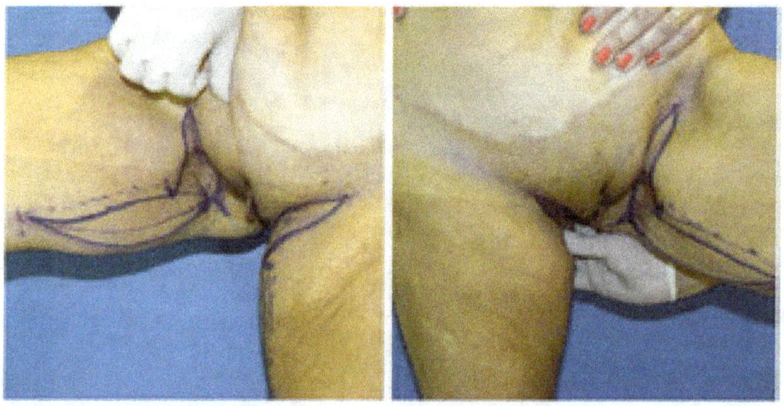

Figure 25. Marking and pinching the defect, the definitive marks are less than original pinch.

The amount of skin and fat excised in the horizontal excess often is less than what we can elevate.

Horizontal excess must be anchored in the Colles fascia just above 2 cm the inguinal crease so the mark in the inguinal region should be 2 cm less than the pinch.

This type of anchoring is strong and the horizontal flap could be suspended by the superficial fascia (**Figure 26**).

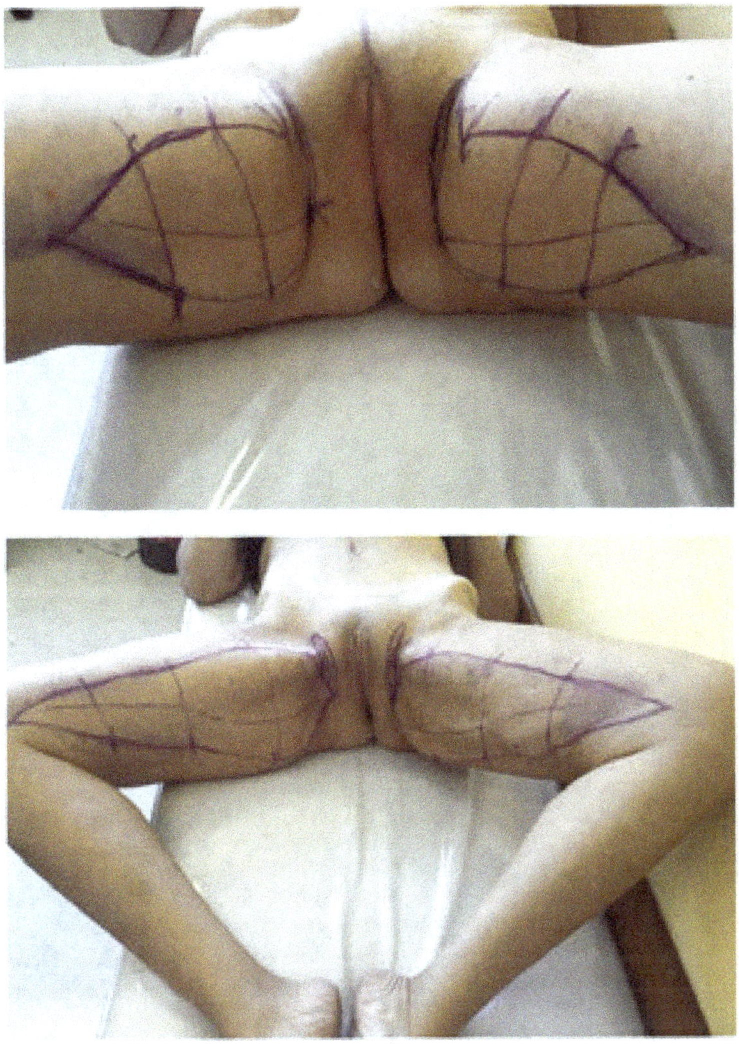

Figure 26. Different patients, different markings, and both improve contour.

4.4.1. Operative technique

- Patient positioned in frog-like position (**Figure 27**).
- Incision made from the distal marking towards inguinal maintaining superficial fascia.
- Sequential to the hatch marks to avoid over resection [4].
- Each hatch mark is accessed closure made from fascia and subdermal.
- Continue at the inguinal incision. Subfascial dissection.
- Do not over resect, suspension of the thigh has to be 2 cm or 3 above the crease to reach the Colles ligament, so marks should be 2 cm less than marked.

- Use polypropylene 0 for anchoring, in a "x" fashion to relax tension in superficial fascia.
- Final closure made, skin glue.
- Drains under closure.

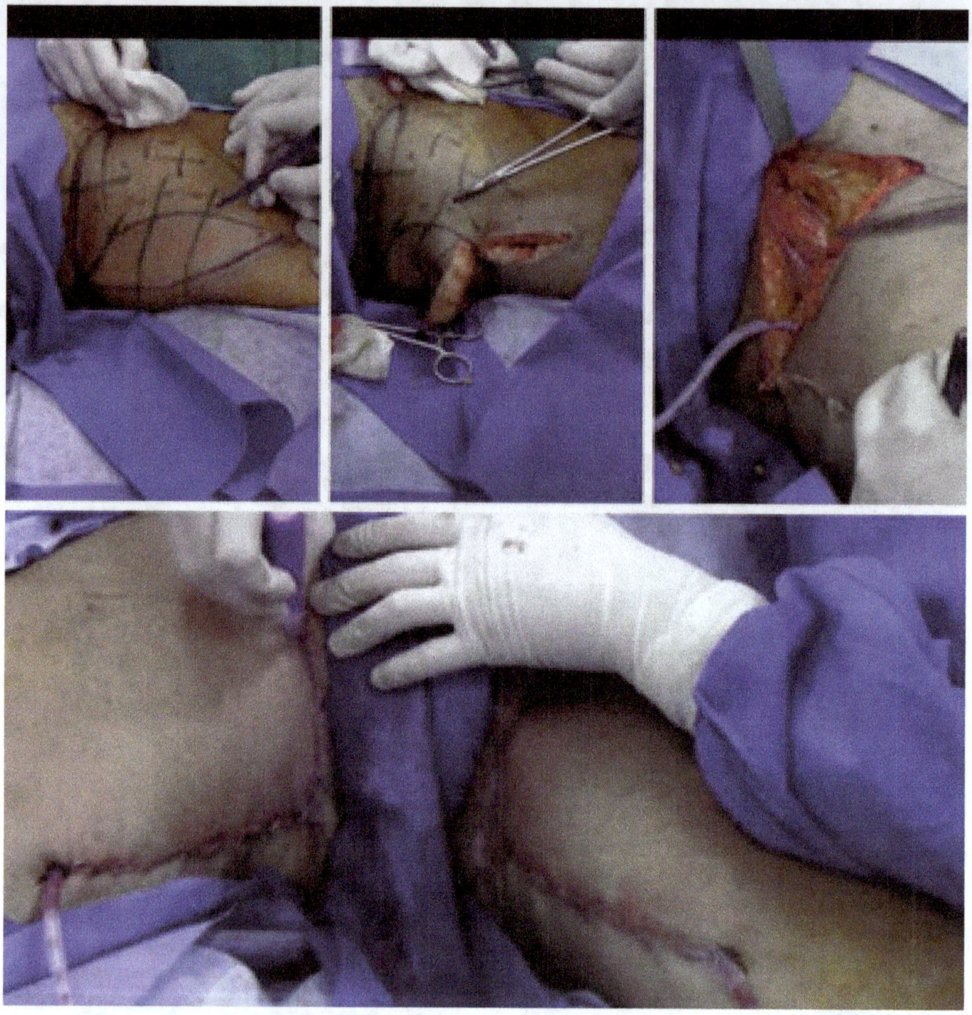

Figure 27. Thigh surgery. Upper right anchoring subfascial tissue to Colles ligament.

4.4.2. Post-op treatment

- Use of compression garments.
- Early deambulation.
- Leave silicone drains until 25 cc/day.

4.4.3. Pre-/post-op Photographs

See **Figures 28** and **29**.

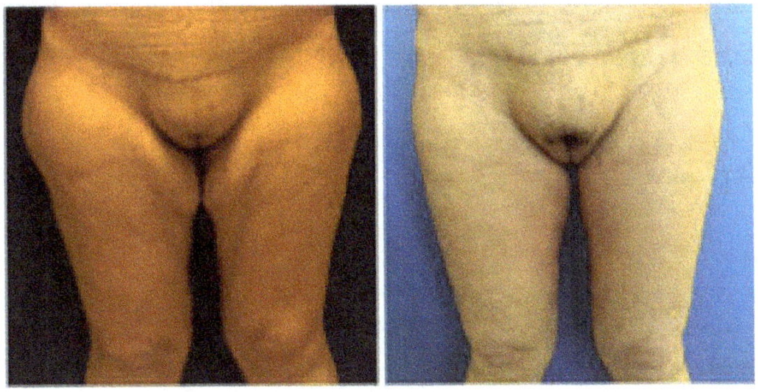

Figure 28. Deformity at inguinal and medial zone. Pre- and post-op.

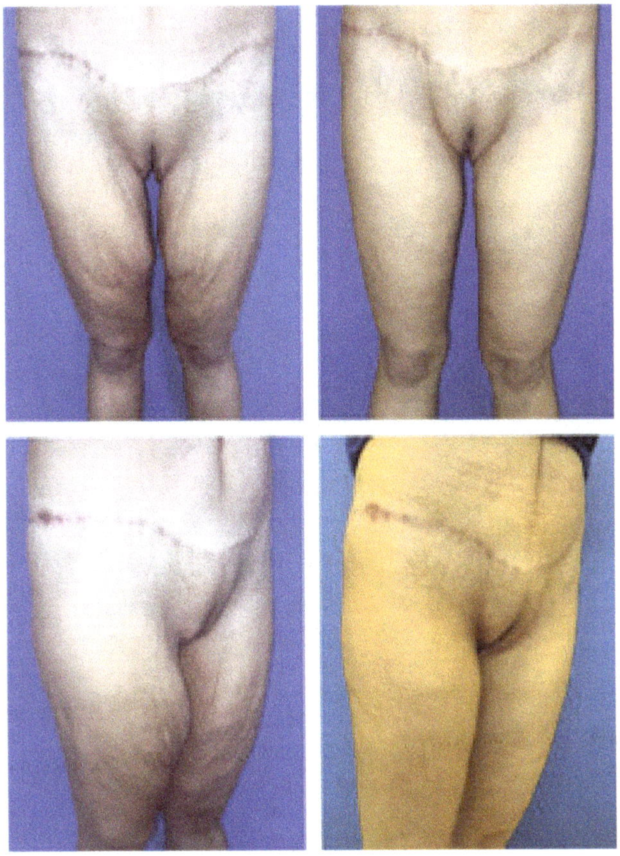

Figure 29. Some patients reach the upper knee so extension of the vertical extension is applied. Pre- and post-op.

5. Discussion

Many techniques have been described through the past century to achieve good contour and aesthetic results. But some of this new postbariatric population with weight loss have contour deformities that never have been shown in past century consultation.

New surgical approach as body lifts, extensive brachioplasty, and thighplasty should be consider as a gold standard for this kind of patients

6. Conclusions

With a comprehensive diagnosis, patient classification, dynamic marking, and postoperative patient management, body contouring has evolved from traditional plastic surgery techniques to a multiple vector correction.

It provides a good contour; skin tension and results are consistent over time, but should consider to:

- Be conservative and do not over resect.
- Plan and mark since these are critical for the surgery.
- Take care of patients' postoperative management, watch out for complications.

Author details

Marcelo A. Cuadrado*, Gabriel Moina and Daniel Moina

*Address all correspondence to: drcuadrado@gmail.com

Hospital Británico de Buenos Aires, Centro de Rinología y Cirugía plástica Dr. Moina, Buenos Aires, Argentina

References

[1] Aly A, Cram A. editors. Body Contouring After Massive Weight Loss. Missouri: QMP Publishing; 2006. 386 p. doi:9781576262115

[2] Ted Lockwood. Superficial fascial system (SFS) of the trunk and extremities: A new concept. Plast Reconstr Surg. 1991;87(6):1009–1018.

[3] Grazer FM. Body contouring. Introduction. Clin Plast Surg. 1996;23(4):511–528.

[4] Cram A, Aly A. Thigh reduction in the massive weight loss patient. Clin Plast Surg. 2008;35(1):165–172.

9

High Definition Liposuction: A Challenge for a Perfect Body Contouring

Javier Soto, Hugo A. Aguilar and
Juan S. Barajas-Gamboa

Abstract

During the last decades, the plastic surgery field has made important advances in terms of clinical results and developing new surgical techniques, minimizing complications and reducing the mortality rates. An innovative and new technique is called High Definition LipoSculture. This is an advanced sculpting technique that creates an athletic and sculpted appearance. The aim of this chapter is to review the principal concepts that involve this technique and describe its clinical application. An electronic literature review was conducted in order to find the most recent medical literature published in this field. Keywords used were plastic surgery, liposuction, body contouring, aesthetic medicine, and surgical procedure. High definition liposuction procedures should be considered revolutionary in the plastic surgery field.

Keywords: plastic surgery, liposuction, body contouring, aesthetic medicine, surgical procedure

1. Introduction

During the last decades, the plastic surgery field has made important advances in terms of clinical results and developing new surgical techniques, minimizing complications and reducing the mortality rates. On the other hand, the revolution of new technologies such as medical devices has opened other alternatives in the current clinical practice [1, 2].

There is no secret about the popularity that plastic surgery procedures have gained even in women and men, as a part of a social-aesthetic revolution that find better bodies and improve personal image. Since its introduction, liposuction has undergone several technical challenges and has improved the clinical outcomes [3, 4].

A wide range of technological advancements has been released to replace traditional methods of suctioning fat: ultrasound, power, laser, and radiofrequency. Each surgical alternative has its own benefits and complications. Different medical device companies across the world are continuously working on the safe surgical instruments for this type of surgical procedures [5]. The dreamed liposuction device has to be in the position to offer different functions at the same time: (1) remove excess of fat, (2) keep safe the surrounded soft tissue, (3) devices allowed to be used under local anesthesia, and (4) device results avoid bruising and swelling [6–8].

An innovative and new technique is called High Definition LipoSculture. This is an advanced sculpting technique that creates an athletic and sculpted appearance. The objective of this procedure is to remove both superficial and deep fat that surrounds muscle groups in order to enhance the visibility of underlying toning and musculature. This technique could be applied in multiple body areas such as abdomen, chest, waist, back, buttocks, arms, flanks, and thighs [2, 4].

The aim of this chapter is to review the principal concepts that involve this technique and describe its clinical application.

2. Background

Obesity, overweight, and metabolic syndrome are a public health issue nowadays. Countries such as the United States report an estimate of 40% of the adult population suffer from this health problem. This spectrum of diseases is associated with high rates of mortality in comparison with cancer, cardiovascular disease, and violent deaths [9, 10].

Recent clinical studies predict that in 2013, more than the 50% of the worldwide population would be facing this reality. Weight loss including strategies such as dietary changes and exercise usually does not achieve the desired weight loss goals. Based on this, bariatric and metabolic surgery has become the treatment of choice for obesity and morbid obesity [11].

The Roux-En-Y gastric bypass still remains the gold standard surgical option for obese patients. In the course of achieving massive weight loss and resolution of comorbidities, bariatric surgery creates quality-of-life problems that are in the medical field of plastic surgeons. Despite the numerous health advantages of bariatric surgery, disgruntled patients complained of disturbing lax skin and subcutaneous tissue [5, 8, 12].

Plastic surgeons learned during the last years that change in body contour with repulsive hanging skin and bizarre rolls of skin and fat. Due to this, High Definition LipoSculture has been presented as a safe and effective option [13].

3. Literature review methods

An electronic literature review was conducted in order to find the most recent medical literature published in this field. Using the keywords such as plastic surgery, liposuction, body contouring, aesthetic medicine, and surgical procedure, the following databases were consulted: Pubmed, Lilacs, Proquest, Cochrane, Ovid, and Google Scholar. With the aim to maximize the number of articles, no date limit in the search was set, and manuscripts in English, Spanish, and Portuguese were considered.

Initially, 87 articles were obtained, of which 25 met the inclusion criteria. However, only 23 were referenced in the current work with a focus on high definition liposuction and body contouring or gave important theoretical contributions.

4. Procedures

4.1. Patient selection

Initially, all the patients are exanimated and evaluated in plastic surgery consultation, and complete medical records are reviewed including previous surgical procedures, current medication use, and recent laboratory analysis. Considering that this type of surgical procedure is created to be a sculpting procedure rather than a debulking technique, an appropriate patients' selection is necessary. A good muscle tone without an excessive amount of fat or skin laxity is expected (body mass index < 30) [3, 14].

Once the physical examination is performed, lipodystrophy throughout the trunk has to be evaluated. Patients are requested to perform various muscle contractions in the clinical assessment to evaluate separately the muscle groups that contribute to the contour of the torso. Finally, skin laxity, elasticity, and quality of tissue are considered [15, 16].

For male patients, there are other aspects to be included in the clinical assessment: the presence of gynecomastia, chest contour, and volume of fat in this area. In the female cases, a comparable estimate is performed: the buttocks, lumbosacral angle, fat disposition in the lateral thighs, and perigluteal area are considered [4, 7, 12].

The physical examination is suggested to include documentation of scars, hernias, and other potential routine findings. Upon completion of the history and physical examination, based on our current clinical guidelines, patients are scheduled for an extra medical examination by the anesthesia department, to have the chance to evaluate other current medical issues ongoing at the same time. Once the patient meets the clinical requirements for this procedure, a final appointment is suggested to show a quick presentation explaining the surgical presentation in details, focused on benefits and potential complications. At the end of this medical visit, patients sign informed consent forms to continue with the medical process of surgery scheduling [17, 18].

4.2. Preoperative care

Patients are requested to be in the ambulatory surgery service 2 h prior to the surgical time. A new medical assessment is conducted to review the general medical status of the patient on the surgery day. Recent laboratory test results, electrocardiograms, and thorax X-rays are reviewed prior to authorizing the patient to be transferred to the operating room. Based on the patients' medical conditions and preferences, epidural or general anesthesia is offered by the anesthesia team.

Preoperative strategies that involve medication such as thromboembolism prophylaxis included low-weight heparin, intravenous corticosteroids, analgesics, and antibiotic prophylaxis are administrated with the main goal to keep the patient in the best condition possible and avoid potential clinical complications.

4.3. Surgical technique

4.3.1. Ultrasound evaluation

Performing an abdominal ultrasonography, the abdominal muscle groups are evaluated. The median, paramedian, and lateral muscle layer planes in the iliac fossae and flanks are comparatively evaluated and demarcated, the boundaries of the rectus muscles, rectus fascia, especially in the supraumbilical region and the contour of the superior oblique with the superficial fascicule close to the iliac edge and correlated with anterior rectus on each side (**Figure 1**).

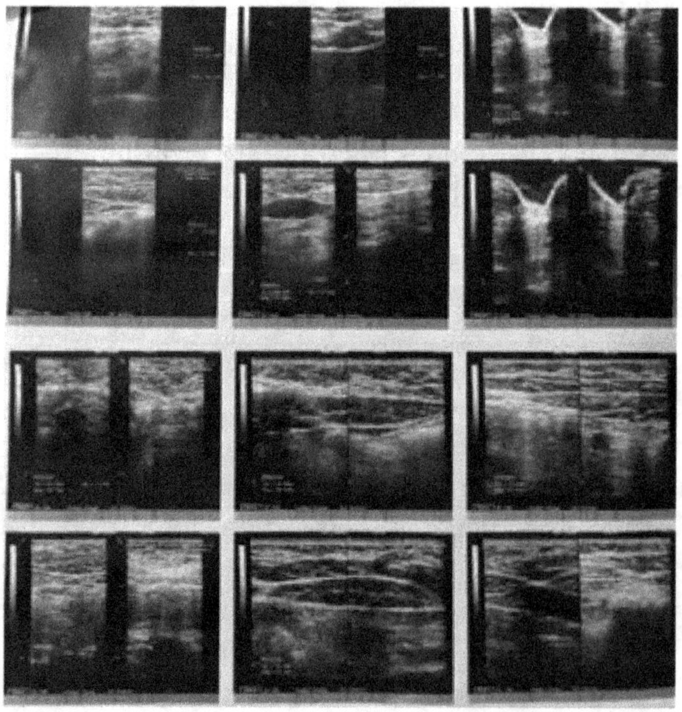

Figure 1. Initial ultrasound evaluation.

4.3.2. Preoperative marking

Once the patients arrive into the operating room, the first step is the surgical marking (**Figure 2**). This is performed with the patient initially in supine and in the upright standing position. It is essential to identify and understand the superficial anatomy and topography. Erroneous marking will lead to deformities and abnormal appearance and affects clinical outcomes [19].

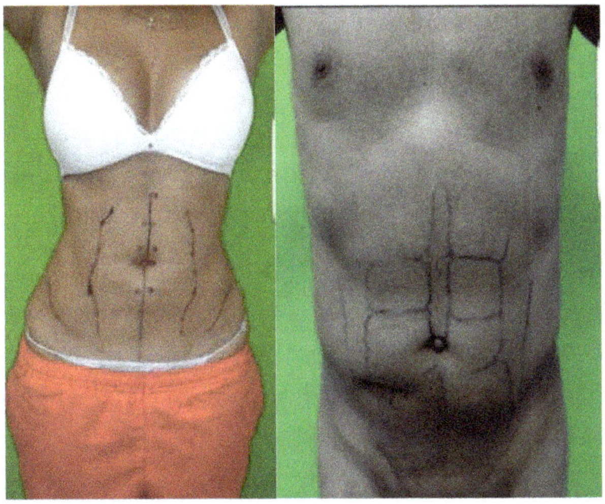

Figure 2. Preoperative marking.

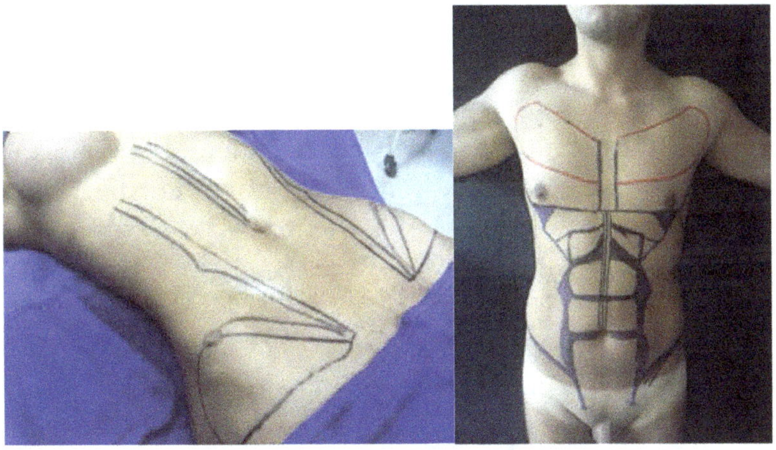

Figure 3. Preoperative marking.

The surface anatomy differs between men and women patients. In women, the transversal lines in the rectus abdominis muscle are not aesthetically desired. In men, the landmarks marked are the pectoralis major, serratus anterior, rectus abdominis, external oblique, iliac crest, and inguinal ligaments and the relationship between those structures. In women, the landmarks are the serratus anterior, rectus abdominis, external oblique, iliac crest, and inguinal ligaments. Other anatomical areas of care comprise the lateral and posterior torso (**Figure 3**) [19, 20].

4.3.3. *Surgical technique*

Under general or epidural anesthesia and previous asepsis and antisepsis, on sterile surgical fields, plastic surgeon initiates the procedure. Infiltration is performed with Klein solution, with tumescence technique. It starts with deep fat liposuction with power-assisted liposuction (PAL). After obtaining the redundant fat tissue and achieve a uniform surface, ultrasound-assisted liposuction (UAL) system is used following anatomical landmarks for 3–5 min per zone. Later, a lipoaspiration is performed with PAL system fat tissue surface along anatomical landmarks. Finally, a foam dressing is placed along the lines of the marking.

4.3.4. *Postoperative care*

Patients are required for a hospital stay at least 48–72 h postoperatively. Pain control, prophylaxis antibiotic, and antiinflammatory medications are given in order to improve the patients' comfort and avoid infections in the operative site. In some cases, open drains are placed both in female and male patients in the sacral area and inguinal area, respectively.

Other postoperative interventions are the use of mild-compression garment, stockings to prevent deep vein thrombosis, and an abdominal band for 4 weeks. Supplementary care includes lymphatic drainage massages and adjunctive external ultrasound (1-h session once a day for 10 days). Patients are scheduled for postoperatively follow-up at 1, 15, 30, and 90 days, respectively. Alarm signs and general recommendations are given for all the patients in order to reduce postoperative complications. The duration of the cosmetic results will be associated with the patient care in terms of healthy life styles and adequate medical follow-up. There is no accurate data describing failed procedures in the follow-up period [21].

5. Clinical results

There are limited clinical studies published in the current medical literature showing extensive series with appropriate and considerable follow-up; however, the level of satisfaction in

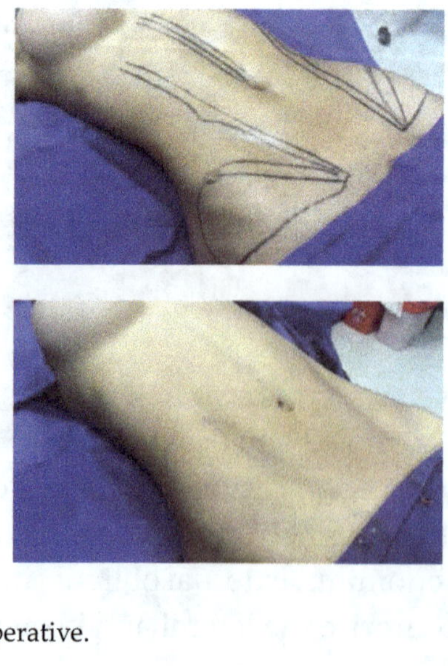

Figure 4. Clinical results: pre- vs. postoperative.

patients is surely high. In 2007, Dr. Hoyos published a study describing the experience in 306 patients using this surgical approach. In 306 subjects enrolled in the trial, 257 (84%) reported satisfactory results. In our clinical experience that include near to 80 patients, our level of patient satisfaction reached 90% (**Figures 4** and **5**) [3, 7, 12].

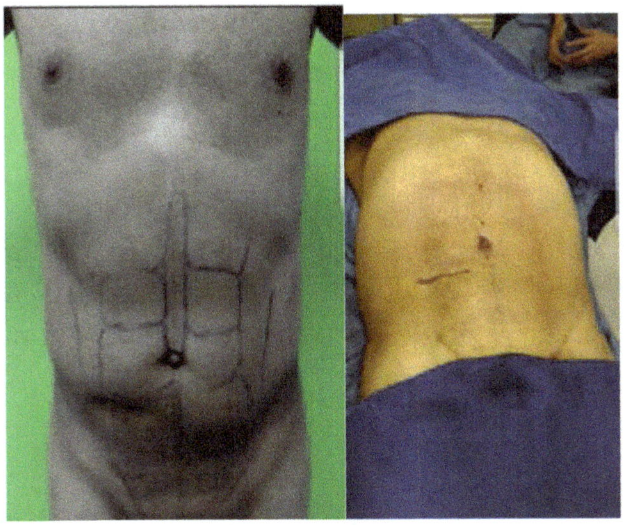

Figure 5. Clinical results: pre- vs. postoperative.

6. Potential complications

As expected in any surgical procedure, based on its nature, patients are exposed to clinical risk, some related with the anesthesia and other associated directly with the surgical technique. In the first group, one could find abnormalities in the cardiac rhythm, obstruction of the airway, allergic reactions, and bronchoaspiration. In the second group, one could find bleedings, low blood pressure, blood clots, pulmonary embolism, deep vein thrombosis, damage in neurovascular structures, hypothermia, and burning with surgical instruments and medical devices [5, 7, 21].

7. Future directions

Researchers and surgeon scientists devoted to improve the clinical outcomes in this surgical field are exploring new alternatives to develop new techniques and surgical approaches with minimal invasion. On the other hand, minimize tissue morbidity, decrease hospital stay and recovery time, and increase skin contraction/tightening are points to improve [22].

These priorities have led the medical and technical industry to develop new devices focused on noninvasive body contouring and nonsurgical adipose reducing techniques. A new medical approach called "High-Intensity Focused Ultrasound"(HIFU) is now available, which delivers high-intensity ultrasonic energy to the deep subcutaneous tissue, producing heat capable of ablating adipose tissue and thermally modifying collagen. Cosmetic outcomes so far are very promising [23].

Other alternative that has been used by experts in this field is the cryolipolysis. This technique refers to use cold exposure to induce subcutaneous fat necrosis secondary to inflammatory reaction/cascade that affects the adipose tissue directly. Clinical studies have proven good clinical results in terms of reduction in the subcutaneous fat deposits and minimal complication rates [6, 7, 14].

Furthermore, radiofrequency devices are designed to use optical energies to treat directly the dermis and hypodermis. This technology allows to target principally the water located in the dermal layer; however, the target is controlled by thermal stress leading to dermal tightening and contraction. At the same time, in the same physical process, there is an activation of the dermal fibroblast to stimulate the new collagen formation. The utilization of bipolar radiofrequency in the hypodermis maximizes fat cell metabolism; devices such as BodyFx™, Invasix use this type of principles [8, 17, 23].

8. Conclusion

High definition liposuction procedures should be considered revolutionary in the plastic surgery field. They are more complex, difficult, and need a special learning curve. The procedures require surgeons to understand how the anatomical configuration skin-fat-muscle-skeletal structures help equally in the 3D superficial topography either in woman or in male human contouring. New technologies and novel medical devices coming up will lead in the future minimal scar procedures with better clinical outcomes.

Author details

Javier Soto[1*], Hugo A. Aguilar[2] and Juan S. Barajas-Gamboa[3]

*Address all correspondence to: Javier.soto@doctor.com

1 Plastic Surgery Department, FOSCAL International, La Riviera Clinic, Aqua SPA Beauty & Health, Bucaramanga, Colombia

2 Plastic Surgery Department, Santander University Hospital (HUS), Bucaramanga, Colombia

3 Surgery Department, Autonomous University of Bucaramanga (UNAB), Bucaramanga, Colombia

References

[1] Manzaneda C, Raúl M. Lipomarcación de alta definición: reporte de dos casos/high definition lipomarking: report of two patient. Horiz Méd. (Impresa) 2015;15(2):70–75, abr.

[2] Leclère FM, Moreno-Moraga J, Mordon S, Servell P, Unglaub F, Kolb F, Rimareix F, Trelles MA. Laser-assisted lipolysis for cankle remodelling: a prospective study in 30 patients. Lasers Med Sci. 2014;29(1):131–136.

[3] Hoyos A, Perez M. Arm dynamic definition by liposculpture and fat grafting. Aesthet Surg J. 2012;32(8): 974–987.

[4] Baer PC, Kuçi S, Krause M, Kuçi Z, Zielen S, Geiger H, Bader P, Schubert R. Comprehensive phenotypic characterization of human adipose-derived stromal/stem cells and their subsets by a high throughput technology. Stem Cells Dev. 2013;22(2):330–339.

[5] Mentz H, Gilliland M, Patronella C. Abdominal etching: Differential liposuction to detail abdominal musculature. Aesthet Plast Surg. 1993;17(4):287–290.

[6] Hoyos AE, Millard JA. Vaser-assisted highdefinition lipoplasty.Aesthet Surg J. 2007;27:594–604.

[7] Klein JA. Tumescent technique for local anesthesia improvessafety in large-volume liposuction. Plast Reconstr Surg. 1993;92:1085–1098; discussion 1099–1100.

[8] Kim YH, Cha SM, Naidu S, Hwang WJ. Analysis of postoperative complications for superficial liposuction: a review of 2398 cases. Plast Reconstr Surg. 2011;127:863–871.

[9] Matarasso A, Levine SM. Evidence-based medicine: liposuction. Plast Reconstr Surg. 2013;132(6):1697–1705.

[10] Garcia O Jr, Nathan N. Comparative analysis of blood loss in suction-assisted lipoplasty and third-generation internal ultrasound-assisted lipoplasty. Aesthet Surg J. 2008;28(4): 430–435. doi: 10.1016/j.asj.2008.04.002.

[11] Commons GW, Lim AF. Treatment of axillary hyperhidrosis/bromidrosis using VASER ultrasound. Aesthet Plast Surg. 2009;33(3):312–323. doi: 10.1007/s00266-008-9283-y. Epub 2009 Jan 3.

[12] Nagy MW, Vanek PF Jr. A multicenter, prospective, randomized, single-blind, controlled clinical trial comparing VASER-assisted lipoplasty, and suction-assisted lipoplasty. Plast Reconstr Surg. 2012;129(4):681e–9e. doi: 10.1097/PRS.0b013e3182442274.

[13] de Souza Pinto EB1, Abdala PC, Maciel CM, dos Santos Fde P, de Souza RP. Liposuction and VASER. Clin Plast Surg. 2006;33(1):107–115, vii.

[14] Matarasso A. Discussion: a multicenter, prospective, randomized, single-blind, controlled clinical trial comparing VASER-assisted lipoplasty and suction-assisted

lipoplasty. Plast Reconstr Surg. 2012;129(4):690e–1e. doi: 10.1097/PRS.0b013e31824c9047. No abstract available. PMID: 22456383

[15] Swanson E. Improved skin contraction after VASER-assisted lipoplasty: is it a change we can believe in? Plast Reconstr Surg. 2012;130(5):754e–756e. doi: 10.1097/PRS.0b013e318267d96a. No abstract available.

[16] Schafer ME, Hicok KC, Mills DC, Cohen SR, Chao JJ. Acute adipocyte viability after third-generation ultrasound-assisted liposuction. Aesthet Surg J. 2013 Jul;33(5):698–704. doi: 10.1177/1090820X13485239. Epub 2013 May 29.

[17] Hurwitz DJ, Ayeni O. Body contouring surgery in the massive weight loss patient. Surg Clin North Am. 2016;96(4):875–885. doi: 10.1016/j.suc.2016.03.011. Review.

[18] Hurwitz DJ. Body contouring surgery for women in comprehensive body contouring: theory and practice [Chapter 4]. New York: Springer; 2016. pp. 63–179.

[19] Song AY, Jean RD, Hurwitz DJ, et al. A classification of contour deformities after massive weight loss: the Pittsburgh rating scale. Plast Reconstr Surg. 2005;116(5):1535–1544.

[20] Hurwitz DJ. Aesthetic refinements in body contouring in the massive weight loss patient: trunk. Plast Reconstr Surg. 2014;134:1185–1195.

[21] Klopper EM, Kroese-Deutman HC, Berends FJ. Massive weight loss after bariatric surgery and the demand (desire) for body contouring surgery. Eur J Plast Surg. 2014;37(2):103–108.

[22] Tremp M, Delko T, Kraljevic M, et al. Outcome in body contouring surgery after massive weight loss: a prospective matched single-blind study. J Plast Reconstr Aesthet Surg. 2015;68:1410–1416.

[23] Hurwitz DJ. Single stage total body lift after massive weight loss. Ann Plast Surg. 2004;52(5):435–441.

10

Fat Grafting in Body Contouring

Marco Romeo, Ayman Elmeligy and
Khalid Elsherbeny

Abstract

Fat transfer had been used since the first decades of the twentieth century for body contouring and reconstruction. Since then, a lot of controversies and ongoing research regarding indications, harvesting and transplantation technique had been a concern for plastic surgeons. More recently, the use of fat as a source of stem cells had been the major point of research joining both the aesthetic and the regenerative advantages. Body reshaping using fat graft is nowadays a common non-invasive resource in the surgeon's armamentarium popularized as body sculpturing merging the benefits of liposuction and lipofilling to improve the aesthetic of virtually all the regions of human body. In this chapter, the role of fat grafting in aesthetic body contouring will be discussed. The association of stem cells is exposed to give the reader the possibility to better understand this option of treatment. Fat harvesting/grafting techniques are explained and the authors' preferred choice is exposed. Lipofilling details are discussed per area of the body with practical tips and pitfalls for the experienced or the newbie surgeon. A final summary on complications will remind all the possible incidences that may occur in the short- and long term after surgery.

Keywords: lipofilling, fat grafting, aesthetic, stem cells, body contouring

1. Introduction

1.1. The history of fat grafting

History of fat grafting is rather fascinating, yet quite controversial with all that it carries within its corners, from frustrations to adventurous experimentation.

The first attempt to use fat in human auto-transplantation was dated to **1889** by **Van der Meulen**, The procedure consisted of grafting an omentum and fat auto-graft between diaphragm and liver.

The first described free fat grafting attempt was recorded by Gustav Adolf Neuber, a German surgeon in 1893. Neuber used small fat grafts in order to fill facial defects in a 20-year-old man. According to Neuber, he had less success when he tried to use larger grafts, saying that 'grafts larger than an almond would not give good results'.

In 1895, Viktor Czerny (1842–1916) reported excising a lipoma and grafting it into a breast defect to establish symmetry following a unilateral partial mastectomy [1].

Gersuny in 1900 proposed paraffin injections. They became commonly used for post-syphilis saddle noses. Paraffin injections gave amazing results initially; however infections, paraffinomas, migration and pulmonary embolism were major complications of the procedure [2].

In 1912, Holländer proposed the technique of fat injection, but there was a high rate of reabsorption. He harvested adipose tissue from patients and mixed it with fat from rams. This mixture was injected as a fluid at body temperature. Patients had a painful rash afterwards for 2–3 days, but he reported a good outcome.

Lexer in 1919 also described fat grafting in his textbook, to correct sequelae of facial trauma, hemifacial microsomia, microgenia, breast asymmetry, and post-traumatic hand stiffness. He also described the use of fat to restore gliding tissue around tendons in Dupuytren disease [3].

Gillies in 1920, showed in his book, patients treated with fat grafting after facial injuries.

Peer in 1950, demonstrated that about 50% of fat cells died after transplantation and were replaced with fibrous tissue and stressed that survival of fat grafts was **dependent on early neovascular anastomoses** (new blood vessels), and stated that 50% of the adipose cells in free fat grafts survive.

Studies and research work in the past decades focused more on the pathology of obesity and the role of genetics on fat cells in obese people.

The general acceptance among researchers is that the number of adipocytes is fixed in adults.

Smith in 1971 described the fibroblast-like cells grown on tissue culture.

The adipocyte precursors studied in tissue culture was more profoundly investigated by Van in 1976, proved that fat tissue was more dynamic than historically thought it was.

It was Roncari who studied the morphology and maturation of cultured adipocytes in a culture system that he developed in 1978 [4].

Liposuction technique was invented by Fischer in 1974.

It was not until the era of liposuction in 1978 when the French physicians Illouz and Fournier further developed the procedure utilizing blunt cannulas for suction lipoplasty that made the process of fat extraction more reliably predicted.

By the early eighties, liposuction became quite popular in the United States. Klein, a dermatologist, invented the tumescent technique for liposuction that allowed patients to have liposuction performed totally under local anaesthesia with less bleeding and with much smaller cannulas.

Ellenbogen started using fat pearls in the reconstruction of facial defects [5] and in 1988, Chajchir described favourable results, emphasising cautious handling of adipocytes, rinsing of the lipoaspirate to eliminate dead cells and grafting into a well-vascularised bed [6].

In the nineties, Sydney Coleman from New York described standardized techniques for fat extraction, processing and injection of fat grafting [7, 8].

1.2. Fat potential and differentiation capacity

In 2001, a group of researchers from the University of Pittsburgh described the implications of adipose tissue in cell-based regenerative therapies.

This was quite a revelation for the scientific community, as up until that time adult mesenchymal stem cells (MSCs) were predominantly thought of as a bone marrow product.

As it turns out, adipose tissue is a much more prolific source of MSCs than bone marrow.

By volume, mesenchymal stem cells are actually 300–500 times more abundant in adipose tissue compared to bone marrow tissue.

Comparison of multi-lineage cells from human adipose tissue and bone marrow is given in Ref. [9].

Adipocytes derived from stem cells (SC) under the right stimulation could differentiate into different lineage like endothelial cells, fat cells, epithelial cells, neuronal cells, chondrocytes, myocytes and osteocytes.

Adipocytes also secrete more than 100 proteins (adipokines) and growth factors that regulate: angiogenesis, inflammation and apoptosis.

Growth factors include: vascular growth factor, liver growth factor, platelet and epidermic growth factors.

Fat grafting has truly opened new frontiers for plastic surgeons and other medical specialties.

Its power is only yet to be understood and it is clear that adipose tissue will be a pillar of regenerative medicine treating a huge spectrum of diseases like DM, Autism, Parkinson's disease, multiple sclerosis and others [10].

1.3. The fate of fat

The old, general concept of fat grafting was that the surgeon had to overfill the grafted area of about 40% of its volume since there will be resorption of 10–60%, some said up to 90%.

There was no proper understanding of the mechanism of survival and fate of grafted fat cells.

Today, research revealed the fate of grafted adipose tissue showing that three different zones will demarcate after 4 weeks of grafting, by name these zones are:

1. The outer surviving zone: the most superficial; several rows of fat cells that are clearly in direct contact with the vascularized recipient tissues of the host.

2. The intermediate regenerating zone: with a thickness from 600 to 1200 μm, which shows both surviving adipocytes along with dead.

3. The inner necrotic zone: with necrotic cells, inflammatory cells, fibrosis, oil drops and rare adipocytes.

At the outermost surviving zone, the cells are quite close to vascularity and the adipocytes tend to survive in a process quite similar to the physiology of skin grafts, called the diffusion/angiogenesis theory that suggests that donor adipocytes survive by oxygen diffusion at the recipient site during the initial days after grafting, with eventual micro-angiogenesis and formation of a viable blood supply.

At the regenerating zone, the fat cells do not succeed to survive; however the adipose-derived stem cells (pre-adipocytes) experience ongoing adipogenesis that increased rapidly after grafting and peaked at 4 weeks and full remodelling was completed by 12 weeks.

The necrotic zones will eventually be absorbed, filled with fibrous tissue, or become a problematic cyst.

Grafted fat tissue undergoes degeneration within 1 week, while regeneration reaches its peak at 4 weeks. Regeneration takes place by adipose tissue-resident progenitor cells. Phagocytosis and cicatrisation occur in the regenerating and necrotic zones, predominantly by M1 and M2 macrophages respectively.

The stabilization process appears to persist for a long time after failed regeneration. The size of the necrotizing zone depends mainly on the size of the graft and the micro-environment into which it is placed. Eventually, necrotic zones will be absorbed, filled with fibrous tissue, or become a problematic cyst. Liposuction and reinjection procedures could be improved by preparing grafts with better viability and in an appropriate size, maximizing the contact surface of the grafts by ideal distribution, and placing the grafts in areas with high vascularity. Stabilization of the grafted fat may not occur until several months after complete regeneration at 3 months. This emphasizes the importance of long-term follow-up to thoroughly evaluate the clinical results of microfat grafting [11].

There are opposing theories about cell survival: The Hofer's theory versus the scaffold or matrix theory.

According to Hofer, all or most of the transplanted adult adipocytes are destined to die, acting as a non-viable scaffold, through which macrophages penetrate and through which stem cell–mediated angiogenesis and adipogenesis occur.

Cytokine induced cell-cell signalling between living and dying, and between the donor and recipient cells, is thought to play a role in this process [12, 13].

According to the scaffold matrix theory of Khouri and Rigotti, overcrowding of injected cells reaches a critical interstitial fluid pressure of 9 mmHg; therefore, in a tight recipient space fat droplets will merge into fat lakes, which is thought to interfere with capillary blood flow and hence oxygen diffusion leading to apoptosis and cell death.

In clinical setting, fat injections larger than 0.16 cm in radius will have a region of central necrosis.

2. Fat grafting technique

Fat grafting is promising, but clinical outcomes are not always predictable due to the variability of degree of fat resorption, which is highly dependent on surgeon's technique.

Fat-grafting procedure is divided mainly to three main steps:

1. Fat Harvesting
2. Fat Processing
3. Fat Grafting

Most surgeons believe that fat, as autologous tissue, can be considered the ideal soft-tissue filler because it is abundant, readily available, inexpensive, compatible, and can be harvested easily. If fat grafts are manipulated correctly, structural fat grafting represents a safe, long-lasting and natural-appearing method for soft-tissue augmentation in patients.

To obtain long-term survival of transplanted autologous fatty tissue, the harvested and processed fat grafts must remain viable before implantation. In 1994, Coleman first described his technique, which uses a syringe, cannula and centrifuge, for structural fat grafting [7].

He later refined and popularized his technique for fat-graft harvesting and processing with patented instruments and a centrifugation protocol, often referred to as the Coleman technique [14].

2.1. Harvesting

A number of techniques have been used for fat harvesting, these include conventional liposuction (syringe with vacuum suction), power-assisted liposuction (specialized cannula with mechanized movement), hand-held syringe liposuction (syringe with manual suction; Coleman technique) and internal ultrasound and LASER-assisted liposuction (specialized cannula that transmits ultrasound or LASER within the body syringe liposuction). A number of studies have compared conventional liposuction with suction- or power-assisted liposuction. Leong et al., upon comparing syringe liposuction to pump-assisted liposuction found no differences in cell viability, cell metabolic activity or adipogenic responses of cultured mesenchymal precursor cells processed from pump or syringe lipoaspirates [15, 16].

In contrast, Pu et al. demonstrated that syringe liposuction yields a greater number of viable adipocytes and sustains a more optimal level of cellular function within fat grafts than conventional liposuction. However, normal histologic structure was maintained in fat grafts obtained by both methods [17].

2.2. Infiltration

For fat aspiration, the donor site is infused with tumescent solution, consisting of a local anaesthetic (LA) (lidocaine, ropivacaine, prilocaine or bupivacaine) for pain relief and epinephrine for haemostasis in Lactated Ringer's solution or normal saline. The most currently used LA for liposuction and Autologous Fat Graft (AFG) is lidocaine and that is on this molecule that literature is the most abundant. Indeed, a survey from the American Society for Aesthetic Plastic Surgery concluded that: for adipose tissue harvest, 40% of surgeons use tumescent solution containing 50 mL of 1% xylocaine + 1 mL epinephrine 1:1000 in 1 L normal saline, which corresponds to 0.5 mg/mL of lidocaine, about 30% of them use a mixture of 0.5% xylocaine with epinephrine and 22% use 1% xylocaine epinephrine mixture. The remaining 8% of American physicians use epinephrine alone or other solution [18].

Several studies [19–21] have examined the effect of the local anaesthetic or epinephrine on fat viability. Oren in a study published in the journal of drugs in dermatology in 2005 stated that neither lidocaine nor adrenaline had long-term unfavourable results on the grafted fat cells.

According to authors' experience, the use of LA should be avoided under general anaesthesia (tumescent solution with diluted epinephrine only), preferably using regional or spinal anaesthesia to avoid injection of local anaesthetics.

2.3. Donor site preference

Whether there is an optimal donor site for fat grafting or not remains to be established.

In several studies, various authors showed that fat from the lower abdomen and medial thighs consist of a higher concentration of adipose-derived stem cells compared to the fat from the upper abdomen, trochanteric region, knee and flank [22].

However, other studies reported no influence of the donor site on fat viability [23, 24].

Among adrenergic receptor subtypes that regulate lipid mobilization, the alpha-2-adrenergic receptor is involved in the inhibition of fatty acid mobilization from adipose tissue and that can explain why some areas are more resistant to fat mobilization, the so called genetic fat areas, like abdomen for the men and trochanteric areas for women.

In our experience, the genetic fat theory had a clinical correspondency, with volumes of fat less susceptible to reduction with diet and exercise. The genetic fat expresses alpha-2 receptors that are more stable with metabolism and are anti-lipolytic. So it is usually useful to ask the patient about his resistant fat areas as a guide to the donor site, usually trochanters, lower abdomen and love handles in most people.

2.4. Optimal lobular size: choice of harvesting cannula

The size of cannula is debated among physicians. Some researchers stated that larger cannulas allow harvesting of bigger fat lobules with a higher survival rate [25].

Others stated that smaller cannula sizes theoretically create less donor site trauma and allow for removal of smaller sized lobules of fat, which may improve flow characteristics and reduce trauma during reinjection. An important consideration besides cannula size is cannula hole size and number of holes. A 12-gauge cannula with 6–8 side holes 2 × 1 mm in size can extract a significant amount of fat despite its small calibre.

The summation of the surface area of the individual openings on a 12-gauge, 12-hole cannula approaches or exceeds the surface area of the opening of a classic 10 mm one-hole cannula. This results in better tissue flow with less trauma in the donor area. In addition, each hole selects for lobules of a small, uniform size, which are more likely to flow easily through the injection cannula during the grafting phase of the procedure thus, there is no need for further processing or syringe transfers. The hole sizes on the aspiration cannula approach the size of the hole on the injection cannula. This ensures 'equalization' of hole sizes for more efficient fat flow [26].

In our experience midsize cannulas (3 and 4 mm) are a good compromise between too fine instruments (2 mm) and aggressive tools (5 or 6 mm).

Using wider-diameter cannulas (2.5 mm) may however be preferred as they have been shown to potentially improve fat-graft survival and reduce fat- graft resorption compared with small-diameter cannulas (1.6 or 2 mm).

The size of the needles does not appear to affect cell viability, at least when using 14-, 16-, and 20-gauge needles (Erdim et al) [27]. However, for any given needle size, it appears that fat viability is influenced by the shear stress, which is a function of the flow rate. Thus, fat injected at a slow rate (low shear stress) results in better fat-graft retention than fat injected at a fast rate (high shear stress) [25]

In the author's practice, nowadays with evolving of microfat and nanofat techniques, harvesting allows injection with ease using 0.7 and 0.9 mm diameter injection cannulas and needles as common practice without much worry about friction and sheer stress especially in areas of the face and hands where tiny injectors are needed.

2.5. Negative pressure

The literature regarding the isolated effects of negative pressure suggests that adipocytes can be suctioned below 700 mmHg without undue trauma according to Shiffman [28].

Claims of syringe suctioning as being safer than machine suctioning should be carefully considered. While a standard liposuction machine can generate up to one atmosphere (760 mmHg) of negative pressure, a 60-cc syringe connected to an in-line manometer can also generate nearly one atmosphere of negative pressure. It is likely that absolute pressure and not the source of this pressure is the key variable in adipocyte trauma and its effect of adipocyte viability [26].

The author's experience agrees with the aforementioned literature about keeping a low suction pressure at the level of 700 mmHg to maintain the viability of fat cells.

2.6. Processing

The harvested fat is processed in order to eliminate tumescent fluid, blood, cell fragments and oil (from disrupted adipocytes) [29].

Processing aims to retain viable adipocytes in a concentrated form which is believed to enhance the graft taken [16].

Filtration, centrifugation and sedimentation (decantation) are the most commonly used fat processing methods.

2.6.1. Filtration

The filtration technique uses a platform for concentrating fat cells and separating cells from fluids, oil and debris. Examples of platform used for filtering fat include filters or strainers with defined pore size, gauze, metal sieve, mesh and operating room cloth. During centrifugation process, the syringe containing the aspirate is placed in a centrifuge at a specified speed and time.

During the sedimentation process, the syringe containing the lipoaspirate is allowed to sit for decantation to occur under the effect of gravity.

A modification of this technique includes washing the lipoaspirate with 1–3 times the volume with normal saline or Lactated Ringer's solution and then left to decant under gravity. In all techniques, centrifugation, sedimentation and washing, the lipoaspirate is separated into three zones: an upper oil zone, a middle purified concentrated fat layer, and a lower aqueous zone consisting of blood and washing liquids. In the centrifugation technique, in addition, a pellet is seen at the bottom of the centrifuge.

2.6.2. Centrifugation

The Coleman technique is the most widely used centrifugation protocol in which the lipoaspirate is centrifuged at ~1200 × g (3,000 rpm) for 3 minutes.

In agreement with Coleman, Kurita et al. evaluated the effect of six centrifugation speeds (from 0 to 4200 ×g for 3 minutes) on fat aspirates and graft taken from nude mice and concluded that centrifugation at more than 3000 ×g significantly damaged adipose-derived stem cells and recommended 1200 ×g as an optimized centrifugal force for obtaining good short- and long-term results in adipose transplantation [30].

Some studies concluded that lower centrifugal forces than in Coleman's protocol may be more adipocyte-friendly.

Hoareau et al. subjected fat tissue to soft (100 ×g/1 min and 400 ×g/1 min) and strong (900 ×g/3 min and 1800 ×g/10 min) forces and examined the grafts viability. Strong centrifugation resulted in 3-fold more adipocyte death than soft centrifugation suggesting that soft centrifugation (400 × g/1 min) seems to be the most appropriate protocol for the reinjection of adipose tissue.

Yet, others suggest that centrifugation has no effect on adipocyte viability as in Pulsfort et al. Pulsfort, using eight different centrifugal forces (up to 20,000 ×g) found no significant differences in the viability of centrifuged adipocytes. Furthermore, no apoptotic changes revealed during cultivation of isolated adipocyte after centrifugation. However, higher centrifugal accelerations were better in cleansing lipoaspirates from oil and cell debris, than lower centrifugal forces.

The authors do not advocate centrifugation forces above 5000 rpm for more than 5 minutes and more than 1200 G finding that it carries the risk of destruction to fat cells.

2.6.3. Sedimentation

Sedimentation is the oldest and the cheapest way to treat fat before injection. The most advanced purification techniques seem to have replaced decantation but some studies still support this simple filtration process also with higher amount of live pre-adipocytes [31].

Condé- Green showed that cell count, per high-power field, of intact nucleated adipocytes was significantly higher in decanted lipoaspirates while centrifuged samples showed a greater majority of altered adipocytes. On the other hand, the MSC concentration was significantly higher in washed lipoaspirates compared to decanted and centrifuged samples. However, the pellet collected at the bottom of the centrifuged samples had the highest concentration [32].

The authors wash adipose tissue grafts and recommend that if centrifugation is used, the pellet containing mesenchymal stem cells should be added to the concentrated adipose phase to augment graft take.

2.7. Fat placement

Although there is no standardized fat placement technique, the Coleman technique is the most widely used. Fat grafts, in this technique, are injected using a blunt Coleman infiltration cannula attached to a 1 mL syringe while withdrawing the cannula. Different syringe sizes (3 and 10 mL) as well as various cannula tip shapes, lengths, gauges and curves can be used depending on the volume of fat to be placed and the recipient site [33].

2.7.1. Types of fat grafting

Different sizes of fat graft obviously reflect the mean lobular size of each type.

Macrofat grafting: as the name implies, represents the largest lobular size and is the size obtained with a standard (3 mm and above) mostly Mercedes type liposuction cannula with large side holes (2 × 7 mm). This kind was mostly the standard practice since the start of fat grafting, indifferently injected to all parts of the body including the face. Probably that was the reason why patients previously had complications like lumpiness and cyst formation due to the unsuitable grafted lobular size to the delicate areas of the face like tear trough.

Macrofat grafting is best indicated in areas that need large volume transfers like buttocks and breasts. Macrofat graft contains both viable adipocytes and adipocyte derived stem cells (ADSCs).

Blunt injection cannulas ranging from 0.7 to 0.9 mm are usually used, with very good results, for microfat grafting, usually performed in the facial area. The fat particles need to be sufficiently small in order to provide a smooth injection through these fine cannulas. If the fat particles are too large, passage through the fine injection cannula would be difficult. As a result, disrupted injection will follow, which may lead to an unequal lipofilling with irregular fat deposits.

Trepsat used a multi-perforated harvesting cannula of 2 mm with 1-mm side holes and 19-gauge injection cannulas, to provide fat grafts with smaller particles for microfat grafting procedures at the lower eyelid. To harvest fat for injection of other parts of the face, a multi-perforated liposuction cannula of 3 mm in diameter with 2-mm side holes was used [34, 35].

According to the authors' practice, the smaller lobular fat-graft size obtained with a (Tonnard) or (Sorensen) microfat harvester cannulas that are multi-port 2-3 mm cannulas (19-gauge) with sharp or bevelled 6–12 side holes of 1 mm in diameter. These are best mounted to a 10 mm luer lock tip syringe for a controlled low pressure microfat harvesting. Microfat-grafts were best used to fill the face, hands and delicate areas as tear trough. Microfat contains both viable adipocytes and adipocyte derived stem cells.

The radius of the fat particle is inversely proportional to its contact surface. This means that for the same volume of injected fat, reducing the diameter by half will double the contact surface. A larger contact surface means better contact with the capillaries in the recipient area and thus a better graft survival rate with less need for overcorrection. The authors do not advocate overfilling with microfat grafting. Microfat grafts due to their micro lobular size are easily injected with 0.7–0.9 mm micro-cannulas injected into different tissue layers in columns of fat pearls.

Aspirated fat has to be processed mechanically to provide a liquid fat emulsion, which is called nanofat. This is to ensure a smooth fat injection through 27-gauge sharp needles [34]. Using a nanofat processing procedure, a yield of 1 ml of nanofat per 10 ml of lipoaspirate can be expected.

For production of nanofat, the lipoaspirated fat is mechanically emulsified after rinsing by shifting the fat between two 10-cc syringes connected to each other by a female-to-female Luer-Lock connector. After 30 passes, the fat changes into an emulsion. At the end of the fragmentation process, the fat becomes liquid and has a whitish appearance. After emulsification process, the fatty liquid is again filtered over the sterile nylon cloth and the effluent is collected as nanofat. Nanofat does not add much volume as its filling capacity is pretty limited since it mostly lacks the viable adipocytes. However, nanofat grafts are rich in ADSCs that are capable of skin rejuvenation as in areas like perioral skin, glabellar skin, sun-damaged skin at the breast cleavage, dark eye hallows and scars. Nanofat is injected using a 23-gauge needle mounted to 1-cc syringe. The effect of nanofat usually appears with a delay of 4 weeks to 3 months.

Increased collagen, elastin synthesis and remodelling are the presumed mechanisms for this regenerative effect on improved elasticity. Stem cells rather than grafted adipocytes most likely trigger these effects. Presumably, the nanofat sample analysis revealed that adipocytes were destroyed during the emulsification process.

Another form of microfat graft, called SNIF (sharp needle intradermal fat injection), through which a 1 ml syringe is injected to the superficial dermal plane with a 23-gauge needle. SNIF is a cheaper and more effective filler for wrinkles in patients willing to have long-term results and would accept the process of fat harvesting and the post-operative swelling.

2.8. Tips and pitfalls

The authors carry on the microfat harvesting and injection technique for purpose of fat injection of the face, hands, scars and breasts. In case of buttocks augmentation, macrofat harvesting and injection techniques are utilized as described formerly in the literature.

Our main steps are:

Harvesting site choice. Selecting area for fat harvesting depending on genetic fat theory asking the patient about his areas of fat deposits that are least affected with metabolism during weight loss. In case of face treatment, the planned amount is usually around 50–100 cc; however in buttocks it could range up to 1 litre. Infiltration: Tumescent technique is carried in a 1:1 ratio of infiltration to aspirate ratio. For every 1000-cc of normal saline, 1ml adrenaline, and 10 cc of sodium bicarbonate. Usually, regional or spinal anaesthesia is utilized or other wise 20 cc of 1 % lidocaine is to be added to the 1 litre solution.

Harvesting. Usually waiting around 10 minutes from the start of infiltration to start suctioning the first infiltrated area. 2 mm microfat harvester cannulas with 6 –12 (1 mm) holes are used. More than one type of microfat cannula harvesters is used. We prefer in our practice the bevelled smooth edged side holes better than cannulas with sharp bevelled edged holes since the sharp edges were found to cut more readily into the connective tissues opening tissue planes together so instead of suctioning from tunnels, changes to spaces and that leads to losing suction pressure fast after a while, especially while using syringe suction which necessitates harvesting other areas to get the needed amount of fat.

Lipoaspiration with a low suction pressure (under 700 mmHg) either using 10-cc syringes for harvesting of microfat or suction assisted motors for larger volumes as for macrofat grafting of the buttocks for augmentation.

Processing. It is carried out with a process of decantation where the fat is collected in syringes standing upright in a metal rack for the fat to sediment into an oil layer (top), fatty layer (middle) and fluid (lower) layer with remains of tumescent fluid and blood.

Decantation. The process is carried with suction of the oil layer with 23-G needle until purification and eliminating the bottom fluid portion. Adding plasma-rich platelets to the purified aspirate in a ratio of 1:9 is an optional step.

Preparing for injection by transferring the filtered, activated microfat into individual 1-cc syringe with a 0.7 or 0.9 mm micro-injector cannulas in case of microfat placement and in 2mm injectors for macrofat placement as in larger volumes as the buttocks.

Placement of the fat should be carried out in many columns of fat pearls with multi-strokes or retrograde filling in different tissue layers, never in one bolus neither in an over correction.

3. Stem cells and fat grafting

Stem cells are present in many tissues of the human body.

The most common source of SC is the bone marrow, which is a relatively complicated location to perform a non-invasive harvesting procedure. Adipose tissue is a natural source of stem cells, which are at the edge of modern research for tissue regeneration, thanks to the easy, non-invasive harvesting and abundant availability of MSCs. Therefore, fat grafting has started to be considered not just a treatment to achieve morphologic improvement but a procedure of regenerative medicine. Beside the large availability of ADSCs, it has been demonstrated that ADSCs express CD3, CD14, CD19, CD34, CD44, CD45, CD73 and CD90 similar to cord tissue MSCs (CT-MSCs) [36], that confirms the same biological quality. ADSCs have been successfully extracted and used in many studies to seed specific tissues to obtain differentiation and local proliferation [37].

On the other hand, out of laboratory, most of the actual clinical applications do not use ADSCs alone but along with their adipose medium due to the easy, inexpensive harvesting and injection (liposuction/lipofilling) process.

Thus, concentration of MSCs is relevant to biological effect and various methods of concentration of cells inside adipose tissue have been invented. All commercially available system demonstrated to be effective but the concentration of MSCs can be quite heterogeneous [38].

Celution® (Cytori Therapeutics, Inc., San Diego, Calif.) demonstrated to be the most effective in concentrating MSCs (2.41 × 105 cells/g) also bringing endothelial cells.

These devices are a promising advance in reconstructive surgery to treat difficult wounds or irradiated tissues. The biggest downside is the elevated cost of maintenance, which limits their use in aesthetic field.

In private practice, an efficient purifying system of adipose tissue (i.e. Puregraft® or centrifugation) has the right balance between cost and effectiveness.

In our experience, high concentration of stem cells has been used in perioral treatment of sclerodermia to enhance tissue regeneration. It is authors' belief that stem cells may be of great help when active regeneration is needed but that aesthetic uses of MSCs may not justify the high processing price.

4. Applications and indications to fat grafting

Fat grafting has relevant roles both in reconstructive and aesthetic fields; for the purpose of this book, only the latter will be discussed.

Lipofilling has become more and more popular, plus the indications are growing broader each year. Therefore, it is hard for the surgeon to have clear guidelines to choose the right technique for the right patient.

In 2007, the American Society of Plastic Surgery (ASPS) [29] developed evidence-based indications to the use of fat grafting supported by strong literature data.

The first applied criterion is safety. Despite some heterogeneity of fat processing among physicians (infiltration, harvesting, processing and fat layering), the overall risk is low. Considering the mild anaesthesia needed, anaesthetic complications are barely reported, which allows including a wider group of potential patients according to general health conditions and comorbidities. Infections, seroma and hematoma are reported but mostly treated conservatively [39, 40].

Doubts related to cancer (mostly breast) due to the biological role of fat and stromal cells have been cleared by several studies [41, 42], although in specific cases, like breast injection, a mammography or ultrasound are recommended.

In aesthetic field the most popular indications include facial and hand rejuvenation, breast and buttocks augmentation, scar revision and less commonly penis and calf enlargement; the most important are discussed in this chapter.

Beside safety, there are some relative limits to aesthetic fat grafting, which include adipose tissue availability, associated risk factors to fat survival, for example smoking, patient permission to possible multiple sessions (therefore, higher costs) and expectations.

In conclusion, standardization of fat manipulation and careful choice of patients can contribute to satisfactory results from both parts.

5. Scar correction

Bad scarring represent either a functional and aesthetic trouble that often needs revision, although surgery (excision and z-plasty) alone may not solve the problem; for example, post-radiotherapy scarring often involves wide areas, which are not amenable of direct excision.

Scar depression and adherence to deep planes are common features of abnormal scarring that come along with pain and potential functional limitation.

For the reasons mentioned before about ADSCs, fat grafting plays a double role in scar revision: mechanical and biological.

In fact, fat layering corrects depressed scars, detach adherences and can release trapped nerves and tendons.

On the other hand, ADSCs enhance local regeneration and improve vascularity, which can become particularly relevant in unstable scars.

Timing is important, if there is room for ordinary surgical revision (for example a z-plasty), fat grafting may anticipate surgery to improve tissues quality. Moreover, various sessions may be required and it must be discussed with the patient when planning surgery.

In any case, it is wise to wait at least 6 months of scar maturation before attempting any correction. Further sessions may come at an interval of 3–6 months.

5.1. Technique tips and pitfalls

Anaesthesia and amount of fat to be transferred cannot be standardized, as the clinical scenario is always different.

The first problem the surgeon will encounter is the stiffness of the scarred tissues, which makes difficult to create the funnels with a blunt cannula: remember that excessive strength pushing the cannula through will lead to poor control of trajectory and potential perforation of superficial and deep organs with high-risk consequences.

Therefore, a V-shaped cannula is the ideal tool to safely create the passages to infiltrate fat. It is possible to use either a simple dissector or a sharp cannula to dissect and infiltrate at once.

In our experience, the latter is better, so you can infiltrate in a retrograde fashion each new tunnel without creating false planes.

Superficial subcutaneous scarring may be treated with percutaneous release (rigottomy) with a thick 14–16 G needle.

It is important to try to create a three-dimensional network of tunnels in all directions to neutralize all the vectors of scarring and improve the result.

6. Facial rejuvenation

Facial aging is a complex phenomenon that includes all soft tissues and bones of the face.

A careful assessment must be made to address separately the loss of volume, the vertical displacement of soft tissues and worsening of skin texture [9, 10].

Volume loss mostly depends on soft tissues atrophy and secondarily on bone resorption.

As a matter of fact, when the bones profile becomes too visible it gives a skully aspect, which is instinctively recognized as aged.

Fat grafting is an excellent long lasting alternative to temporary hyaluronic acid (HA) filling.

Like HA, fat is used to correct nasolabial folds, marionette lines, and cheek prominence, tear trough, lip volume, jaw line and the temporal zone to restore a youthful oval face.

6.1. Technique tips and pitfalls

Fat grafting can be carried out as an outpatient procedure under sedation and local anaesthesia with or without nerve blocks.

Care must be taken to respect the principles of micrografting; a 1mm cannula is probably the best to retain more fat. On the other hand, the amount of resorption rate in the face is lower than other parts of the body; therefore overfilling is equally a potential mistake. The most critical areas of the face are the tear trough (TT) and the lips.

TT assessment must clarify whether there is a problem of a deep anatomical groove or an excess of eye bags near the lower lid, in the second case a blepharoplasty is indicated against lipofilling.

Moreover, due to the thin skin of this area, one must avoid injecting too superficially to avoid permanent visible and palpable lumps; an inexperienced surgeon should not perform TT correction as his/her first procedure.

Lips enhancement is technically easier and equally rewarding for the surgeon and the patient but may suffer of delayed complications if the patient gains weight with deformities and distortion of the lip due to asymmetric adipose tissue expansion. This point must be discussed with the patient prior to surgery and possibly included in the consent form.

7. Hand rejuvenation

While face ageing has always been a concern for people, hand ageing awareness is a more recent discovery in our culture.

Hands more than anything else speak about us, our job, our hobbies and our lives.

With time subcutaneous tissues thin out making visible tendons, bones and veins, which give the typical 'skeleton hand' appearance perceived as aged.

Fat graft helps to restore the subcutaneous layers hiding the over mentioned structures [43].

7.1. Technique tips and pitfalls

The treatment can be performed as an outpatient procedure; thanks to the limited harvesting the procedure can be performed under mild sedation, local anaesthesia and nerve blocks at the wrist.

Once fat has been prepared with the preferred method, it can be injected through tiny access points in the second, third and fourth we space with a 1 and 2 mm cannula sliding dorsally in the superficial compartment immediately in the subcutaneous space. The correct plane of injection is above the dorsal veins, nevertheless it is advisable to aspirate before injecting in a retrograde fashion to avoid fat embolism.

The linear pattern in between the metacarpal bones can be enough for mild correction, cross-linear infiltration is indicated when major resurfacing is indicated, it is important to respect the micro-tunnelling principle, excessive lipofilling may lead to involuntary dissection of the plane with confluence of all the fat with fat necrosis/resorption.

The amount of fat depends on the correction we want to achieve, usually between 15 and 25-cc of fat per hand is enough.

Lipofilling can be safely combined with superficial peeling in the same session (30% trichloroacetic acid gave good results in the authors' experience) or laser to erase age marks and dyschromia.

A light bandage may be placed after surgery for a couple of days; no special care is needed afterwards.

8. Body contouring: gluteal augmentation using fat graft

The beauty of the buttock area is a difficult subject to address since racial and aesthetic preferences plays a major role in identifying the definition of an aesthetically pleasing buttock. There are some consensuses about the characteristics of a beautiful buttock area, which includes rounded shape, smooth projecting curves, short intergluteal crease and intragluteal crease that reach mid-thigh. The waist hip ratio (WHR) plays a crucial role in determining the upper extent of buttock and thus the back-to-buttock interface. Toledo [44] mentioned this ratio as 0.6 in South Americans and 0.7 in European females. In an attempt to understand the deformities in the buttock area, Murillo [45] had divided the buttock into A-direct areas (gluteus maximus, iliac, trochanteric and ischiorectal), B-indirect areas (sacral, femoral) and C-the border line area (gluteofemoral). We like to use a simple classification based in our mind, the WHR and the end shape we want to reach. This classification represents the buttock area and influencing areas around they are eight areas as shown in **Figure 1**. Based on these descriptions and deformities, there are four shapes of buttocks (triangular, trapezoidal, round and square) as given in **Figure 2**. Mendieta [46] describes point A, B and C. The foundation of this area is the pelvic skeletal system, which eventually share in forming the overall shape of buttocks, Caldewell-Moloy [47] described skeletal pelvis into gynecoid, anthropoid, platypelloid and android. We find this classification although explains different shapes of buttock area

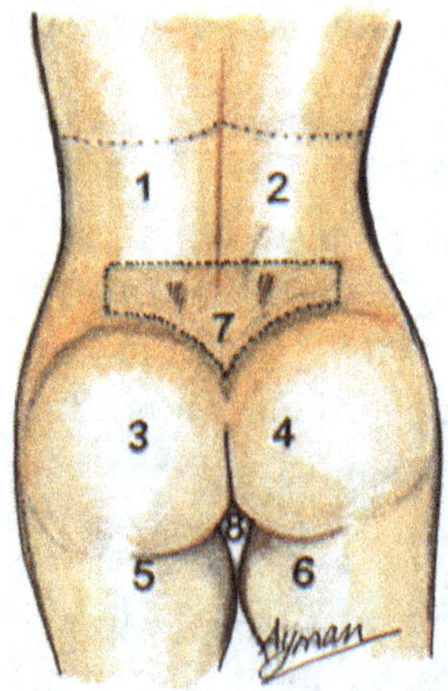

Figure 1. The buttock area and influencing areas around (1,2) bilateral symmetric waist area, (3,4) bilateral symmetric buttock area, (5,6) bilateral symmetric thighs, (7) sacral area, (8) diamond shaped area.

yet from practical point is irrelevant since there is no technique that involves bone remodelling for buttock reshaping.

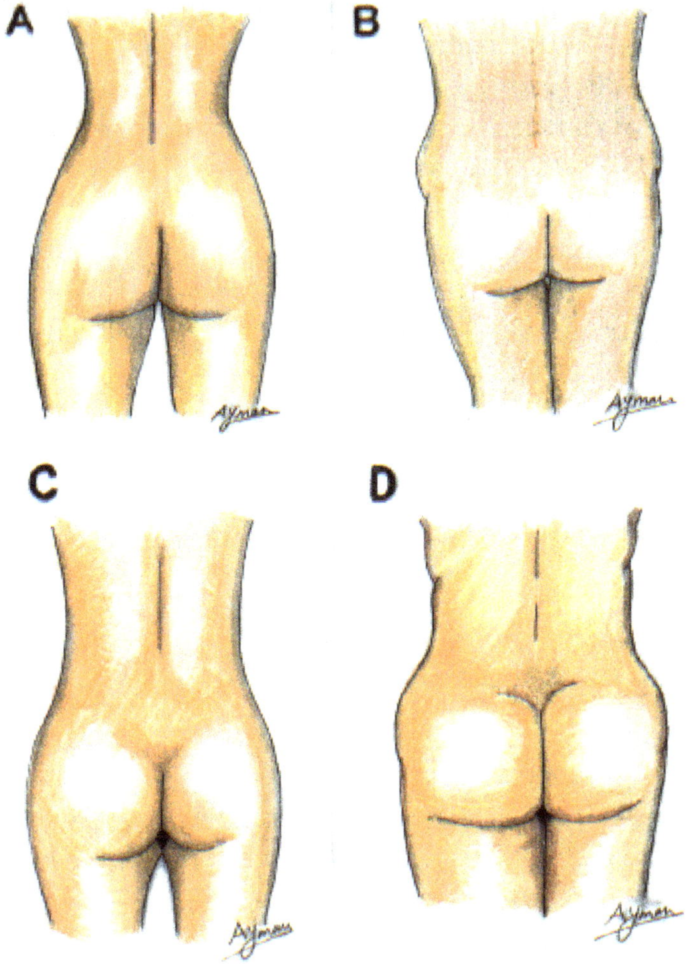

Figure 2. The four common shapes of buttocks A—triangular; B—trapezoidal; C—rounded; and D—square.

8.1. Technique tips and pitfalls

The key idea to reach the final shape of the buttock that is agreed upon with the patient is to remove and add fat in areas based on clinical analysis. The patient is instructed to shave related areas and take a shower the night before operation. Marking are done before operation while patient is standing in front of a mirror to double check the patient's will and opinion. Two colours are used in drawing areas to be injected and liposuctioned with estimate amount of fat to be added or removed on both sides. Although the choice of epidural anaesthesia is given, most patients pick up general anaesthesia. Scrubbing of patient is done after anaesthesia and towelling follows, the solution used is 500-cc Lactated Ringer's solution with adrenaline concentration (1/100000). Injection is done on a 1:1 ratio based on the amount of liposuction. The method used for liposuction is the conventional one using a 5-mm cannula and syringe .The amount depends on degree of deformity putting in mind to obtain an aesthetic WHR. The fat to be injected is decanted, usually we wait for 10 minutes and watery fluid is thrown and fat is taken to be injected .The buttock injection is done using same cannula in more than one plane avoiding intra-muscular injection. The average amount per side injected is 700cc, this is followed by gentle massage to settle injected fat and redistribute it evenly, suturing of incisions are done, the patient is encouraged to walk next day, have a shower and wear elastic garments for 4-6 weeks. A follow-up after 5 days and then every 10 days for one month to check on current condition and exclude any complications is carried out. Fat grafting in buttocks has two main issues that plastic surgeons do differ about; the first is resolution of the fat injected and longevity of the grafts injected. In our technique, we believe that intra-muscular injection can produce more complications than the postulated benefit of increase survival of fat grafts and, hence increase projection. Some authors reported the increased survival of fat when injected intra-muscular, moreover this may be lethal and carry a mortality rate as described by Czerny [48]. Lexer [6] had demonstrated using MRI scan, the survival of fat grafting in buttocks conforming role of fat grafting to increase buttock projection. The other point is the choice of buttock implant rather than fat injection, in the Ref. [7] high complications as regard to augmentation of buttocks as exposure and infection are reported. This may even necessitate removal of implant with corrective operation later on.

9. Body contouring: breast reshaping using fat graft

The word 'reshaping' is a more accurate description than 'augmentation' simply using fat grafts is one of techniques which result in ending up with an aesthetically pleasing breast and not only increasing the size of pre-existing breast. The history of breast augmentation dates back to more than a century. Many techniques were used; some worked, others did not. Substances that were used were paraffin, petroleum jelly and silicon [49]. The use of fat grafts had been used very early with a lot of changes to reach the final form we are using now. Berson [50] used dermofascial grafts with uncertain results. Complications like fat necrosis and major degree of resorption had been described by Watson [10] when injecting fat graft in the breast. Coleman [51] reported successful fat grafting in some of cases in 2007 . In 2009, the ASPS fat graft task force stated that, 'Fat grafting may be considered for breast augmentation and correction of defects associated with medical conditions and previous breast surgeries; however, results are dependent on technique and surgeon expertise' [29].

9.1. Indications

In our experience, fat grafting has been used in various scenarios of breast surgery, from aesthetic to reconstruction.

For those patients, who do not want implants, primary breast augmentation in patients suffering from small sized breast and wish for modest increase about one cup. Sequential fat injections can increase the total amount injected reaching more than a one-cup size.

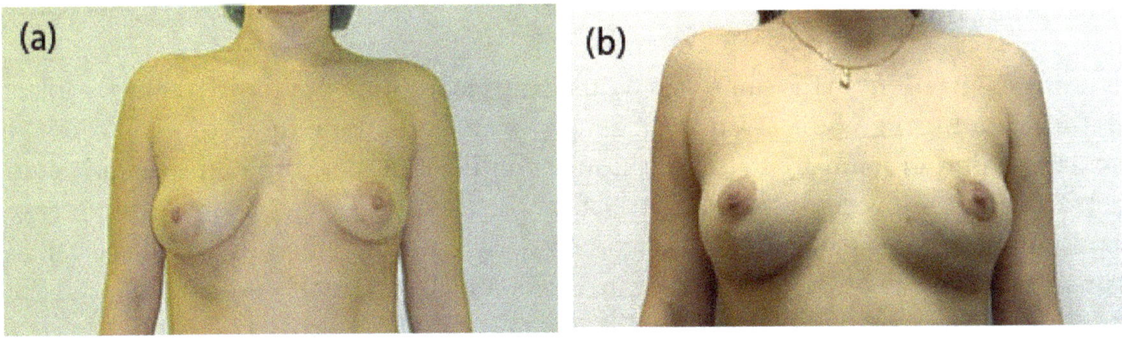

Figure 3. (a and b) Tuberous breast case treated with right mastopexy and left side lipofilling (two sessions) rigottomy and areola downsizing.

In association with silicone implants, fat injection could be used for masking apparent edges of breast implant or correction of associated wrinkles; it is an effective non-invasive procedure to correct visible rippling.

When implant explanation is required and the patient want to downsize the breast a combination of fat grafting and decreasing the pocket by sutures is usually a good choice for reaching the patient's goal.

Congenital breast deformity cases with tuberous breast where release of constricted base and fat injection would give a nice suitable breast size and shape when implant is not desired by patient or strictly necessary thanks to enough breast glandular volume (**Figure 3a** and **b**).

Breast reconstruction cases that had resultant defect after lumpectomy or skin sparing mastectomy or breast reduction asymmetry could benefit from localized fat injection to correct contour of breast or recreate the whole breast (**Figure 4a** and **b**).

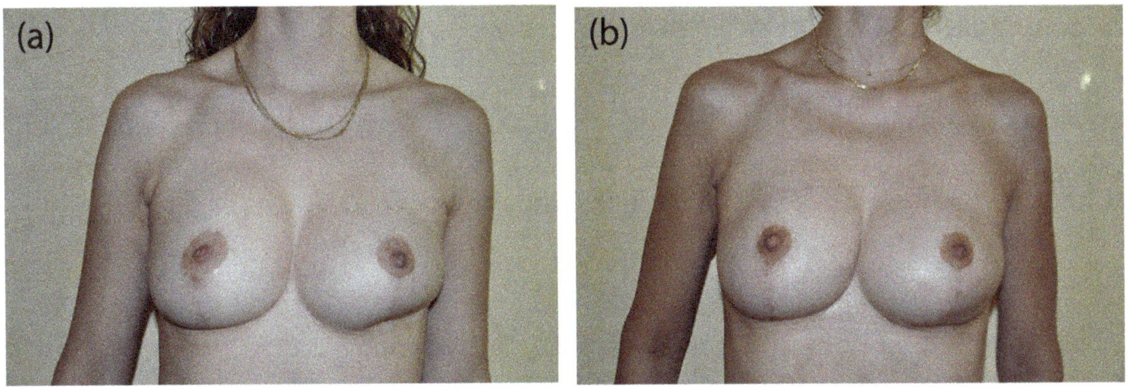

Figure 4. (a and b) Breast reshaping using fat graft after surgery complication. Two to three sessions may be needed.

Fat injection in breast had been used in combination with what is called the Brava system in cases of small breasts with very tight skin envelopes .The Brava system is an apparatus that induce external expansion to the skin to create a well-shaped cavity to be injected with fat thus forming a nice shaped breast. The apparatus is used for 3–4 weeks before surgery then breast-reshaping using fat injection is done.

9.2. Technique tips and pitfalls

Harvesting of fat is done in the same way we use in gluteal augmentation, as regard to injection, the fat is placed using blunt cannula 17 gauge, injection is done in all levels but not intra-muscular putting in mind that superficial injection plays a major role in the final shape of breast. The amount injected is about 300–400-cc per breast. In cases of depressed scars, a v-shaped cannula is used to separate skin from underlying tissue. Incisions used are usually in inframammary crease or periareolar. All incisions are closed by 4/0 prolene, padding and a well-fitting bra are used while the patient is on table. In 1895, Czerny [48] had a 1 year stable result after lipoma transfer. In 1919, Lexer [3] had described positive results after fat grafting to all area including breast. In 1995 Coleman [52] had positive predictable results with their technique. In our experience fat injection in breast is a reliable technique with the potential to increase breast volume and reach an aesthetic shape even without using the Brava system (Brava, Inc., Miami, FL, USA), this can be done by multiple procedures specially in patients needing to increase the size more than one cup. We find the Brava technique helpful in cases with severe tight skin, we also used decanting only in fat preparation with no centrifuge with optimum results .it is obvious that although there are many indication for fat grafting in breast it is mainly for ' breast reshaping', rather than augmentation on the other hand breast prosthesis are still having a more popular and reproducible results but in breast augmentation. One point, which is still controversial, is the safety of fat injection especially in the breast.

The ASPS Task Force recommendations regarding fat grafts specified the high-risk patient who carries the BRCA-1, BRCA-2 gene and if they or their families have history of breast cancer. We agree on that and follow such recommendations, but the subject especially with the introduction of fat derived stem cells should be further studied.

10. Complications of fat grafting

Fat transfer is a widely used procedure now with a wide range of indications and the surgeon being acquainted with complications and dealing with it is of utmost importance. We should remember that this procedure includes complications of liposuction as well as fat transfer. A resume of complications that can happen shortly after procedure within a week and late complications will help the reader to recognize and manage them.

Infection. Although rare nowadays, still it can be seen in some cases. The primary goal is to prevent it from happening as dealing with infected fat grafts is troublesome and usually results in deformity. This can be done by the presence of sterile operating room and instrumentation, using of prophylaxis antibiotics, proper screening of patient for HIV and hepatitis B and C.

Embolism. It may be due compression on the venous system as in calf injection with resultant thrombus formation and produce a serious complication like pulmonary thromboembolism that either resolves or result in an increased pulmonary infarction and hypertension. Accidental injection of air in subcutaneous tissue with opening of big veins like the ones present in the neck could be lethal and mimic picture of massive pulmonary embolism

Blindness. It can take place in cases where fat injection is done around the orbit either by directly injecting fat into veins or by penetrating the eye capsule with formation of thrombus and resultant in central retinal vein occlusion. This can be avoided by using blunt cannula and marking of any veins apparent, also injection while withdrawing the cannula. Not only blindness had been described but also brain insults in the form of infarction had been recorded [53].

Skin necrosis. This can happen from severe infection or over-injection with resultant oedema and too much compression, there is no definite volumes that is fixed, each individual varies from the other yet average amount injected depends on laxity of skin and under-injection is always better than over-injection as there is the chance to inject more later but it is difficult to treat skin necrosis.

Haematoma and seromas. This can happen occasionally. As regard to haematoma, this can be avoided by proper pre-operative management and evaluation stopping smoking for 4 weeks and non-steroidal medications for 1 week would protect against unwanted bleeding. The uses of blunt cannula and avoid injury of seen veins. Compression is the main line of treatment and in the case of seroma, persistence aspiration and compression is done

Nerve injury. Depending on the site, facial nerve branches may be affected in injection of face or dorsal nerves in cases of hand injection. The injury could be permanent or transient with recovery depending on degree and type of injury [54].

Absorption (excessive). The rate of absorption depends a lot on atraumatic technique used in harvesting as well as areas where fat is harvested from, like upper abdomen and upper back. The rate of absorption varies from 0–50%. Some authors had prescribed over-correction by 30% [55]. This is suitable in areas like buttocks and breast but surely not the face in our opinion.

Asymmetry. Since fat injection is done on both sides of body, for example breasts gluteal area and hands, symmetrical injection should be done unless there is asymmetrical obvious difference, sometimes a combined liposuction and fat injection to reach symmetry is done. Minimal asymmetry can be accepted, as it is not obvious except for the patient only.

Cysts and mass formation. Cysts of various sizes can occur after fat injection it is mainly oily cyst, it can occur in any site but more common with increased fat injection. Various treatments had been described triamcinolone injection [56], aspiration and compression in big cysts. Hypertrophy of part of injected fat leads to formation of localized mass or sometimes generalized hypertrophy of the whole injected area. In order to avoid this, over-injection of fat is not recommended and the proper amount and plane of injection should be done. Fat also may migrate when over-injection is done and has been reported in the forehead where authors used botulinum toxin in association with fat injection [57].

Calcifications. Calcifications in breast are the most ones that invite worries yet for an experience radiologist both the size and form are quite different. Micro-calcifications from fat necrosis are Peri-parynchymal and do not exhibit multi-density, rod-like, punctate or branching spicule [58].

Acknowledgements

Thanks to Dr. Carlos Oaxaca for contributing with clinical images of his own cases.

Author details

Marco Romeo[1*], Ayman Elmeligy[2] and Khalid Elsherbeny[2]

*Address all correspondence to: doctor@drmarcoromeo.com

1 University Autonoma of Madrid and Fundación Jimenez Diaz, Madrid, Spain

2 Department of Plastic Surgery, Ain Shams University, Cairo, Egypt

References

[1] C. S. Hultman and S. Daiza, "Skin-sparing mastectomy flap complications after breast reconstruction: review of incidence, management, and outcome," *Ann. Plast. Surg.*, vol. 50, no. 3, pp. 249–255; discussion 255, 2003.

[2] R. Gersuny, "About subcutaneous prosthesis," *Ztschr Heilk*, vol. 21, p. 199, 1900.

[3] E. Lexer, "*The free trasplants*". Enke, Stuttgart, Germany, 1919.

[4] D. A. Roncari and R. L. Van, "Promotion of human adipocyte precursor replication by 17beta-estradiol in culture," *J. Clin. Invest.*, vol. 62, no. 3, pp. 503–508, 1978.

[5] R. Ellenbogen, "Free autogenous pearl fat grafts in the face – a preliminary report of a rediscovered technique," *Ann. Plast. Surg.*, vol. 16, no. 3, pp. 179–194, 1986.

[6] A. Chajchir, I. Benzaquen, and A. Arellano, "Comparative study on lipoinjection and other methods," *Med. Cutánea Ibero-Latino-Americana*, vol. 16, no. 6, pp. 489–496, 1988.

[7] S. R. Coleman, "Facial recontouring with lipostructure," *Clin. Plast. Surg.*, vol. 24, no. 2, pp. 347–367, 1997.

[8] S. Coleman, "The technique of periorbital lipo infiltration," *Oper Tech. Plast. Reconstr. Surg.*, vol. 1, no. 2, pp. 120–126, 1994.

[9] D. A. De Ugarte, K. Morizono, A. Elbarbary, Z. Alfonso, P. A. Zuk, M. Zhu, J. L. Dragoo, P. Ashjian, B. Thomas, P. Benhaim, I. Chen, J. Fraser, and M. H.

Hedrick, "Comparison of multi-lineage cells from human adipose tissue and bone marrow," *Cells. Tissues. Organs*, vol. 174, no. 3, pp. 101–109, 2003.

[10] P. Gir, G. Oni, S. A. Brown, A. Mojallal, and R. J. Rohrich, "Human adipose stem cells: current clinical applications," *Plast. Reconstr. Surg.*, vol. 129, no. 6, pp. 1277–1290, 2012.

[11] H. Kato, K. Mineda, H. Eto, K. Doi, S. Kuno, K. Kinoshita, K. Kanayama, and K. Yoshimura, "Degeneration, regeneration, and cicatrization after fat grafting: dynamic total tissue remodelling during the first 3 months," *Plast. Reconstr. Surg.*, vol. 133, no. 3, pp. 303e–313e, 2014.

[12] D. Del Vecchio and R. J. Rohrich, "A classification of clinical fat grafting," *Plast. Reconstr. Surg.*, vol. 130, pp. 511–522, 2012.

[13] S. O. P. Hofer, K. M. Knight, J. J. Cooper-White, A. J. O'Connor, J. M. Perera, R. Romeo-Meeuw, A. J. Penington, K. R. Knight, W. A. Morrison, and A. Messina, "Increasing the volume of vascularized tissue formation in engineered constructs: an experimental study in rats," *Plast. Reconstr. Surg.*, vol. 111, no. 3, pp. 1186–1192; discussion 1193–1194, 2003.

[14] S. R. Coleman, "Hand rejuvenation with structural fat grafting," *Plast. Reconstr. Surg.*, vol. 110, no. 7, pp. 1731–1744; discussion 1745–1747, 2002.

[15] D. T. W. Leong, D. W. Hutmacher, F. T. Chew, and T. C. Lim, "Viability and adipogenic potential of human adipose tissue processed cell population obtained from pump-assisted and syringe-assisted liposuction," *J. Dermatol. Sci.*, vol. 37, no. 3, pp. 169–176, 2005.

[16] A. Gabriel, M. C. Champaneria, and G. P. Maxwell, "Fat grafting and breast reconstruction: tips for ensuring predictability," *Gland Surg.*, vol. 4, no. 3, pp. 232–243, 2015.

[17] L. L. Q. Pu, S. R. Coleman, X. Cui, R. E. H. Ferguson, and H. C. Vasconez, "Cryopreservation of autologous fat grafts harvested with the coleman technique," *Ann. Plast. Surg.*, vol. 64, no. 3, pp. 333–337, 2010.

[18] M. R. Kaufman, J. P. Bradley, et al. "Autologous fat transfer national consensus survey: trends in techniques for harvest, preparation, and application, and perception of short- and long-term results," *Plast. Reconstr. Surg.*, vol. 1, no. 119, pp. 323–331, 2007.

[19] O. Shoshani, J. Berger, L. Fodor, Y. Ramon, A. Shupak, I. Kehat, A. Gilhar, and Y. Ullmann, "The effect of lidocaine and adrenaline on the viability of injected adipose tissue – an experimental study in nude mice," *J. Drugs. Dermatol.*, vol. 4, no. 3, pp. 311–6, 2005.

[20] M. Keck, M. Zeyda, K. Gollinger, S. Burjak, L.P. Kamolz, M. Frey, and T. M. Stulnig, "Local anesthetics have a major impact on viability of preadipocytes and their

differentiation into adipocytes," *Plast. Reconstr. Surg.*, vol. 126, no. 5, pp. 1500–1505, 2010.

[21] A.C. Girard, M. Atlan, K. Bencharif, M. K. Gunasekaran, P. Delarue, O. Hulard, C. Lefebvre-d'Hellencourt, R. Roche, L. Hoareau, and F. Festy, "New insights into lidocaine and adrenaline effects on human adipose stem cells," *Aesthetic Plast. Surg.*, vol. 37, no. 1, pp. 144–152, 2013.

[22] M. Zhu, Z. Zhou, Y. Chen, R. Schreiber, J. T. Ransom, J. K. Fraser, M. H. Hedrick, K. Pinkernell, and H.C. Kuo, "Supplementation of fat grafts with adipose-derived regenerative cells improves long-term graft retention," *Ann. Plast. Surg.*, vol. 64, no. 2, pp. 222–228, 2010.

[23] K. Li, J. Gao, Z. Zhang, J. Li, P. Cha, Y. Liao, G. Wang, and F. Lu, "Selection of donor site for fat grafting and cell isolation," *Aesthetic Plast. Surg.*, vol. 37, no. 1, pp. 153–158, 2013.

[24] K. Small, M. Choi, O. Petruolo, C. Lee, and N. Karp, "Is there an ideal donor site of fat for secondary breast reconstruction?," *Aesthet. Surg. J.*, vol. 34, no. 4, pp. 545–550, 2014.

[25] J. H. Lee, J. C. Kirkham, M. C. McCormack, A. M. Nicholls, M. A. Randolph, and W. G. Austen, "The effect of pressure and shear on autologous fat grafting," *Plast. Reconstr. Surg.*, vol. 131, no. 5, pp. 1125–1136, 2013.

[26] Daniel Del Vecchio and Hetal Fichadia (2012). Autologous Fat Transplantation — A Paradigm Shift in Breast Reconstruction, *Breast Reconstruction — Current Techniques*, Prof. Marzia Salgarello (Ed.), ISBN: 978-953-307-982-0, InTech, Rijeka, Croatia

[27] M. Erdim, L. E. Teze, A. Numanoglu, and A. Sav, "The effects of the size of liposuction cannula on adipocyte survival and the optimum temperature for fat graft storage: an experimental study," *J. Plast. Reconstr. Aesthet. Surg*, vol. 62, no. 9, pp. 1210–1214, 2009.

[28] M. A. Shiffman and S. Mirrafati, "Fat transfer techniques: the effect of harvest and transfer methods on adipocyte viability and review of the literature," *Dermatolog. Surg.*, vol. 27, no. 9, pp. 819–826, 2001.

[29] K. A. Gutowski, "Current applications and safety of autologous fat grafts: a report of the ASPS fat graft task force," *Plast. Reconstr. Surg.*, vol. 124, no. 1, pp. 272–280, 2009.

[30] M. Kurita, D. Matsumoto, T. Shigeura, K. Sato, K. Gonda, K. Harii, and K. Yoshimura, "Influences of centrifugation on cells and tissues in liposuction aspirates: optimized centrifugation for lipotransfer and cell isolation," *Plast. Reconstr. Surg.*, vol. 121, no. 3, pp. 1033–1041; discussion 1042–1043, 2008.

[31] R. Khater, P. Atanassova, Y. Anastassov, P. Pellerin, and V. Martinot-Duquennoy, "Clinical and experimental study of autologous fat grafting after processing by centrifugation and serum lavage," *Aesthetic Plast. Surg.*, vol. 33, no. 1, pp. 37–43, 2009.

[32] A. Condé-Green, N. F. Gontijo De Amorim, and I. Pitanguy, "Influence of decantation, washing and centrifugation on adipocyte and mesenchymal stem cell content of

aspirated adipose tissue: a comparative study," *J. Plast. Reconstr. Aesthetic Surg.*, vol. 63, no. 8, pp. 1375–1381, 2010.

[33] S. R. Coleman, "Structural fat grafts: the ideal filler?," *Clin. Plast. Surg.*, vol. 28, no. 1, pp. 111–119, 2001.

[34] P. Tonnard, A. Verpaele, G. Peeters, M. Hamdi, M. Cornelissen, and H. Declercq, "Nanofat grafting: basic research and clinical applications," *Plast. Reconstr. Surg.*, vol. 132, no. 4, pp. 1017–1026, 2013.

[35] P. S. A. Nguyen, C. Desouches, A. M. Gay, A. Hautier, and G. Magalon, "Development of micro-injection as an innovative autologous fat graft technique: the use of adipose tissue as dermal filler," *J. Plast. Reconstr. Aesthet. Surg.*, vol. 65, no. 12, pp. 1692–1699, 2012.

[36] M. S. Choudhery, M. Badowski, A. Muise, and D. T. Harris, "Comparison of human mesenchymal stem cells derived from adipose and cord tissue," *Cytotherapy*, vol. 15, no. 3, pp. 330–343, 2013.

[37] J. M. Gimble, A. J. Katz, and B. A. Bunnell, "Adipose-derived stem cells for regenerative medicine," *Circ. Res.*, vol. 100, no. 9, pp. 1249–1260, 2007.

[38] J. A. Aronowitz and J. D. I. Ellenhorn, "Adipose stromal vascular fraction isolation: a head-to-head comparison of four commercial cell separation systems," *Plast. Reconstr. Surg.*, vol. 132, no. 6, p. 932e–939e, 2013.

[39] J. Haik, R. Talisman, J. Tamir, J. Frand, E. Gazit, J. Schibi, A. Glicksman, and A. Orenstein, "Breast augmentation with fresh-frozen homologous fat grafts," *Aesthetic Plast. Surg.*, vol. 25, no. 4, pp. 292–294.

[40] L. Hang-Fu, G. Marmolya, and D. H. Feiglin, "Liposuction fat-fillant implant for breast augmentation and reconstruction," *Aesthet. Plast. Surg.*, vol. 19, no. 5, pp. 427–437, 1995.

[41] J. Y. Petit, V. Lohsiriwat, K. B. Clough, I. Sarfati, T. Ihrai, M. Rietjens, P. Veronesi, F. Rossetto, A. Scevola, and E. Delay, "The oncologic outcome and immediate surgical complications of lipofilling in breast cancer patients: a multicenter study—Milan-Paris-Lyon experience of 646 lipofilling procedures," *Plast. Reconstr. Surg.*, vol. 128, no. 2, pp. 341–346, 2011.

[42] F. De Lorenzi, V. Lohsiriwat, and J. Y. Petit, "In response to: Rigotti G, Marchi A, Stringhini P et al. 'Determining the oncological risk of autologous lipoaspirate grafting for post-mastectomy breast reconstruction,' Aesth Plast Surg 2010; 34: 475," *Aesthetic Plast. Surg.*, vol. 35, no. 1, pp. 132–133, 2011.

[43] N. Villanueva, S. M. Hill, K. H. Small, and R. J. Rohrich, "Technical refinements in autologous hand rejuvenation," *Plast. Reconstr. Surg.*, vol. 136, no. 6, pp. 1175–1179, 2015.

[44] L. S. Toledo, "Gluteal augmentation with fat grafting the Brazilian buttock technique: 30 years' experience," *Clin. Plast. Surg.*, vol. 42, no. 2, pp. 253–261, 2015.

[45] W. L. Murillo, "Buttock augmentation: case studies of fat injection monitored by magnetic resonance imaging," *Plast. Reconstr. Surg.*, vol. 114, no. 6, pp. 1606–1614; discussion 1615–1616, 2004.

[46] C. G. Mendieta, "Classification system for gluteal evaluation," *Clin. Plast. Surg.*, vol. 33, no. 3, pp. 333–346, 2006.

[47] H. A. Caldwel and W. Moloy, "Natomical variations of female pelvis and their effect in labor with a suggested classification," *Am. J. Obs. Gynecol.*, vol. 26(4), no. 26, pp. 479–505, 1933.

[48] V. Czerny, "Plastic replacement of the mammary gland by a lipoma" *Zentralbl Chir*, vol. 27, p. 72, 1895.

[49] M. Thorek, "Plastic surgery of the breast and abdominal wall," *Plast. Surg. Breast Abdom. Wall*, vol. 120, no. 1, p. 85, 1942.

[50] M. I. Berson, "Derma-fat-fascia transplants used in building up the breasts," *Surgery*, vol. 15, no. 3, pp. 451–456, 1914.

[51] S. R. Coleman and A. P. Saboeiro, "Fat grafting to the breast revisited: safety and efficacy," *Plast. Reconstr. Surg.*, vol. 119, no. 3, pp. 775–785; discussion 786–787, 2007.

[52] S. R. Coleman, "Long-term survival of fat transplants: controlled demonstrations," *Aesthetic Plast. Surg.*, vol. 19, no. 5, pp. 421–425, 1995.

[53] O. Thaunat, F. Thaler, P. Loirat, J. P. Decroix, and A. Boulin, "Cerebral fat embolism induced by facial fat injection," *Plast. Reconstr. Surg.*, vol. 113, no. 7, pp. 2235–2236, 2004.

[54] J. I. Park, "Preoperative percutaneous facial nerve mapping," *Plast. Reconstr. Surg.*, vol. 101, no. 2, pp. 269–77, 1998.

[55] M. A. Shiffman, "History of Autologous Fat Transfer," in *Autologous Fat Transfer*, Berlin, Heidelberg: Springer, 2010, pp. 3–4.

[56] G. Johnson, "Autologous fat graft by injection: ten year experience," *Am. J. Cosmet. Surg.*, vol. 9, 61–65, 1992.

[57] E. A. Coleman, S. J. Min, A. Chomiak, and A. M. Kramer, "Posthospital care transitions: patterns, complications, and risk identification," *Health Serv. Res.*, vol. 39, no. 5, pp. 1449–1465, 2004.

[58] M. Bircoll, "Autolougus fat transplantation:an evaluation of microcalcification and fat cell survivability following (AFT) cosmetic breast augementation," *Am. J. Cosmet. Surg.*, vol. 5, pp. 283–288, 1988.

11

Pneumodissection: Enhancement of the Receptor Area before Fat Grafting

Guillermo Blugerman, Diego Schavelzon,
Gabriel Wexler, Marcelo Lotocki,
Victoria Schavelzon and Guido Blugerman

Abstract

Introduction: Fat grafts have become a frequent procedure among plastic surgeons due to their versatility for different pathologies. Different techniques have been described about graft enhancement to increase survival; in this chapter, with CO_2 pneumodissection, a technique for improving the biological conditions of the receptor area is exposed. Already known effects of carboxitherapy, such as vasodilation, enhanced Bohr effect and neoangiogenesis, are applied to increase the chance of graft survival. Tissue pneumodissection reduces the fat infiltration pain, thus reducing the sedation requirements.

Materials and methods: Carbon dioxide is infiltrated in the subcutaneous tissue with a needle before grafting procedure. The amount of CO_2 injected varies according to the recipient area. Sixty patients treated in past 15 months were included in the study. Patients were followed up every week for the first month, 3 and 6 months postoperative.

Results: Grafts survived in all 40 patients according to clinical observation and follow-up. Sedation requirements were minimal. Special interest is the use of this technique when a scar is adherent to deep planes and skin elasticity is reduced.

Keywords: fat graft, carboxitherapy, receptor area, graft survival, lipofilling, fat graft enhancement, pneumodissection

1. Introduction

The introduction of grafts and/or fillers within the subcutaneous tissue implies the creation of tunnels or planes of dissection within tissue. However, this is not without some significant degree of trauma to the dermis and hypodermis cellular structure and the fragile microcirculation and nerves found within these layers.

In addition, the struggle of the instrument against the resistance of these solid cellular tissues produces pain by transecting nerve endings or compression of the pressure sensors and/or direct distension of these fragile receptors within the skin.

Until now, the only possible solution to reduce these effects was the application of local anesthesia of different modalities, that is, blockades, infiltration or tumescent anesthesia. This implies the introduction of a set volume of liquid and chemicals, which modify the tissue composition both physically and chemically. This alteration to the biophysical composition of the host tissue and the direct limitation of surround tissue elasticity and expandability makes for a suboptimal graft host environment. The ideal environment for graft uptake includes contact with living tissue for nutrition, abundant vascularization in living tissue and consistent blood flow through this vascular net. These characteristics provide for nutrition of the graft and also remove free radicals, toxic for the grafts. We propose a new technique of pneumodissection using carbon dioxide in the gas state to expand and dissect tissue planes while preserving delicate microcirculation at the site, enhancing the host area conditions and decreasing pain to the patient.

2. Characteristics of carbon dioxide

Carbonic acid gas, is also known as carbon dioxide, carbonic anhydride and dry ice in its solid phase, is composed of one carbon atom and two oxygen atoms, with a chemical formula of CO_2.

Its properties have stamped its use as an industrial material as may be seen in fire extinguishers and welding gas. Commercially, it is added to carbonated beverages, including beer and champagne, and its solid form, known as "dry ice," has been used as a refrigerant and as an abrasive in dry ice blasting.

Within the living cell, a series of reactions in the effort to generate energy in the form of adenosine triphosphate (ATP) produces one of the main by-products of aerobic respiration, that is, carbon dioxide gas (CO_2). Within the presence of oxygen, each molecule of glucose produces 6 molecules of carbon dioxide, 6 molecules of water and up to 30 molecules of ATP. This CO_2 is then excreted through diffusion from the cells into the blood stream, whereby its binding to hemoglobin ensures its passage to the lungs for exhalation.

Due to the increased solubility of carbon dioxide over oxygen in plasma, each time blood circulates through the body, 4 vol% of carbon dioxide is removed from the tissues and delivered to the lungs to be exhaled. However, this can increase 10 times during physical exercise.

3. Uses of carbon dioxide gas in medicine

Carbon dioxide was first described in 1648 by the chemist Jan Baptist van Helmont upon observing the mass discrepancy when burning charcoal within a closed vessel. He surmised that the difference in mass of the ash to the original charcoal had been transmuted into an invisible substance, which he referred to as a "gas" or "spiritus sylvestre." Following Jan Helmont, much work was carried out on the niche properties of carbon dioxide in the 1700s and 1800s with Adrien-Jean-Pierre Thilorier in 1835, describing solid carbon "snow" CO_2.

Carbon dioxide's high purity of 99.9% and nontoxic properties makes it suitable for therapeutic use. Most commonly employed in insufflation gas for minimal invasive surgery (laparoscopy, endoscopy and arthroscopies) [1–4] in order to enlarge body cavities, protect and facilitate manipulation of intra-abdominal structures.

Possessing no hypersensitivity response, regardless of the volume used, it has been used as a contrast medium in angiography and venograms [5–7]. Its applicability as a supercritical fluid state has been marketed within the medical sterilization realm and also when temperatures of −60°C are reached its therapeutic use in cryotherapy or as local analgesia by external application onto the skin surface.

In 1964, Kumar Patel from the USA invented the CO_2 laser, which is still available and which is one of the most useful varieties of medical, surgical, industrial and military applications.

Other uses have, in the addition to pure oxygen in medical grade oxygen, to help provoke breathing and stabilize the O_2/CO_2 balance within blood.

The uses of carbon dioxide gas on the surface and in the depth of the human body have proven to be highly safe and beneficial in different areas of medicine and surgery. The history of therapeutic use of carbon dioxide gas by either percutaneous or subcutaneous injection, otherwise known as carboxitherapy, began in 1932 at a thermal waters station in the Spy of Royat, France. There, a group of cardiologists utilized CO_2 on patients with peripheral and functional artheropathies (artherosclerotics, Buerger, Raynaud) with significant success. In 1940, Jean Baptiste Romuef [8], a respected cardiologist published his 20-year experience with carboxitherapy. By the mid-1980s, over 400,000 patients had been treated at Royat providing carboxitherapy as not only an efficient therapeutic method but also a safe one.

The known therapeutic effects of CO_2, such as arterial and capillary vasodilation, enhancement of Bohr and lipolytic effect, increased sympatholytic action and with experimental work demonstrating its neoangiogenetic effect means that its use continues to expand within the realms of its therapeutic properties to medicine. There is abundant bibliography that describes the utilization of carbon dioxide gas in patients with chronic obstructive artery disease and gangrene who were treated with CO_2 injection with significantly good results [9–13].

Also acting on vascular pathologies, in 2002, Toryama et al. [14] showed an excellent improvement in the peripheral circulation in patients with critical ischemia, with a reduction of 83% of amputation cases.

For several decades, we have used the subcutaneous injection of carbon dioxide gas to improve local circulation of the skin and subcutaneous tissues, to produce detachment of fibrous tissues and to promote the formation of new collagen in the treated areas [15]. It is also used in its cryogenic state to perform procedures in cryosurgery.

4. Physiological effects

4.1. Stimulation of blood circulation

Blood circulation is locally increased with pneumodissection due to a vasodilator effect and a neoangiogenic effect. Vasodilation is produced through two main mechanisms:

- Inflammation
- Acidification

The inflammatory response to an "aggression" is immediate. It physically acts to destroy, dilute or block the offending agent, but, in turn, this triggers a series of events at the vascularized connective tissue level, including plasma, in cells circulating in the blood vessels and in the extravascular components of connective tissue, with the objective to heal and rebuild the damaged tissue. Acute phase inflammatory mediators, such as histamine, bradykinins and prostaglandins, produce vasodilation to increase to the local blood flow in order to deliver white blood cells to the insulted area. Changes in microcirculation occur, increasing the vascular permeability to cells and proteins.

Histological aspects in the repair process demonstrated the proliferation of small newly formed blood vessels and fibroblasts [16].

Inside the body, carbon dioxide reacts with water producing carbonic acid. This reaction acidifies the local medium where $CO_2$is injected. The local increase of H+ stimulates vasodilation. In this way, carbon dioxide directly in microcirculation of the vascular connective tissue, promoting vasodilation [17, 18] and an increase in the venous and lymphatic drainage. According to researchers, this can be a reflection of the increase in parasympathetic activity by the decrease in sympathetic activity in these tissues. In addition to that, the persistence of clinical improvement or "temporary cure" of the blood vessel conditions can be explained by the neoangiogenesis [19], due to the formation of angiogenic factors, and vascular endothelial growth and fibroblast growth triggered by hypercapnia tissue.

With carboxitherapy, through the infusion of CO_2, it is demonstrated that a persistent vasodilation is identified during assisted laparoscopy, which leads to a significant rise in the concentration of oxygen (O_2) in the local body cavity. Studies with Doppler flow monometry have demonstrated the action of the carboxitherapy in improving blood flow locally.

4.2. Bohr effect

The affinity of hemoglobin for oxygen depends on the pH of the medium; the acidity stimulates the release of oxygen thus reducing this affinity. In addition to the acidity, the increase in the concentration of carbon dioxide (CO_2) as described in the oxygen-hemoglobin dissociation curve also lowers the oxygen affinity. The presence of higher levels of CO_2 and protons (H+) in the capillaries of tissues in active metabolism promotes the release of O_2 of hemoglobin, the reciprocal effect occurs in the capillaries of the alveoli of the lungs and the high concentration of O_2 releases CO_2 and H+ of the hemoglobin. This relationship is known as Bohr effect [20, 21].

There is a consensus among authors about the existence of a significant increase in the concentration of oxygen (O_2) locally after subcutaneous infusion of CO_2 demonstrating an increase in the partial pressure of O_2. These authors [22, 23] have reported that a decrease in affinity of hemoglobin for oxygen in the presence of carbon dioxide gas leading to more oxygen delivery to the cells, which would boost the metabolism of tissues in the region being treated (potentiation of the Bohr effect).

4.3. Role of CO_2 in connective tissue

Carboxitherapy produces a "mechanical trauma" post the insertion of the insufflation cannula and the direct trauma of the CO_2 gas insufflating between tissue planes and creating a form of pneumodissection. This pneumodissection produces an inflammatory process and the consequent migration of fibroblasts to the region of insufflation, leading to the subsequent proliferation of fibroblasts and therefore the synthesis of collagen and activation of other extracellular matrix proteins such as fibronectin and glycoprotein, which are essential in the biological processes such as adhesion and cell differentiation, tissue repair, serving as a substrate for fibrinolytic enzymes and clotting.

Histological studies of the tissues treated with carboxitherapy have found an increase in the thickness of the dermis, as evidenced by the increased stimulus of neocollagenases. There is total preservation of the connective tissue layers, including its vascular and neurovascular structures as evident within these collagen fibers.

5. Carbon dioxide gas as pneumodissector of tissues—carboxitherapy

Insufflating gases within tissue is not an innovative idea in current medicine. Ivån Goni Moreno, an Argentinean surgeon from the early 1900s, is credited with his operation of introducing progressive preoperative pneumoperitoneum for the repair of large hernias in 1940. Moreno progressively placed large amounts of room air preoperatively into the peritoneal cavity over a period of weeks. With this technique, the patient became adjusted to an increased intra-abdominal pressure and tolerated the sudden reduction of the viscera during the repair, free from respiratory distress.

Currently, with the widespread of laparoscopic procedures, insufflation with carbon dioxide is widespread in all therapeutic and diagnostic laparoscopy as utilized in general, gynecological and urological surgeries.

Due to carbon dioxide's high degree of diffusion, this gas is rapidly absorbed and eliminated, leaving only the vasodilator effect (pneumodissection) in the tissues, without the increased risk of fatal air embolism.

Subcutaneous infiltration of CO_2 began to be used for aesthetic purposes in the 1970s in France, with the object of treating cellulite and localized areas of adiposities in the subcutaneous tissue. More recent work of Brandi et al. [24, 25] showed measurable reductions in maximum circumference of abdomen, thigh and knee regions with the transcutaneous administration of CO_2 and improved skin irregularity after repeated sessions of carboxitherapy.

6. Theory behind the use of carboxitherapy for pneumodissection during fat grafting

The ideal conditions for adipose (fat) grafting within tissue includes (1) ease of dissection of tissue planes with the advancement of the infiltrating cannula, (2) the ability to layer this fat by placing minimal amounts of adipocytes in multiple tunnels in order to maximize contact with the surrounding tissues therefore increasing the grafts survival rate, (3) good vascularization and oxygenation of tissue recipient site, (4) minimal trauma to reduce the risk of bruising, (5) the absence of vasoconstriction, (6) the absence of toxic chemicals in the recipient tissue and (7) good elasticity of the adjacent tissues to comply with the additional volume. The use of carbon dioxide gas as a pneumodissector of the tissue planes may be the one way to achieve these ideal conditions in the host tissue.

The resistance of the tissues to the advancement of a needle or cannula is predetermined by the density of cell structures and fibrosis of the tissue area on the body. Some of the causes of pain during the introduction of fluids and grafts into tissues are due to the compression of pressure receptors (baroreceptors) and also by the stretching of the nerve endings by direct mechanical pressure from the advancing cannula or needle. Also, the pH of the solutions being injected produces pain and burning. The slow insufflation of the carbon dioxide in its gaseous state by percutaneous injection produces tissue plane dissection, which subsequently decreases the tissues' overall resistance while increasing its three-dimensional space, yet preserving the neurovascular characteristics of that tissue by pneumodissecting these structures away with the advancement of the needle/cannula and therefore decreasing the possibility of direct pain.

7. Clinical experience

The pneumodissection flow and the total volume of gas infiltrated subcutaneously are controlled with CARBOTECH F650 from Axt Medical Systems®, with complete control over the speed and volume of CO_2 gas infiltrated (**Figure 1**).

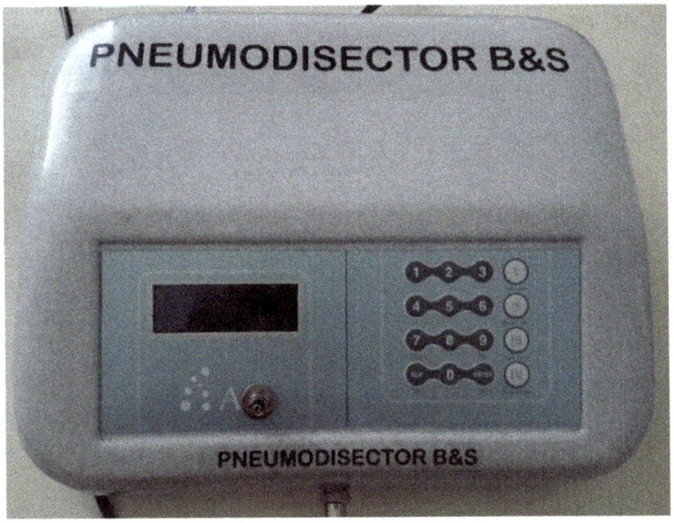

Figure 1. Pneumodissector console.

The pneumodissector console is connected to the pure carbon dioxide gas tank. The CO_2 is injected under the control of the surgeon for speed of flow, time of injection and overall administered dose through a disposable tube with 25G needle attached through luer-lock. This needle is then inserted directly under the skin of the patient within the designated site.

The flow of CO_2 through the pneumodissector is fixed at 80 ml per minute. Insufflation between 100 and 1000 ml per area depending on the procedure to be carried out and the site on the body to be performed is undertaken. CO_2 easily distributes to all of the injected area and its surrounding tissue (**Figure 2**).

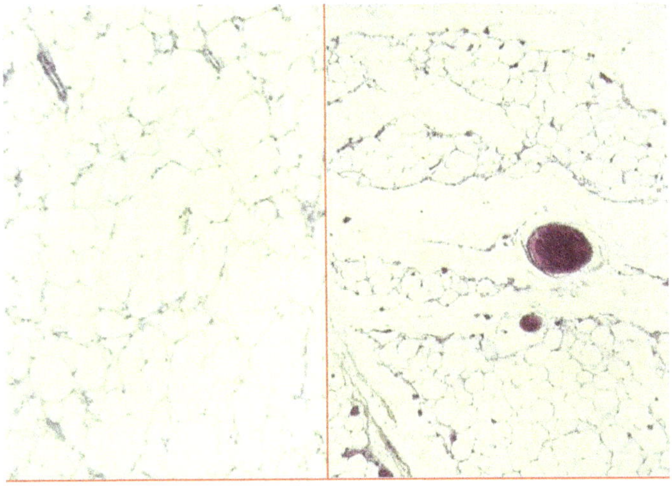

Figure 2. Histology of pneumodissected tissue (hematoxylin-eosin). Left, Normal subcutaneous tissue. Right, Subcutaneous tissue after pneumodissection, note the air spaces between septums and vessels.

During the past 12 months, we have used the pneumodissection technique intraoperatively prior to the grafting of adipocytes at various quantities in 60 patients (**Table 1**).

Area	Amount injected (cc)	Volume of CO_2 infused (cc)
Breast	210	333
Breast	600	707
Breast	560	765
Buttocks	400	580
Buttocks	700	765
Buttocks	800	1000
Buttocks	480	580
Buttocks	550	595
Buttocks	840	843
Buttocks	780	865
Buttocks	440	564
Buttocks	620	789
Buttocks	680	721
Arms	240	469
Arms	225	342
Facial	26	45
Facial	54	89
Facial	32	48
Facial	38	74
Facial	49	107
Buttocks	200	378
Buttocks	680	731
Buttocks	250	379
Buttocks	540	763
Buttocks	780	893
Buttocks	300	389
Breast	150	333
Breast	400	586
Breast	520	555
Breast	460	632
Breast	380	509
Hand	40	100
Hand	50	104
Hand	40	132
Genitalia	30	105
Abdomen	12	40
Abdomen	20	57
Abdomen	10	58
Thigh	180	287
Calf	110	215
Breast	250	380
Breast	550	647
Breast	610	805
Buttocks	450	640
Buttocks	650	700
Buttocks	840	999

Area	Amount injected (cc)	Volume of CO_2 infused (cc)
Buttocks	430	520
Buttocks	600	700
Buttocks	780	900
Buttocks	700	800
Buttocks	445	507
Buttocks	635	885
Buttocks	600	651
Arms	200	461
Arms	221	302
Facial	22	41
Facial	55	91
Facial	30	44
Facial	34	70
Facial	45	101

Table 1. Patients table. Details of volume of fat grafted and CO_2 infused.

Areas of both the body (abdomen, buttocks, arms, breast, and legs) and face have been successfully pneumodissected prior to fat grafting with clinically superior results compared to commonly used hydrodissection technique (**Figures 3–11**).

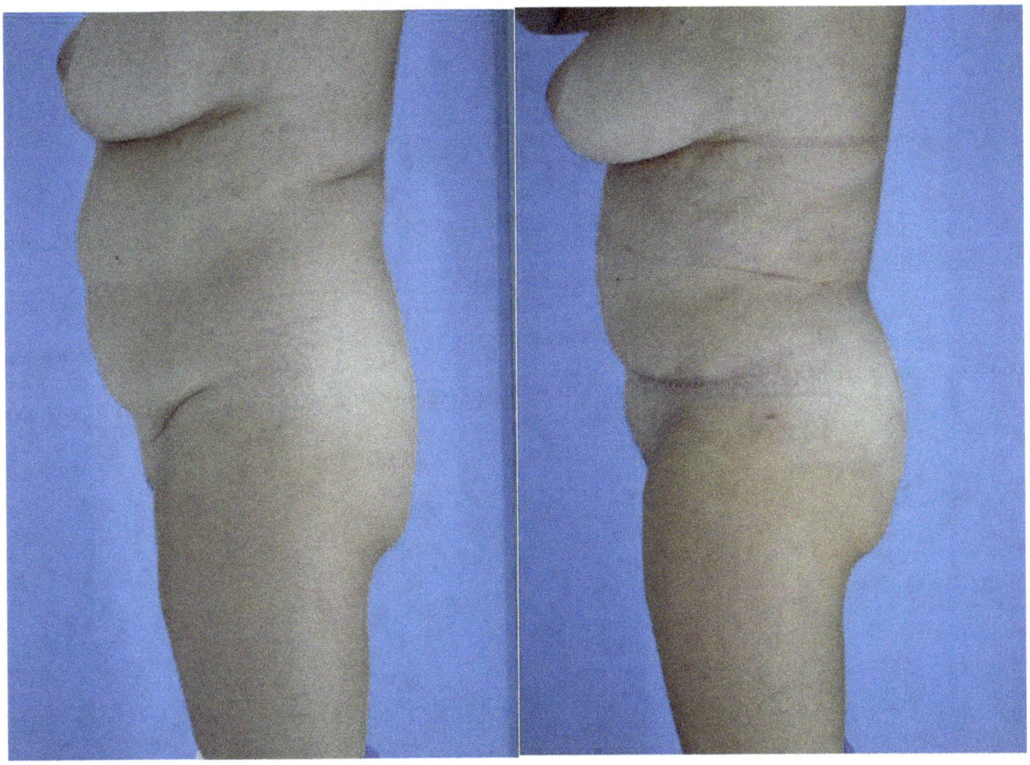

Figure 3. Patient with abdominal flaccidity, lipodystrophy and gluteal hypoplasia. Preoperative (left) and 3 months postoperative of TULUA, liposuction and pneumodissection-assisted fat grafting to gluteal area in the subcutaneous plane (right).

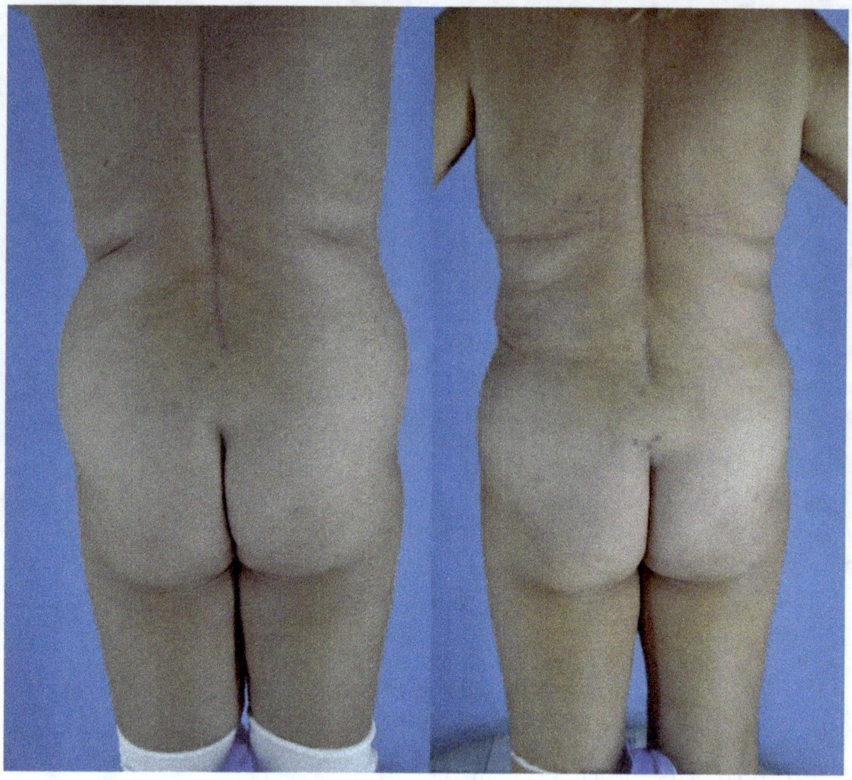

Figure 4. Patient with abdominal flaccidity, lipodystrophy and gluteal hypoplasia. Preoperative (left) and 3 months postoperative of TULUA, liposuction and pneumodissection-assisted fat grafting to gluteal area in the subcutaneous plane (right).

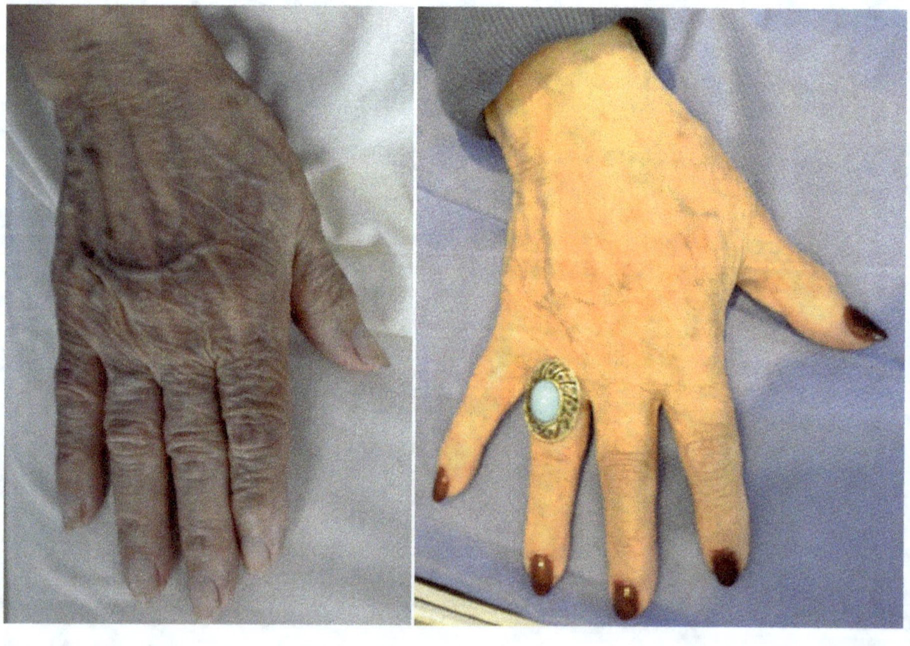

Figure 5. Patient with hand aging. Note skin quality, flaccidity and prominence of vascular network (left). Three months postoperative of pneumodissection-assisted fat grafting in hands in the subcutaneous plane (right).

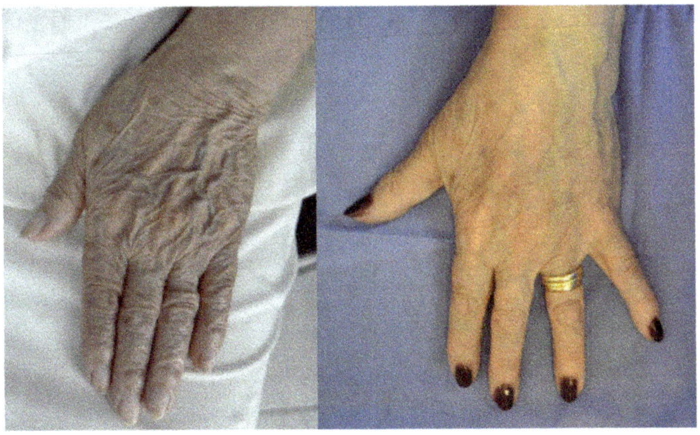

Figure 6. Patient with hand aging. Note skin quality, flaccidity and prominence of vascular network (left). Three months postoperative of pneumodissection-assisted fat grafting in hands in the subcutaneous plane (right).

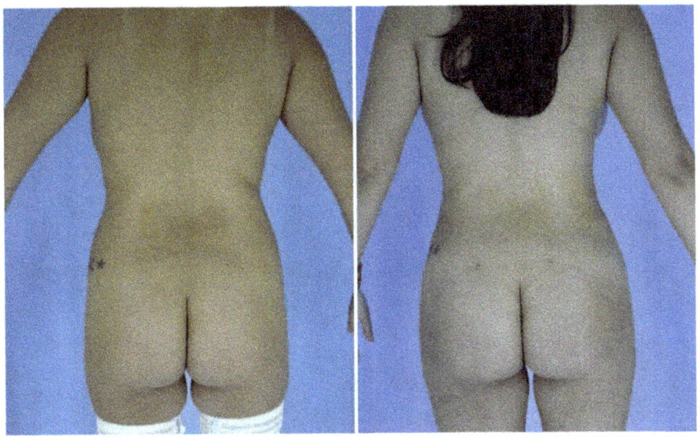

Figure 7. Patient with gluteal hypoplasia (left). After 3 months of pneumodissection-assisted fat grafting in the gluteal area in the subcutaneous plane (right).

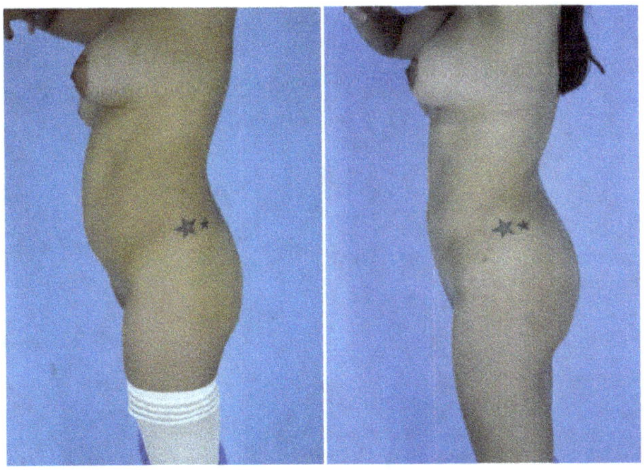

Figure 8. Patient with gluteal hypoplasia (left). After 3 months of pneumodissection-assisted fat grafting in the gluteal area in the subcutaneous plane (right).

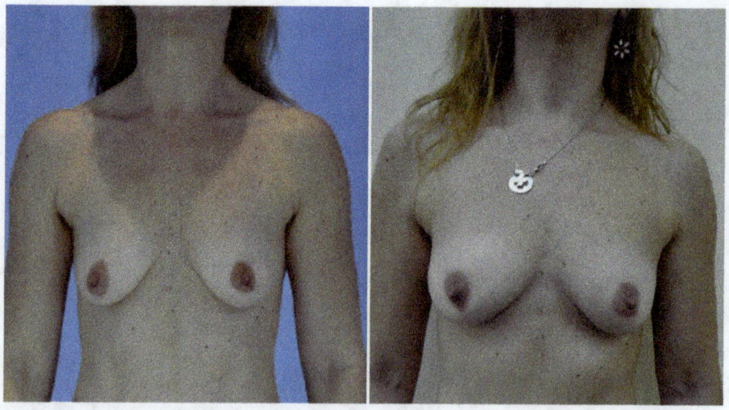

Figure 9. Patient with breast hypoplasia (left). After 3 months of pneumodissection-assisted fat grafting in breasts in the subcutaneous plane (right).

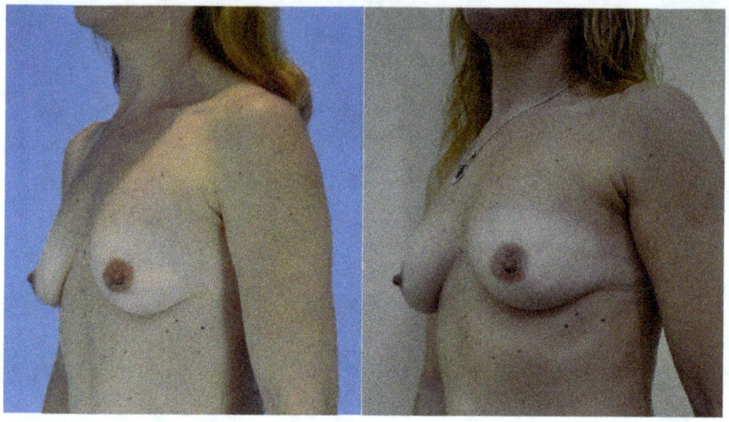

Figure 10. Patient with breast hypoplasia (left). After 3 months of pneumodissection-assisted fat grafting in breasts in the subcutaneous plane (right).

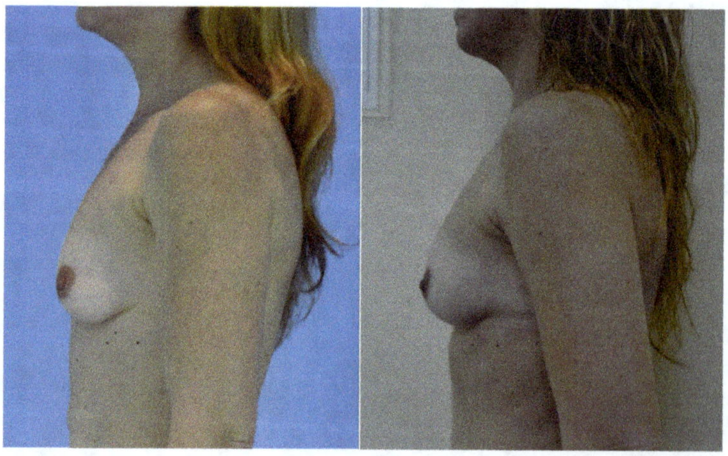

Figure 11. Patient with breast hypoplasia (left). After 3 months of pneumodissection-assisted fat grafting in breasts in the subcutaneous plane (right).

Upon pneumodissection of the tissue planes, the subsequent ease with which the introduction and advancement of the infiltrating cannula allows for ease of larger amounts of grafting tissue (adipocytes) with greater uniformity to be placed, less resistance from normal tissue planes and decrease in both intra- and postoperative discomfort to the patient. There was less bruising of the skin noted within the postoperative period.

8. Complications and adverse events of carboxitherapy

As already mentioned, carbon dioxide gas is a versatile gas utilized within many industries. It is a by-product present in the blood circulation as a consequence of aerobic respiration. Based on current literature, carboxitherapy can be considered as a safe therapeutic treatment, without adverse effects or major complications, both local and systemic.

The amount of gas injected during a therapeutic dose of carboxitherapy is below the volume produced by the body itself. Our body produces 200 cc of CO_2 when at rest and during vigorous exercise this amount may rise to 10 times that value. In addition, the patients in our study subjected to subcutaneous injections of CO_2 show no damage to the connective tissue or its microcirculation.

Therefore, we know that CO_2 works in the affected area and is rapidly eliminated from the body with no possibility of air embolus. However, in our study, minimal complications were noted with the administration of subcutaneous CO_2 therapy. These included and were limited to (1) local pain at the injection site of the 25G needle, (2) small bruising and ecchymosis from the needle entering the dermis, (3) A "cracking sensation" experienced by patients due to the formation of local emphysema that disappears within 30 minutes of the procedure.

9. Contraindications to carboxitherapy

Contraindications to the treatment include acute myocardial infarction, unstable angina, heart failure, hypertension, acute thrombophlebitis, gangrene or localized infections at the site therapy, epilepsy, respiratory failure, renal failure, pregnancy and psychiatric disorder. But in any case, these patients would not be candidates for an elective body contouring surgery. So, in healthy patients with usual comorbidities, there are no contraindications.

10. Conclusion

Carbon dioxide is an abundant gas found in every living species on Earth. Its role in many industries, including medicine, have stemmed from its early discovery in 1648. With respect to its effect on both the skin and subdermal layers, CO_2 has sound physiological principles confirmed through histological studies.

Our technique of pneumodissection prior to adipocyte grafting has worked with these principles in mind. Using CO_2 to establish volume within given tissue planes yet preserving the fragile microcirculation of the tissue is a valuable prerequisite to the survival of the graft.

Author details

Guillermo Blugerman[1*], Diego Schavelzon[1], Gabriel Wexler[2], Marcelo Lotocki[3], Victoria Schavelzon[1] and Guido Blugerman[1]

*Address all correspondence to: drblugerman@gmail.com

1 Centro ByS, Buenos Aires, Argentina

2 Estetica Wexler, Cordoba, Argentina

3 Genesis, Obera, Misiones, Argentina

References

[1] McMahon, AJ, Baxter, JN, Murray, W, Imrie, CW, Kenny, G, O'Dwyer, PJ. Helium pneumoperitoneum for laparoscopic cholecystectomy: ventilatory and blood gás changes. Br J Surg 1994; 81: 1033-1036.

[2] Wolf, JS Jr, Carrier, S, Stoller, ML. Gas embolism: helium is more lethal than carbon dioxide. J Laparoendosc Surg 1994; 4: 173-177.

[3] Yau, P, Watson, DI, Lafullarde, T, Jamilson, GG. An experimental study of the effect of gas embolism using different laparoscopy insufflation gases. J Laparoendosc Adv Surg Tech 2000; 10: 211-216.

[4] Vilos, GA, Vilos, AG. Safe laparoscopic entry guided by Veress needle CO_2 insufflation pressure. J Am Assoc Gynecol Laparosc, 2003 Aug; 10(3): 415-420.

[5] Zwaan W, Kloess W, Kagel C, Kummer-Kloess DR, Matthies-Zwaan S, Schutz RM, Weiss HD. Carbon dioxide as an alternative contrast medium in peripheral angiography, Rofo Fortschr Geb Rontgenstr Neuen Bildgeb Verfahr. 1996; 165(2): 180.

[6] Roberts, MW, Mathiesen, KA, Ho, HS, Wolfe, BM. Cardiopulmonary responses to intravenous infusion of soluble and relatively insoluble gases. Surg Endosc 1997; 11: 341-346.

[7] Lang EV, Gossler AA, Fick LJ, Barnhart W, Lacey DL. Carbon dioxide angiography: effect of injection parameters on bolus configuration. J Vasc Interv Radiol. 1999 Jan; 10(1): 41-49.

[8] Romeuf, JB. Study of subcutaneous injections of thermal gas from Royat. Clermont Ferrand, Imp Moderne, 15 rue du Port 31, Mars 1940.

[9] Ambrosi C, Delanoe G. Therapeutic effect of CO_2 injected subcutaneously in arteriopathies of the limbs. Experimental research (author's transl). Ann Cardiol Angeiol (Paris). 1976; 25(2): 93-98.

[10] Fabry R, Dubost JJ, Schmidt J, Body J, Schaff G, Baguet JC. Thermal treatment in arterial diseases: an expensive placebo or an effective therapy? Therapie. 1995; 50(2): 113-122.

[11] Savin, E, Bailliart, O, Bonnin, P, Bedu, M, Cheynel, J, Coudert, J, Martineaud, JP. Vasomotor effects of transcutaneous CO_2 in stage II peripheral occlusive arterial disease. Angiology 1995; 46(9): 785-791.

[12] Hartman, B, Bassenge, E, Hartman, M. Effects of serial percutaneous application of carbon dioxide in intermittent claudication: results of a controlled trial. Angiology. 1997, 48(11): 957-963.

[13] Castex M, Di Cio A, Lista GA. Plantar ulcer with arterial calcification: results of treatments with carbogen. Revista de la Asociacion Medica Argentina, 30 de diciembre de 1934.

[14] Toryama T, Kumada Y, Matsubara T, Murata A, Ogino A, Hayash H, Nakashima H, Takahashi H, Matsuo H, Kawahara H. Effect of artificial carbon dioxide foot bathing on critical limb ischemia (Fontaine IV) in peripheral arterial disease patients. Int Angiol. 2002; 21(4): 367-373.

[15] Ferreira, JCT, Haddad, MD, Tavares, SAN. Increase in collagen turnover induced by intradermal injection of carbon dioxide in rats. J Drugs Dermatol. 2008;7(3): 201–6.

[16] Colin, C, Lagneaux, D, Lecomte, J. Local vasodilating effects of carbon dioxide on cutaneous blood vessels. J Belge Med Phys Rehabil, 1978; 1(4): 326-334.

[17] Ito, T, Moore, J, Koss, M, Topical application of CO_2 increases skin blood flow. J Invest Dermatol. 1989; 93(2): 259-262.

[18] Schnizer, W, Erdl, R, Schops, P, Seichert, N. The effects of external CO_2 application on human skin microcirculation investigate by laser Doppler flowmetry. In J Microcirc Clin Exp, 1995, 4(4): 343-350.

[19] Hidekazul I, Tatsumi T, Takamiya M, Zen K, Takahashi T, Azuma A, Tateishi K, Nomura T, Hayashi H, Nakajima N, Okigaki M, Matsubara T. Carbon dioxide-rich water bathing enchances collateral blood flow in ischemia limb vía mobilization of endothelial progenitor cells and activation of NO-cGMP system. Circulation 29, 2005; 1523-1529.

[20] Guyton et al. Textbook of Medica Physiology, Rio de Janeiro, Guanabara Koogan, 2002.

[21] Houssay, BA. Human Physiology 5 ed. Rio de Janeiro. Guanabara Koogan, 1984, p. 346-349.

[22] Hartman, BR, Bassenge, E, Pittler, M. Effect of carbon dioxide – enriched water and fresh water on the cutaneous microcirculation and oxygen tension in the skin of the foot. Angiology, 1997; 48(4): 337-343.

[23] Hartmann, B, Drews, B, Burnus, C, Bassenge, E. Increase in skin blood circulation and transcutaneous oxygen partial pressure of the top of the foot in lower leg immersion in water containing carbon dioxide in patients with arterial occlusive disease. Results of a controlled study compared with fresh water. Vasa 1991; 20(4): 382-387.

[24] Brandi, C, D'Aniello, C, Grimaldi, L, Bosi, B, Dei, I, Lattarulo, P, Alessandrini, C. Carbon dioxide therapy in the treatment of localized adiposities: clinical study and histopathological correlations, Aesthetic Plast Surg. 2001; 25(3): 170-174.

[25] Brandi, CD, Aniello, C, Grimaldi, L, Caiazzo, E, Stanghellini, E. Carbon dioxide therapy: Effects on skin irregularity and its use as a complement to liposuction. Aesth Plast Surg. 2004; 28(4): 222–5.

12

Laser-Assisted Liposuction in Body Contouring

Zoran Žgaljardić and Ivonne Žgaljardić

Abstract

Laser liposuction was initially developed as a technique for laser lipolysis. In 1992, Apfelberg was the first to describe the direct action of laser in the adipose tissue. Initially, the technique was developed only for lipolysis of unwanted fat in a small region without suction of dissolved fat. Later, it evolved as laser-assisted liposuction, which is a technique that combines adipocyte disruption with laser beam and suction of the dissolved fat from the treated area with different types of cannulas. The neodymium-doped yttrium aluminum garnet (Nd:YAG) 1064 nm has been introduced as first laser for lipolysis. Blugerman, Schavelzon, and Goldman introduced the concept of the pulsed 1064-nm Nd:YAG system for laser lipolysis. They proved the effect of the laser energy on fatty tissue as well as the on surrounding tissues (dermis, vasculature, apocrine, and eccrine gland). After tissue damage with photo-optical thermal energy, the following histological changes have been noted: (1) adipocyte cells have been disrupted, (2) blood vessels have been coagulated, (3) new collagen has been induced. All those histological changes induce better clinical outcome such as less ecchymosis, less bleeding, smoother, and firmer skin as result of new collagen formation followed by skin retraction. Laser liposuction was developed as a minimally invasive liposuction technique, where energy breaks adipocytes (comparing with traditional liposuction, in which disruption is manual). Wave length of 1064 nm has hemoglobin as a target for its photo-optical energy, and new wave length of 1470 nm has water molecules (H_2O) as a target. Infiltration of the Klein's solution helps laser to dissolving of fatty tissue faster and more energy to accumulate, followed by new collagen formation. Laser-assisted liposuction in all types of lipodystrophies and cellulite can be successfully applied. High definition of the body is a result of the energy as well as the technique of liposuction. Laser liposuction can be applied on the face for fat removal and as a part of face lifting or better to say endolight lifting. Today, we have lot of companies that have developed different liposuction lasers (Nd:YAG; diode) with different wave lengths.

Keywords: laser, liposuction, lipolysis, skin tightening, high-definition

1. Introduction

According to the statistics of the American Society for Aesthetic Plastic Surgery (ASAPS) for 2014, liposuction has been most commonly performed cosmetic surgical procedure [1]. The technique of fat removal using a curette subcutaneously connected to a suction device was created in the 1970 and 1980. Various surgeons concurrently were performing the similar method, but the Italian gynecologist Giorgio Fischer in 1974 presented a prototype machine [2, 3]. Illouz introduced the liposuction technique in 1982 at the Annual Meeting of the American Society of Plastic and Reconstructive Surgeons [4]. Since then, there have been various attempts in improving this technique. With the progress of technology, various methods have been described in addition to traditional suction-assisted liposuction in order to improve the final cosmetic result and diminish complications.

In this chapter, we describe the use of laser energy in traditional suction-assisted liposuction and body contouring.

2. Laser

A laser is a device that emits light through a process of optical amplification based on the stimulated emission of electromagnetic radiation. The term "laser" originated as an acronym for "light amplification by stimulated emission of radiation" [5, 6]. Theodore H. Maiman in 1960 produced the first laser using ruby as a medium that was stimulated using high energy flashes of intense light. Laser light is monochromatic, bright, unidirectional, and coherent [7].

3. Laser-assisted liposuction—history overview

Dr. Leon Goldman is called the father of laser medicine. He was the first to introduce lasers in medicine shortly after the first laser was invented. In 1963, he published first scientific article on the pathology of the effect of the laser beam on the skin [8]. Hukki et al. were first to describe the tissue effects of different Nd:YAG contact laser scalpels on pig skin and subcutaneous fat in 1988 [9]. Dressel was first to perform laser lipolysis procedure in 1990 on a 34-year-old man with abdominal adiposity [10]. Formally, laser-assisted liposuction was first introduced by Apfelberg in 1992 when he described direct action of laser in the fat tissue [11]. In 1994, Apfelberg et al. performed FDA-approved study on fifty-one patients in five plastic surgery centers. Nd: YAG (neodymium-doped yttrium aluminum garnet) laser was used. The 600 μm fiber was enclosed in 4 or 6 mm cannula. The energy used was 40 W. Pulse duration was 0.2 s. The laser fiber was not in direct contact with the tissue [12]. The study showed slight benefit for ecchymosis, pain and discomfort, and edema, but it was not enough for the FDA to approve the technology so in that time, it was abandoned and the development of the technology transferred to South America and Europe.

The current principles for the use of laser energy in laser lipolysis/liposuction were founded by Blugerman, Schavelzon, and Goldman in the early 2000. They were first to describe the effects of laser on adipose tissue and surrounding structures—dermis, vasculature, and interstitial tissue [13–16]. Badin et al. also reported their findings in 2002. They found laser lipolysis to be superior to the conventional suction-assisted liposuction in terms of reduced bleeding, disrupted adipose cell membranes, and introduction of new collagen. Its histological findings correlated with their clinical observation—less ecchymoses, decrease in local adiposity and skin tightening (badin-flaccidity under control) [17].

On 31 October of 2006 FDA-approved a 1064 nm Nd: YAG laser (smartLipo, Cynosure) for the surgical excision, vaporization, ablation, and coagulation of soft tissues. That caused the market to explode and various companies introduced their laser lipolysis machines with various wavelengths as well as the laser source. That also enabled new studies to be performed, and it was followed with a number of articles that advocated the benefits of laser-assisted liposuction.

Around the same time of the FDA approval, laser lipolysis was also approved in Japan where Ichikawa et al. were first to demonstrate the histologic and photonic relationship of energy absorption and lipolysis using a pulsed Nd:YAG laser. Scanning electron microscopy after irradiation showed greater destruction of human adipocytes than in the control. Degenerated cell membrane, vaporization, liquefaction, carbonization, and heat coagulated collagen fibers were observed [18]. In 2005, Badin demonstrated that laser-assisted liposuction produces more major irreversible damage on the adipose cells with less bleeding that the traditional suction-assisted liposuction [19]. In 2007, Mordon et al. represented mathematical model of laser lipolysis. The importance of that article was actually in their conclusion that heat rather than particular wavelength leads to lipolysis and skin tightening. They concluded that the temperature of 48–50°C inside the lower dermis is sufficient to induce skin tightening, which corresponds to external temperature of 38–41°C [20]. Finally, in 2008, McBean and Katz were first to evaluate the skin tightening effect by photographic documentation and measurement. Subjects had 4 × 4 cm temporary India ink tattoos placed at the treatment site and measurements showed 18% decrease in surface area. They also performed histological evaluation that indicated new collagen and myofibroblast compared to the baseline [21]. Until today, various studies have been performed and articles have been published regarding superiority of laser-assisted liposuction but also complications have been described. Therefore, it should be remembered that laser is just a tool in a surgeon's hand and care must be taken to use the maximum from the energy tool but also not to endanger patient's safety.

4. Mechanism of action

Basic mechanism of action in laser lipolysis is photothermal [20, 22]. Targeted tissue absorbs laser energy and converts it into heat. During laser lipolysis and constant moving of the laser beam, two parallel processes occur: absorption and scattering. Absorption occurs momentarily and, in biological tissue, is mainly caused by water molecules, proteins, and pigments.

Absorbed laser light energy converts into heat, thus producing desired thermal damage. The heat acts on adipose cells and the extracellular matrix to produce both reversible and irreversible cellular damage. For low-energy settings, heat generated by the laser alters the balance of sodium and potassium of the cellular membrane, allowing the free transport of extracellular liquid to intracellular space. For higher energy, settings rupture of adipose cells, coagulation of collagen fibers, and small vessels are observed. Cell lipases are liberated in the surrounding area, thus liquefacting the tissue [23–25].

At the same time, scattering occurs. Scattered parts of the laser beam are refracted and finally also absorbed. This effect broadens the final volume of tissue where the absorption and thermal damage finally occur.

In human skin and subcutaneous adipose tissue, scattering predominates over direct absorption for the wavelengths between 450 and 1800 nm [24]. When there is higher absorption, scattering is mitigated, which results in low thermal effect. Considering all of the above, the optimal choice of wavelength for laser lipolysis is one that is scattered as well as absorbed in tissue. As the wavelength increases, the absorption increases also and scattering decreases.

The photothermal process of fat cell disruption occurs with the tissue heated on 50–65°C. Lower temperatures do not result in destruction of adipocytes. Higher temperatures are not advisable due to complications—tissue necrosis and scarring [23, 26]. To achieve skin tightening, temperatures of 48–50°C must be reached within the dermis to induce collagen contraction. Collagen injury from thermal damage promotes collagen remodeling, leading to increases in skin tone and texture. Whenever a controlled, reversible thermal injury is created, the body's response is to release mediators responsible for the healing process. In turn, fibroblasts are stimulated to generate and lay a bed of newly formed collagen [27–29].

Different wavelengths have been selected for laser lipolysis in an attempt to specifically target: adipose tissue, collagen (water), and blood vessels. There are not enough reports in current literature for a final conclusion to be made but some have been made. According to Perlette and Kaminer, the most selective wavelength for adipocyte cell disruption is 924 nm. Since the technology used is not only to diminish the subcutaneous fat layer but also to use it in an optimal way for body contouring which includes the skin during the procedure. The wavelength should be used that manages to disrupt fat cells but also achieves substantial skin tightening. With the wavelengths tested in the report, authors state that the 1064-nm wavelength has lower fat absorption but a better tissue disruption and there for produces better skin tightening effect. In that sense, for the treatment of fragile areas, authors suggest the use of 1320 nm because it has lower penetration and is safer to use [23, 30].

The final result of laser-assisted liposuction/lipolysis is visible after 90 days. For the certain amount of adipose cells that were irreversibly damaged (but not ruptured at the time of the lysis) and were not suction during liposuction, the process of adipocitolysis occurs through macrophage activity and this process takes approximately 90 days.

Also, after the initial thermal effect on the interstitial tissue, healing process is activated and fibroblast is stimulated to form new collagen. Neocollagenesis takes about 3–10 weeks.

5. Advantages of laser-assisted liposuction

The most significant advantage of laser energy in liposuction is the skin tightening effect. The physiology of action has previously been described. Most candidates that undergo liposuction have significant adipose tissue amount and generally have moderate excess of skin. In cases where skin excision is not indicated the amount of skin tightening that evolves from using the laser energy is generally enough to achieve satisfactory result. Therefore, it is always indicated in patients that could result in excess skin after aspirating the subcutaneous fat. Surgeons should also remember that effects of laser energy are prolonged. Skin tightening occurs during several months after the procedure. The patients should also know that definitive result can be seen after several months [21, 27, 30, 31].

During laser-assisted lipolysis/liposuction, smaller cannula sizes are used. The adipose tissue is liquefacted; thus, it takes up less volume and the incision site can therefore be smaller. Smaller cannulas result in less trauma to the surrounding tissue resulting in less pain and discomfort after the procedure that enables the patient to recover faster and return to normal everyday activity. Smaller cannulas also enable to perform liposuction in smaller areas where much more precision is needed. That combined with the uniform liquefaction of the adipose tissue makes perfect combination for treating localized adiposity in thigh and knee area, arms, and submental and facial fat. Also, smaller cannulas can be especially useful in areas like male chest, back, or hips. Those areas are very fibrous; therefore, the fat is trapped in smaller compartments. The smaller is the cannula used for lipolysis and it facilitates fat melting in fibrous locations. In the same time, smaller cannula size diminishes trauma to the surrounding tissue experienced with larger sized cannulas. Only laser lipolysis without aspiration of the liquefied content is described in the literature. Dudelzak, Hussain, and Goldberg reported study with 20 patients that underwent laser lipolysis of extensor arm fat pads. The liquefied fat was removed in 50% of the patients, and the results were observed 6 months after the procedure. Their conclusion was that the results were identical whether or not post-laser lipolysis aspiration was undertaken [32]. Individual case reports can be found describing masses after laser lipolysis alone [33]. Fat necrosis is usually a gradual process that is noticed by the patient or physician as a mass. Radiologically, it can imitate cancer. Complications from necrosis of any kind are in direct correlation with the amount of necrotic tissue. Larger amounts of necrosis create a greater inflammatory response. If the amount of necrotic tissue is too big, in time, macrophages will not be able to resolve all of the necrosis but only that which is placed peripherally and is in contact with the viable tissue. The central part will remain, and the immune system will encapsulate the remaining necrosis [34]. The authors advocate the use of aspiration whenever possible to avoid such complications. Laser lipolysis alone should be reserved only to small treated areas where aspiration could result in irregularities.

Laser-assisted lipolysis/liposuction results in reduced blood loss due to coagulation effect of the laser energy. Abdelaal and Aboelatta conducted a study on 56 patients. Equal amounts of liposuction were performed—traditional-assisted liposuction on one side and laser-assisted liposuction on the contralateral side. Blood loss volumes were calculated from the lipoaspirates by measuring hemoglobin and red blood cell content. Laser lipolysis reduced the blood loss by more than 50% compared to the traditional liposuction [35]. Considering the reduced blood loss, laser-assisted liposuction is indicated in large-volume liposuctions (>5 L of lipoaspirate) to prevent secondary anemia due to blood loss during surgery. Reduced blood loss diminishes the need for postoperative blood transfusions and therefore results in faster recovery. Reduced blood loss is especially important in patients who previously underwent bariatric surgery. In those patients, preoperative anemia is often present [36]. Coagulation of the vessels also contributes to less bruising and edema, which also results in faster recovery and higher patient satisfaction [25].

Many surgeons have noted an improvement of cellulite after laser lipolysis procedures. The causes of cellulite are multifactorial, including changes in fibrous septae within the hypodermis that macroscopically show herniation of subcutaneous fat into the dermis [37]. In 2008, Goldman et al. published a new treatment approach combining subdermal Nd: YAG laser lipolysis and autologous fat transplantation that resulted in significant clinical improvement in cellulite. A majority of patients (84.6%) rated the results of treatment as either good or excellent [38]. In 2016, Petti et al. reported the use of the Nd:YAG laser at a wavelength of 1440 nm, along with an innovative 1000-μm directional side-firing fiber-optic laser system for single stage contouring of the lower body and concluded that both problems could be addressed at a same time with high satisfaction rate using different laser energy that according to their specifications have better effect on fat melting or collagen heating [39]. These findings are in correlation with findings reported by Forman Taub and Friedman [23].

Last, but not least, because the adipose tissue is liquefied, fatty tissue removal should be hastened creating less strain for the surgeon. Aspiration of the liquefied adipose tissue should be smooth, and large surgeon's strength should not be involved.

6. Complications specific to laser-assisted liposuction

Due to photothermal effect of the laser energy and the heat accumulated in the tissue during the procedure, laser burns or skin necrosis can occur. Accumulating the heat in one place which happens if you do not move around the tissue with the fiber fast enough and you remain on one place overaccumulation of the heat will happen in one place and thermal injury will develop. It can start as a blister and in the beginning can appear as a partial skin thickness burn, but you must remember that the damage came from the inside; therefore, it will result in full skin thickness burn and will definitely leave a mark. As it was described before, there is a thin line between the desired effect and adverse event. To avoid this complication when beginning using laser energy in liposuction, the authors suggest to start with lower energy levels and avoid very superficial areas of the subcutaneous tissue to avoid direct dermal as well as dermal vascular plexus injury. An infrared thermometer (some devices are equipped with an internal subcutaneous thermometer) can be used to control the heat. Outside control of the temperature can be done but in reality is unreliable. Some surgeons also advise cold compresses on the treated area to diminish the effect of the laser on the skin [40]. The authors suggest continuous movement of the fiber with contralateral hand on the treated skin area to control the applied energy, and therefore, the accumulated heat to minimize the risk of laser burns.

In cases where laser lipolysis without aspiration is done, fat necrosis may occur. As mentioned before, fat necrosis is possible. In reasonable small amounts, the body is able to process and remove the cellular debris and biochemical by-products of the melted fat cells. In larger amounts, the results are unpredictable with hard nodules, lumps, and uneven scarring. The risk of fat necrosis is diminished with the use of aspiration but is not completely disappeared. As it was mentioned before, the prolonged effect of thermal injury happens in cases where adipose cells' membrane was not disrupted but the cell accumulated enough energy to produce irreversible damage and that kind of tissue was not aspirated subsequently but left inside. During time, adipocitolysis via the macrophages starts. If the area of irreversible damage is larger with no blood flow, then the macrophage delivery to the point of injury is impossible and body starts to localize the process and the fat necrosis present like a mass. To avoid these kind of complications, authors suggest the uniform lipolysis with the laser as well as uniform aspiration following lipolysis.

Overaccumulation of the heat can result in hyperfibortic reaction that can be visible as a strain or palpable or patient can complain of the straining in some of the treated parts especially during movement. These adverse reactions can be treated with injection of the triamcinolone acetonide injections in the strains but mostly resolve during time with compressive massage.

At the beginning of the use of lasers in liposuction, there has been concern regarding the increase of serum lipids due to degradation of the adipose cells. Mordon et al. published an article in 2009. They studied standard lipid profile (total cholesterol, HDL cholesterol, LDL cholesterol, and triglycerides) before the procedure and 1 day, 3 days, 2 weeks, and 1 month after the laser lipolysis procedure. They concluded that serum cholesterol and triglyceride levels remained in the normal range after laser lipolysis. They proposed two hypotheses: fat elimination is so gradual that an increase in circulating lipid levels is not measurable and/or the damaged adipocytes are undergoing apoptosis and being removed by phagocytosis, presumably via activated macrophages [41].

Recently, in August of 2015, Shin and Chang reported a case of a 34-year-old patient that was diagnosed with rhabdomyolysis with acute kidney injury after laser-assisted liposuction. No similar reports until now have been made [42].

7. Description of the technique

Preoperative evaluation of the patient must be done. Pinch test should be performed to evaluate the amount of excess skin and to exclude the need for surgical excision of the excessive skin. Irregularities of the skin should be marked, while patient is standing to avoid losing the 3D relations once the patient is on the operating table. Preoperative photographs should be taken with emphasis on the skin irregularities.

Targeted area should always be larger than the aspiration site to achieve better skin tightening effect and to allow the overlying skin to attach to the infrastructure uniformly. For example, when treating gynecomastia/pseudogynecomastia, laser energy should be applied to whole chest area to achieve better skin retraction and accommodation (see **Figures 1–5**).

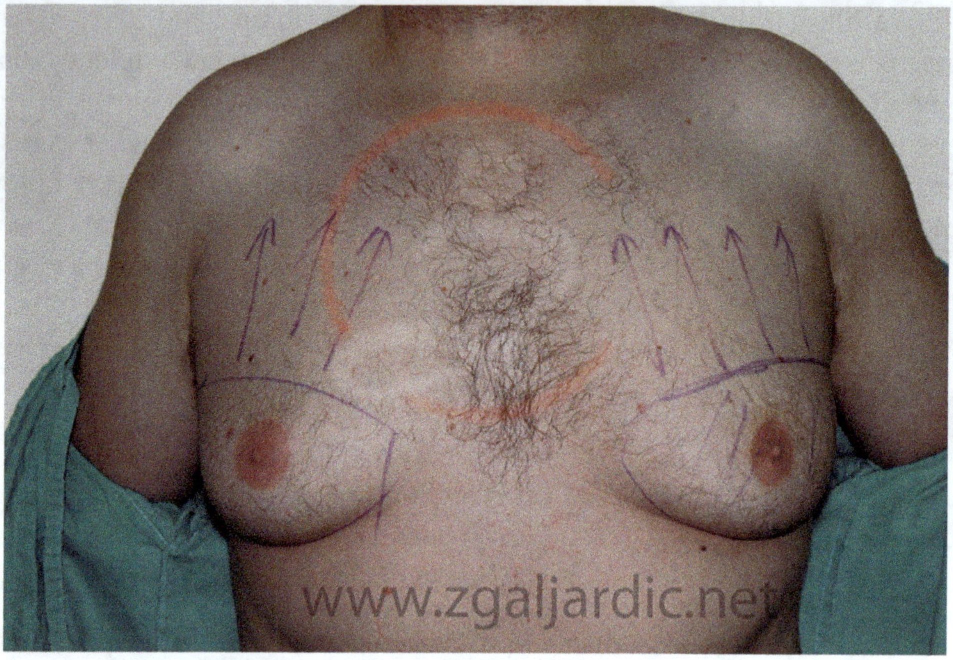

Figure 1. Preoperative markings—case 1.

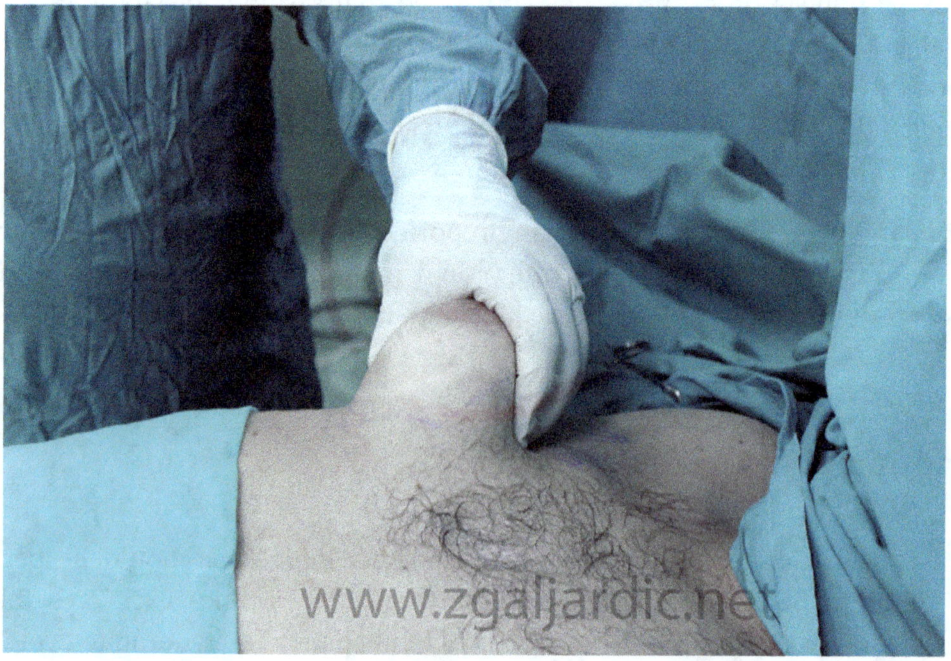

Figure 2. Intraoperative "pinch test" to evaluate the amount of the fat tissue during the procedure—case 1.

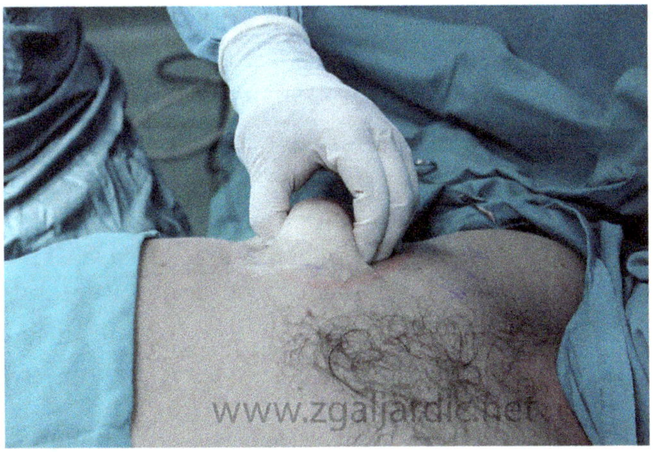

Figure 3. Intraoperative "pinch test" to evaluate the amount of the fat tissue during the procedure—case 1.

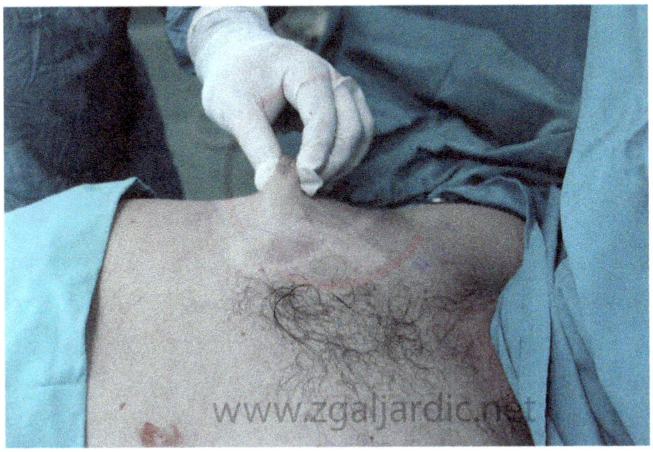

Figure 4. Intraoperative "pinch test" to evaluate the amount of the fat tissue during the procedure—case 1.

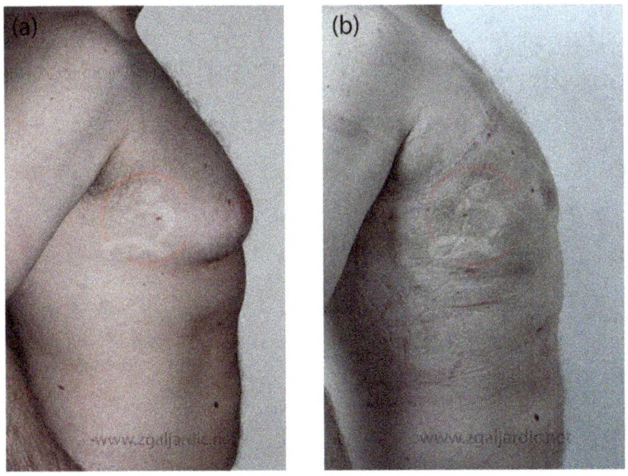

Figure 5. (a) Before photographs—case 1. (b) After 7 days—case 1.

Although there are many advocates of liposuction done solely in tumescent anesthesia, the authors prefer general anesthesia due to their comfort as well as the patients. The authors advise tumescent anesthesia only in cases of localized adiposity in one treated area. Authors also recommend 12- to 24-h observation after the whole-body procedure to administer the loss of intravascular volume as well as to help patients in early postoperative period.

In cases when the whole body (e.g. legs, abdomen, flanks, back) is treated, we recommend the disinfection of the skin in the treated areas should be done while patient is in the standing position and awake to be able to disinfect the whole circumference of the body and once finished patient should be laid down on the operating table previously covered sterilely.

Perioperatively single dose of 2 g cephazoline should be administered and continued orally with second-generation cephalosporin antibiotics.

Infiltration is done with the infiltration pump to minimize the time needed for the infiltration as well to deliver the infiltration uniquely. In case of tumescent anesthesia only standard Klein's solution in used. If the patient is in general anesthesia, only epinephrine can be used (1 ml of 1:1000 on 1 L of normal saline) to avoid the toxicity of lidocaine but still achieve vasoconstriction. Fifteen minutes after the infiltration, the laser lipolysis can be started (that is the approximate time needed for the infiltration process so once the infiltration is done normally you can start the laser lipolysis on the area firstly infiltrated).

The authors use the diode 1470 nm laser for the last 6 years. Energy applied normally is set to 12 W (for abdomen, flanks, back, legs, pseudogynecomastia), 10 W for the arms, and 6 W for the facial area and the submental fat. Pulse wave is continuous. As opposed to other laser wavelengths, which are absorbed by both water and oxyhemoglobin, 1470 nm demonstrates a greater water absorption coefficient. Sliding of the fiber should be smooth without surgeons' strength involvement. Thus, when strength should be applied, one should wait for a second in the place while the laser delivers the energy and the resistance in the tissue should ease up and allow us to slide through the tissue without mechanically disrupting the tissue fibers. Care must be taken all the time to avoid thermal injuries. The authors suggest to always have the opposite hand on the treated area to evaluate the temperature of the area. Devices equipped with internal subcutaneous thermometer can be used to monitor the temperature, or infrared thermometer can be used to measure outside temperature being careful not to exceed 38–40°C. Cold packs on the surface can diminish the temperature on the surface and thus avoiding the thermal injury of the skin. In 2009, Reynaud et al. published a retrospective analysis of 534 procedures of lipolysis using a 980-nm diode laser and calculated mean amount of energy and tumescent fluid infiltration for each location [25]. The lysis should first be done in deep layer parallel to the underlying structures radially covering the whole area available from the incisional site. Once the liquefaction in the deeper layer is achieved, the fiber should be moved to the upper layer starting from the incisional site.

The authors always advise to aspirate the liquefied adipose tissue after lipolysis to avoid complications described before. The aspiration starts with the bigger cannula moving to the smaller once to accelerate the aspiration but to avoid irregularities.

The incisional sites could be left open in large-volume liposuctions to allow the additional drainage.

To achieve the best skin tightening result, the authors advise applying the laser energy in the tissue once more after the aspiration process is done.

Compressive plates as well as the compressive garments should be applied at the end of the procedure to maximize the result. Postoperative instructions are explained later on in the chapter.

8. High-definition liposuction

Small size of the laser fiber enables the use of cannulas of small diameter. That facilitates the melting of the adipose tissue in delicate places so it allows us to melt the fat very superficial under the skin and enclosed in small fibrous compartments. Those specifications allow us to perform high-definition liposuction. It is reserved for the individuals who seek more defined and athletic look but cannot get rid of the small amount of the stubborn unwanted adipose envelope.

Preoperative markings are very important. Surgeon should mark the patient in the standing position. Goal is to mark the borders of the defining muscles such as m. rectus abdominis, m. pectoralis major, m. obliquus abdominis, m. deltoideus especially their tendinous parts. That can be achieved by asking the patient to contract the specific muscles or to perform the movement that emphasizes a specific muscle. During contraction or movement, you should mark the borders of the muscles and their tendinous parts.

Intraoperative process is the same as with the standard laser-assisted liposuction. During laser lipolysis, care must be taken not to make thermal injury of the skin so the movements of the laser fiber should be precise, smooth, and fast moving. Here is when the preoperative markings are important. To achieve highly defined structure, the intention is to apply more laser energy and thus more heat at the area where you marked the tendinous parts. More heat applied over the tendinous parts serves to promote collagen formation in the fibrous septa over the underlying tendinous structure so that those parts macroscopically look defined. Aspiration should be done with small diameter cannulas to ensure precise work and to avoid irregularities that can easily be done in already athlete patient. Postoperatively adhesive bandages can be placed with small amount of pressure on the previously mentioned tendinous parts to guide the healing process in the early postoperative period (7 days).

High-definition laser liposuction is a precise method and should not be performed if you are just beginning to use the laser device. There is no place for mistakes in high-definition liposuction. Too much energy applied subcutaneously can easily make thermal injury of the skin that will leave a mark. Also overaspiration of even small amount of the subcutaneous fat can result in a visible irregularity. You have to remember that individuals seeking high-definition liposuction are highly demanding and seeking only the perfect result. High-definition laser liposuction should be reserved for the physicians who are familiar with the technique.

9. Laser lipolysis/liposuction of the face and neck

Due to the skin tightening effect of the laser energy, the technique has also found its place in contouring face and neck. Submental region, cervicomandibular angle, Periparotid fat, and perinasolabial area are the treated areas. Energy applied in these areas is smaller than in the other parts of the body —6 W. As with the high-definition laser-assisted liposuction, this is not the technique for the beginners.

This technique is useful not only in treating facial adiposity but also for patients seeking facial rejuvenation procedures and with proper indication can replace traditional face and neck lift [43, 44]. There are no long incisions, only incisional places for the laser fiber and subsequently used microcannulas. The results are long lasting and comparable to those of traditional surgery. Recovery time is faster and can be done in tumescent anesthesia.

10. Postoperative instructions

1. Compression garments should be worn for 3 weeks.
2. Compression plates that can be found on the market or should be made at the end of the procedure by individual's structural characteristics (costal arch, iliac crest, sizes of the flanks, back, or chest) of hard, yet flexible material that allows movements (should be dressed up in compresses) should be worn for 7 days during whole day and for the next 2 weeks during the night.
3. In cases of high-definition laser-assisted liposuction adhesive bandages mentioned before are worn for 7 days.
4. Showering of the treated area is allowed after check up on 7th postoperative day only with cold water to avoid vasodilatation and subsequent edema.
5. Peroral antibiotics of second generation of cephalosporin are given during 5 days.

Postoperative measurements are important in obtaining the best result possible. It should be carefully explained to the patient the importance of those instructions as they are in their best interest. They should be explained that all those postoperative measures have important role in their recovery and that they allow us to guide the healing process and that is in their best interest to follow them carefully. Postoperative measurements serve as a tool in obtaining best skin tightening effect and to avoid contour irregularities.

11. Results

The authors have been using laser-assisted lipolysis for the last 10 years. Laser used for the last 6 years was diode 1470 nm laser. 1470 nm has proved to be very safe. This wavelength shows high absorption rate for water molecules and fat cells; therefore, there is no need for high power settings during the procedure. That enables to work faster and also prevents damages to the surrounding tissue. In that way, it diminishes complication rates. During that time, no significant complication specific to laser has been seen. The authors are very satisfied with the results that are achieved with the use of laser in body contouring procedures. Satisfaction rate among the patients treated is extremely high, and they claim the postoperative period to be painless and fast (see **Figures 6–35**).

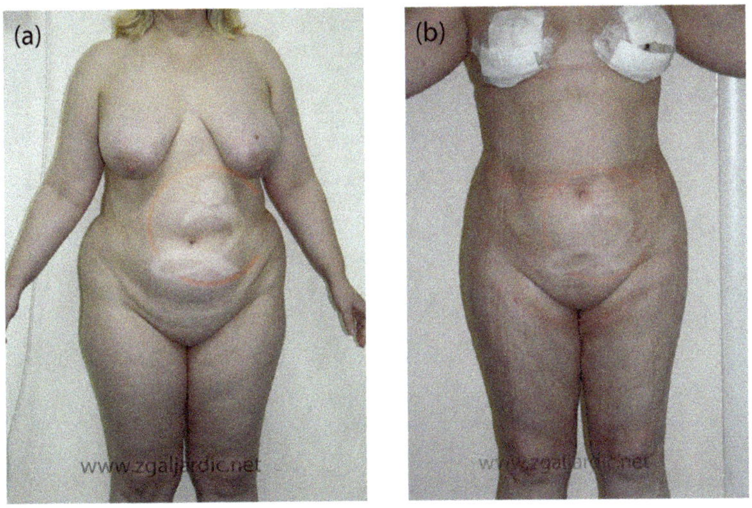

Figure 6. (a). Before photograph(front)- case 2. (b). Case 2(front) after 7 days.

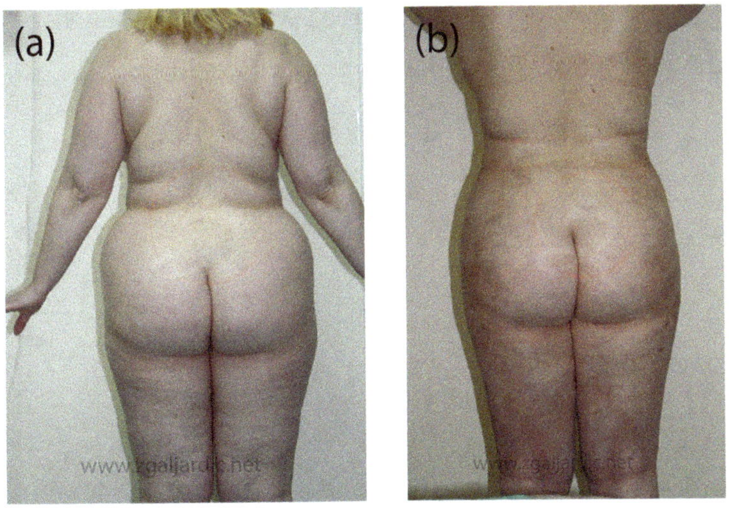

Figure 7. (a). Before photograph(back)- case 2. (b). Case 2(back) after 7 days.

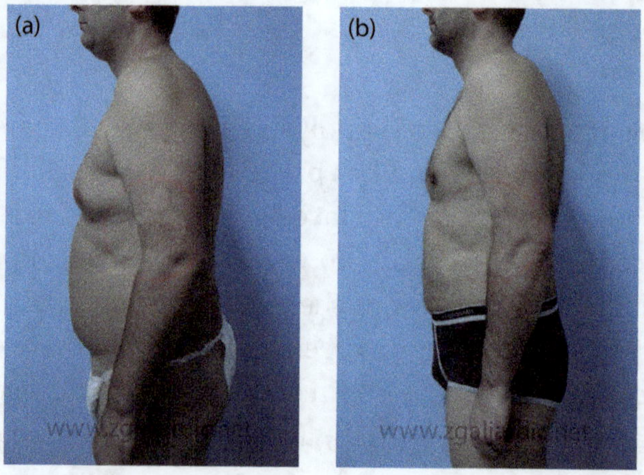

Figure 8. (a). Before photograph- case 3. (b). Case 3- after 3 weeks.

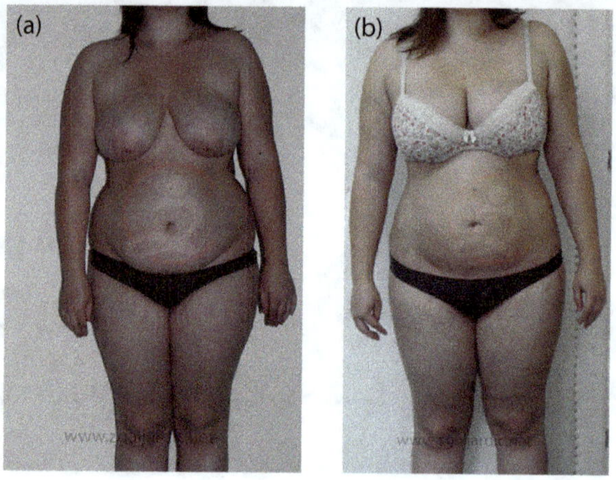

Figure 9. (a). Before photograph (front)—case 4. (b). Case 4 (front)-after 2 weeks.

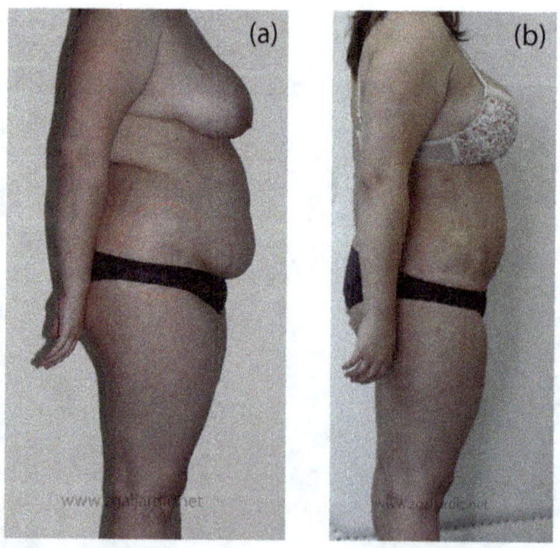

Figure 10. (a). Before photograph (profile)- case 4. (b). Case 4 (profile)- after 2 weeks.

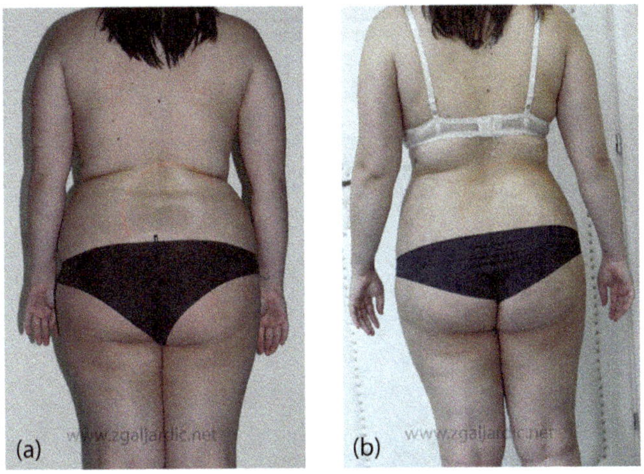

Figure 11. (a). Before photograph (back)-case 4. (b). Case 4 (back)-after 2 weeks.

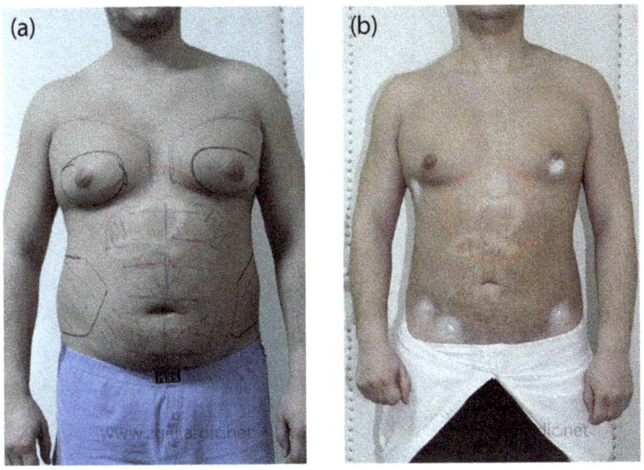

Figure 12. (a). Before photograph (front)-case 5. (b). Case 5 (front)-after 7 days.

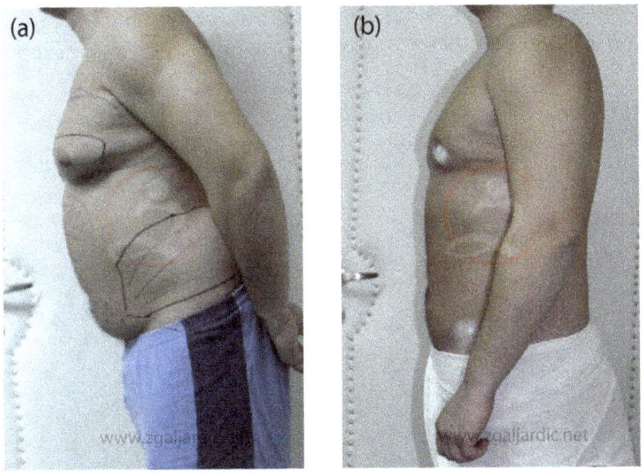

Figure 13. (a). Before photograph (profile)-case 5. (b). Case 5 (profile)-after 7 days.

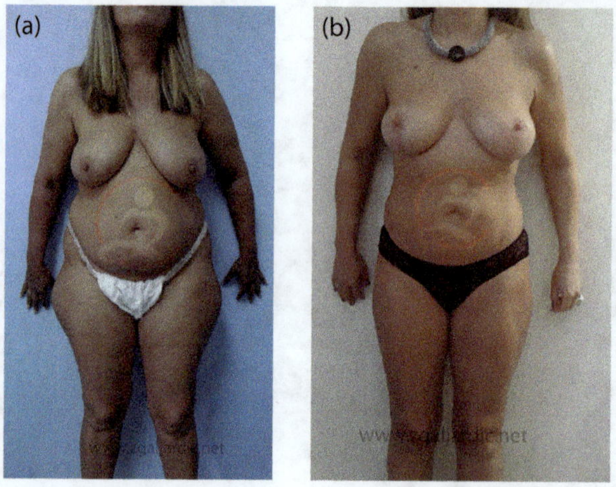

Figure 14. (a). Before photograph (front)- case 6. (b). Case 6 (front)-after 3 weeks.

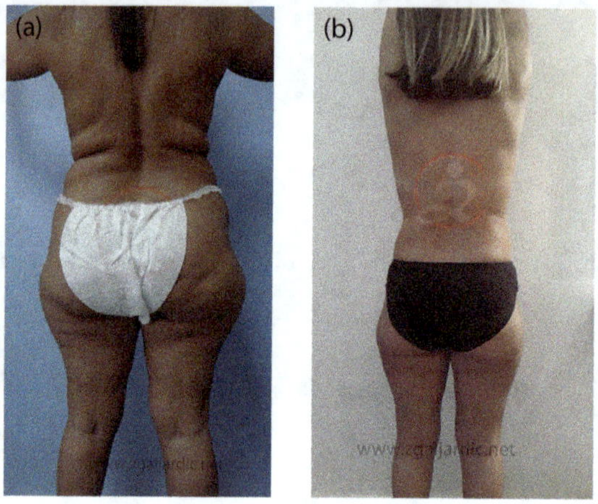

Figure 15. (a). Before photograph (back)- case 6. (b). Case 6 (back)-after 3 weeks.

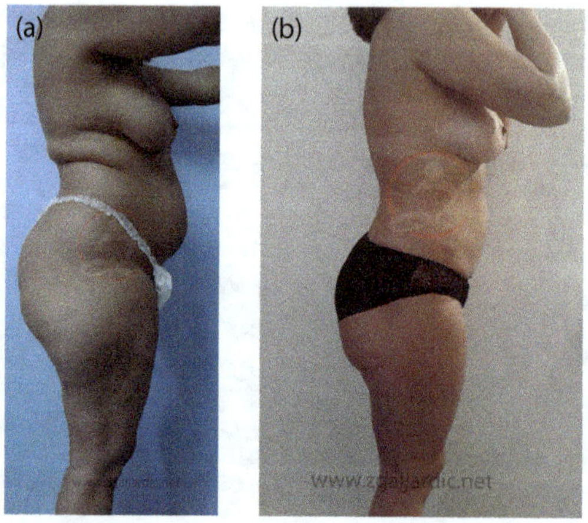

Figure 16. (a). Before photograph (profile)- case 6. (b). Case 6 (profile)-after 3 weeks.

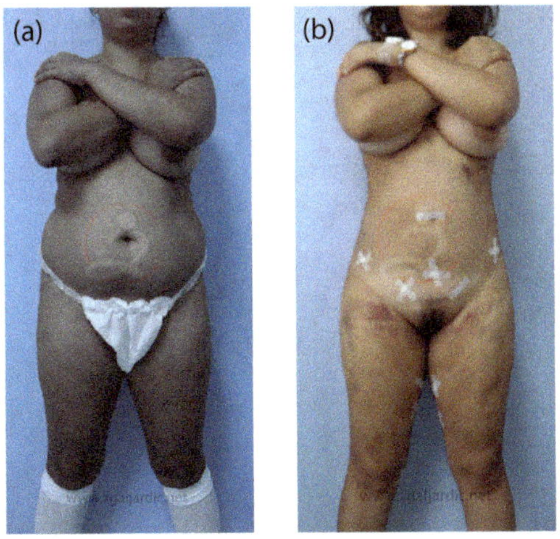

Figure 17. (a). Before photograph (front)- case 7. (b). Case 7-(front)- after 7 days.

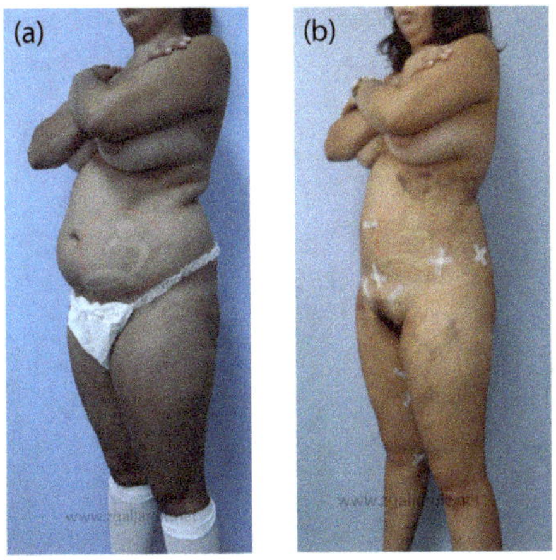

Figure 18. (a). Before photograph (semiprofile)- case 7. (b). Case 7 (semiprofile)- after 7 days.

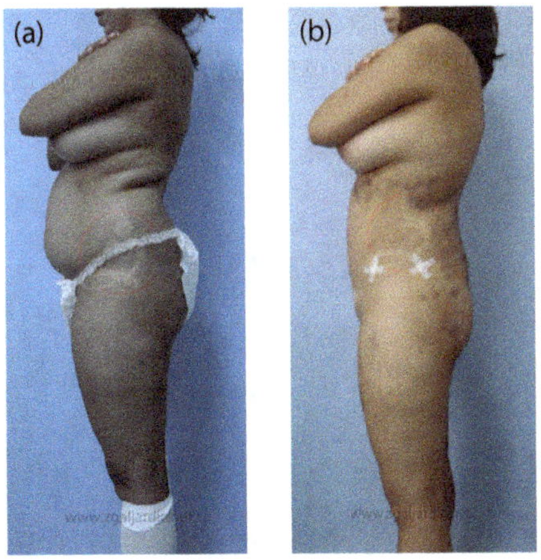

Figure 19. (a). Before photograph (profile)- case 7. (b). Case 7 (profile)-after 7 days.

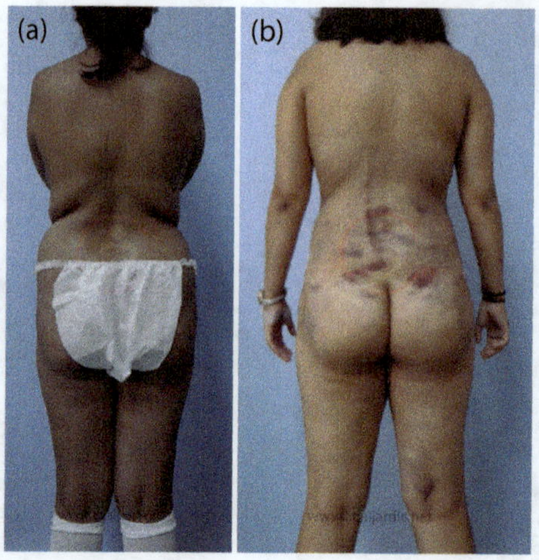

Figure 20. (a). Before photograph (back)- case 7. (b). Case 7 (back)- after 7 days.

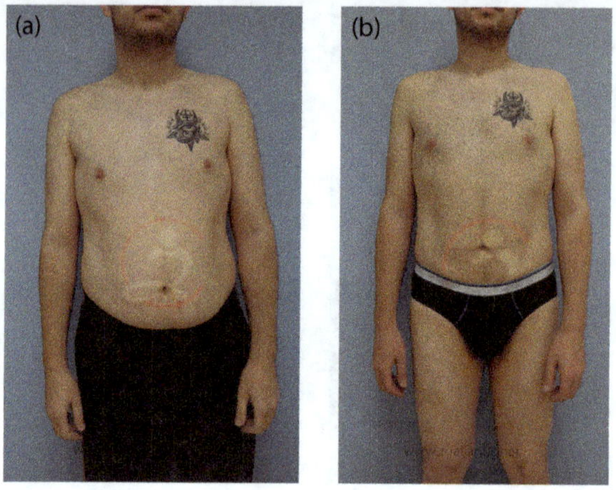

Figure 21. (a). Before photograph (front)- case 8. (b). Case 8 (front)-after 2 weeks.

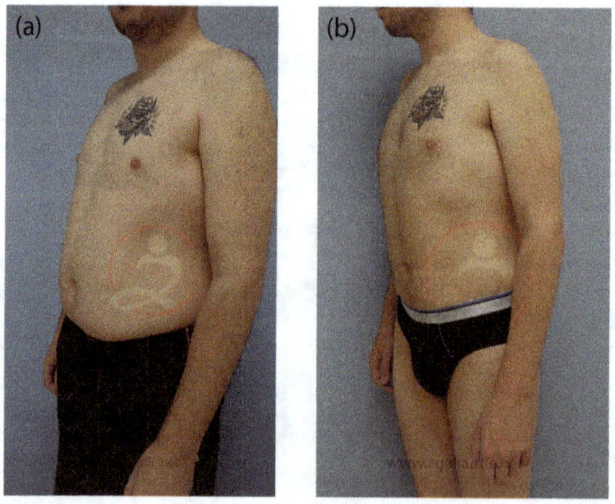

Figure 22. (a). Before photograph (semiprofile)- case 8. (b). Case 8 (semiprofile)- after 2 weeks.

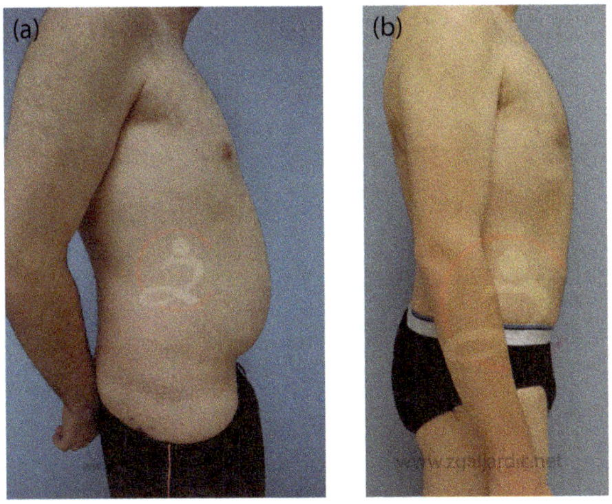

Figure 23. (a). Before photograph (profile)-case 8. (b). Case 8 (profile)- after 2 weeks.

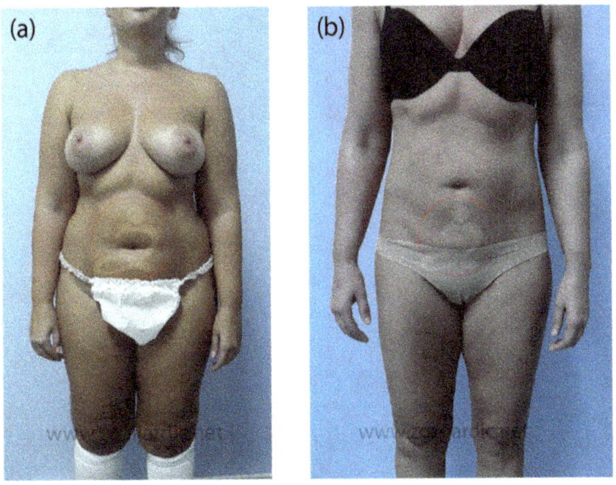

Figure 24. (a). Before photograph (front)- case 9. (b). Case 9 (front)- after 6 weeks.

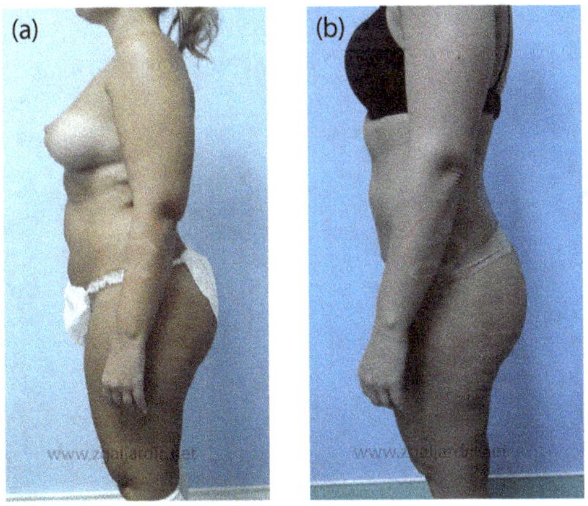

Figure 25. (a). Before photograph (profile)- case 9. (b). Case 9 (profile)- after 6 weeks.

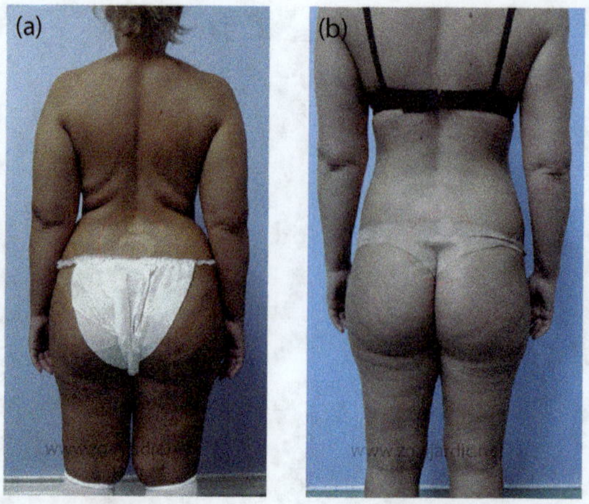

Figure 26. (a). Before photograph (back)- case 9. (b). Case 9 after (back)- 6 weeks.

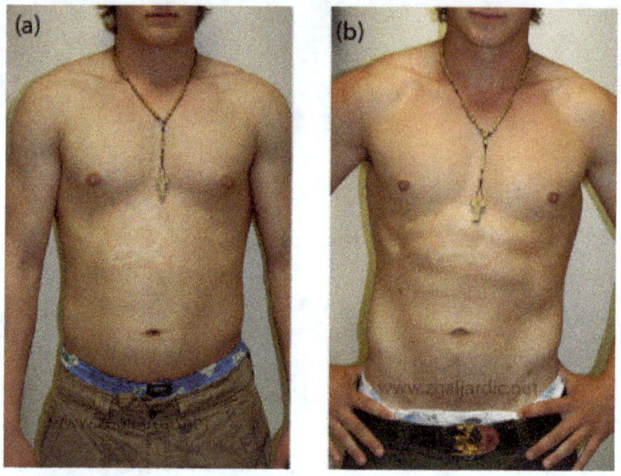

Figure 27. (a). Before photograph (front)-case 10. (b). Case 10 (front)- after 3 weeks.

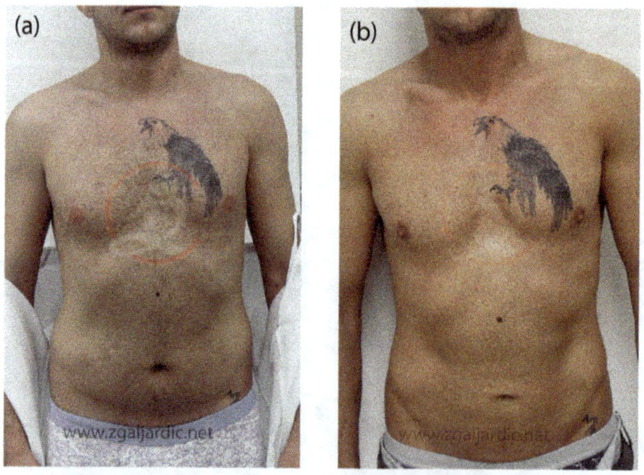

Figure 28. (a). Before photograph (front)- case 11. (b). Case 11 (front)- after 3 weeks.

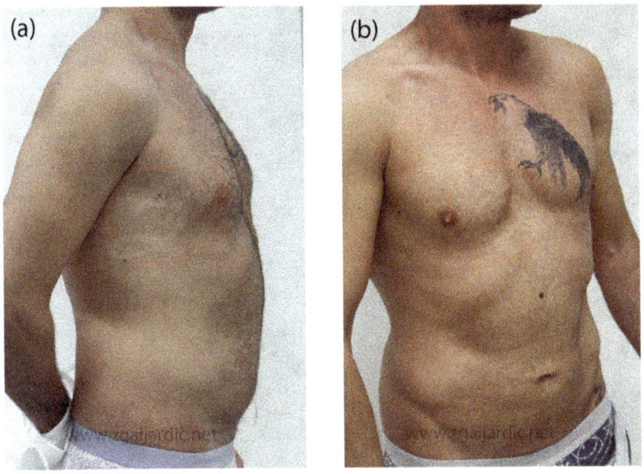

Figure 29. (a). Before photograph (profile)- case 11. (b). Case 11 (semiprofile)- after 3 weeks.

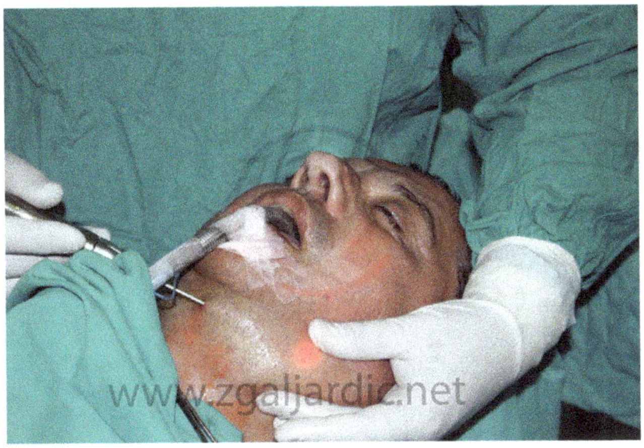

Figure 30. Laser lipolysis of the neck: always be aware of the probe's position to avoid injuries of the marginal nerve.

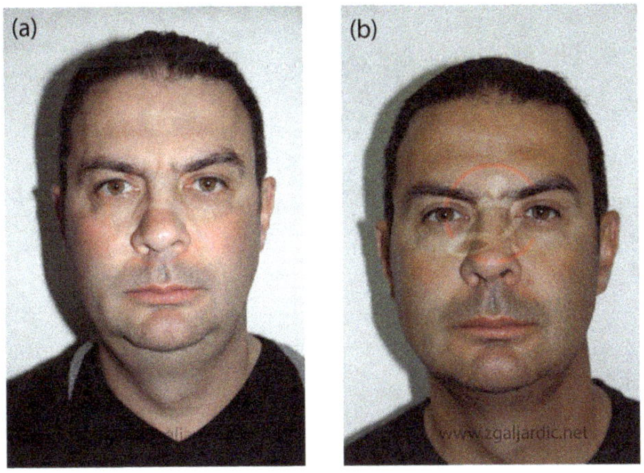

Figure 31. (a). Before photograph(front)- case 12. (b). Case 13 (front)- after 3 weeks.

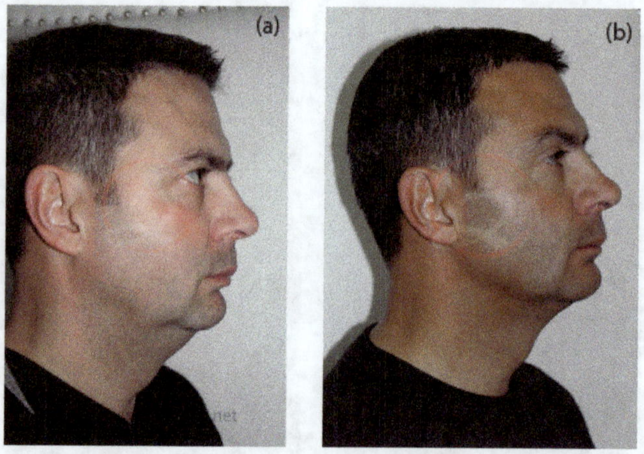

Figure 32. (a). Before photograph (profile)—case 12. (b). Case 13 (profile)- after 3 weeks.

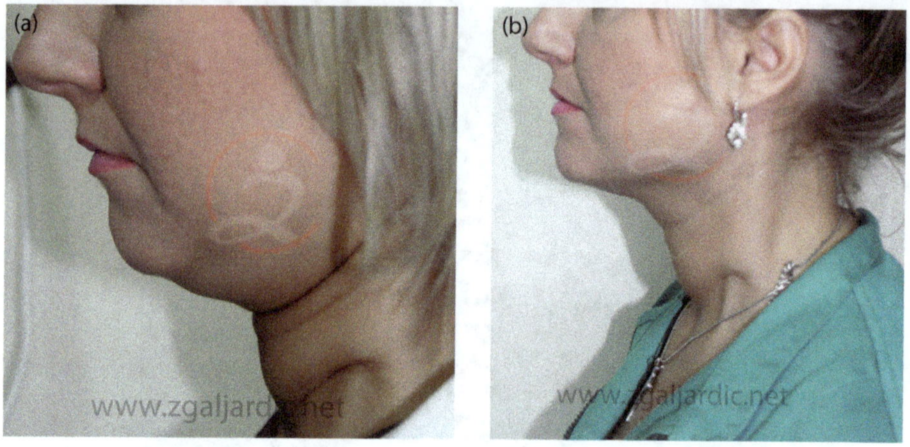

Figure 33. (a). Before photograph (profile)- case 14. (b). Case 14 (profile)- after 1 month.

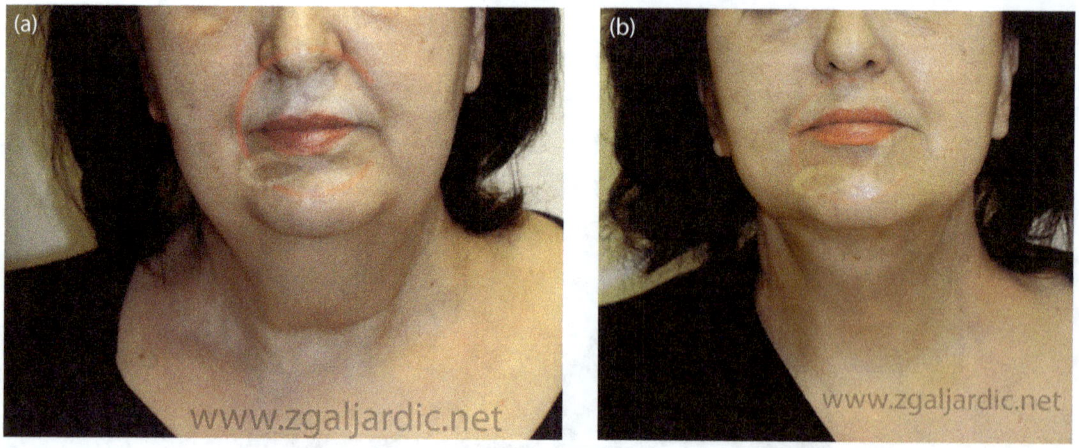

Figure 34. (a). Before photograph (front)—case 13. (b). Case 13 (front)- after one month.

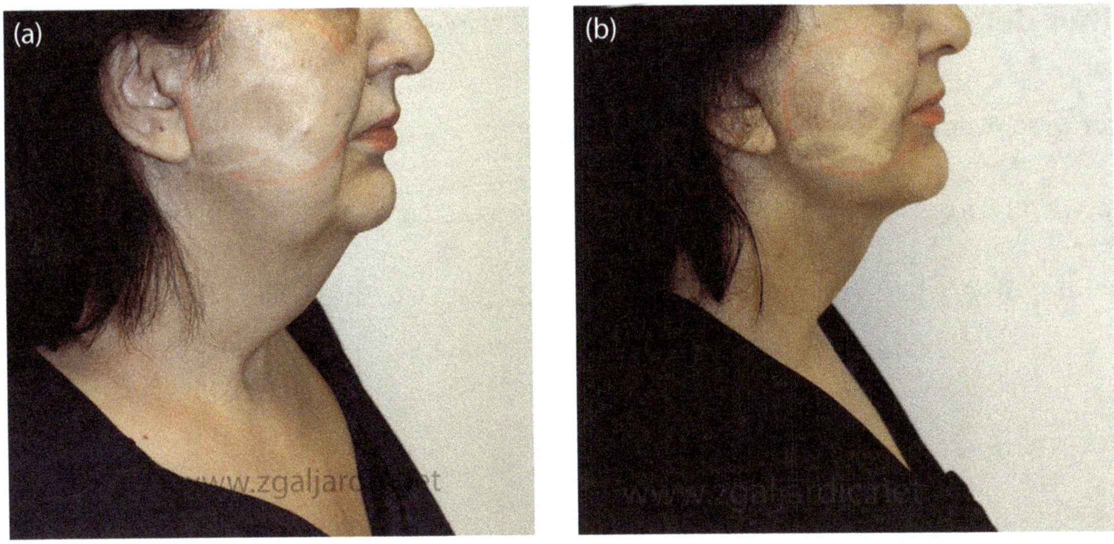

Figure 35. (a). Before photograph (profile)- case 13. (b). Case 13 (profile)- after one month.

12. Conclusion

Laser-assisted liposuction is a big step forward in body sculpting. Since the laser was introduced in this area, various studies have been made and showed its benefits. The superiority of laser-assisted liposuction over traditional liposuction can be summarized as follows:

1. Superior skin tightening effect: changes occur in the tissue after absorption of laser energy due to photothermal effect. That characteristic enables us to treat any area with the excessive adipose tissue and modest skin laxity with obtaining better cosmetic result.

2. Coagulation of blood vessel: the use of laser reduced the blood loss after the liposuction and also reduces bruising after the procedure. That enables the patient to recover faster which leads to higher satisfaction rate.

3. Disruption of the adipose cells: the lipoaspirate is liquefied that enables the smoother aspect of the treated area.

4. Use of smaller cannulas: after the laser lipolysis has been done, the aspiration can be made with smaller cannulas that allows us to aspirate the areas of the fat that cannot be reached with traditional liposuction.

The specific complications of the laser energy should not be forgotten. Although laser allows us to reach results beyond the results of traditional liposuction, one should always have in mind that technology is just a tool in a physician's hand. The goal is to optimize the amount of energy delivered to the tissue thus maximizing the final result but avoiding possible side effects and complications.

Author details

Zoran Žgaljardić* and Ivonne Žgaljardić

*Address all correspondence to: zoran.zgaljardic@gmail.com

Aestehtic Surgery Center Dr. Žgaljardić Opatija, Zagreb, Croatia

References

[1] The American Society for Aesthetic Plastic Surgery's cosmetic surgery statistics [Internet]. Available from: http://www.surgery.org/sites/default/files/ASAPS-Stats2015.pdf [Accessed: 2016-06-15]

[2] Shridharani SM, Broyles JM, Matarasso A: Liposuction devices: technology update. Med Devices (Auckl) 2014;7:241–251.

[3] Shiffman MA, Aiache AE: Atlas of Liposuction. 1st ed. New Delhi: Jaypee Brothers Medical Publishers (P) Ltd.; 2013. p. 1.

[4] Illouz Y. Liposuction: The Franco-American Experience. Beverly Hills, Calif: Medical Aesthetics, 1985.

[5] Einstein A. On the Quantum Thoery of Radiation. Physikalische Gesellschaft Zürich Miteilungen 1916;18:47–62 published in Physikalische Zeitschrift 1917;18:121–128. Reprinted in Kox AJ et al ., eds. The collected papers of Albert Einstein: The Berlin Years, Writings, 1914–1917, Princeton: Princeton University Press, 1966:381–397.

[6] Einstein A. On a Heuristic Point of View Concerning the Production and Transformation of Light. Annalen der Physik. 1905;17:132–184.

[7] Alster TS. Preface. In: Manual of Cutaneous Laser Techniques. Philadelphia: Lippincott Williams and Wilkins, 2000. p. 11.

[8] Goldman L. Pathology of the effect of the laser beam on the skin. Nature 1963;197:912–914.

[9] Hukki J, Krogerus L, Castren M, Schroder T: Effects of different contact laser scalpels on skin and subcutaneous fat. Lasers Surg Med. 1988:8:276–282.

[10] Goldberg DJ, Berlin AL: Disorders of Fat and Cellulite: Advances in Diagnosis and Treatment. Boca Raton: CRC Press; 2011. p. 103.

[11] Apfelberg, D. Laser-assisted liposuction may benefit surgeons and subjects. Clin Laser Mon. 1992;10:259.

[12] Apfelberg DB, Rosenthal S, Hunstad JP, et al.: Progress report on multicenter study of laser-assisted liposuction. Aesthetic Plast Surg. 1994;18(3):259–264.

[13] Blugerman GB. Abstracts of World Congress on Liposuction Surgery. Dearborn, Michigan: 2000. Laser lipolysis for the treatment of localized adiposity and "cellulite."

[14] Schavelzon DS, Blugerman G, Goldman A, Abstracts of the 10th International Symposium on Cosmetic Laser Surgery. Las Vegas: 2001. Laser lipolysis.

[15] Goldman AG, Schavelzon D, Blugerman G. Laser lipolysis: liposuction using Nd:YAG laser. Revista da Sociedade Brasileira de Cirurgia Plástica. 2002;17:17–26.

[16] Goldman AG, Schavelzon D, Blugerman G. Liposuction using neodimium:yttrium-aluminiumgarnet laser. Abstract in Plast Recontr Surg. 2003;111:2497.

[17] Badin AZ, Moraes LM, Gondek L, et al. Laser lipolysis: flaccidity under control. Aesthetic Plast Surg. 2002;26(5):335–339.

[18] Ichikawa K, Tanino R, Wakaki M: Histologic and photonic evaluation of a pulsed Nd:YAG laser for ablation of subcutaneous adipose tissue. Tokai J Exp Clin Med. 2006;31(4):136–40.

[19] Badin AZ, Gondek LB, Garcia MJ, Valle LC, Flizikowski FB, de Noronha L: Analysis of laser lipolysis effects on human tissue samples obtained from liposuction. Aesthetic Plast Surg. 2005;29(4):281–6. Epub 2005 Jul 19.

[20] Mordon SR, Wassmer B, Reynaud JP, Zemmouri J: Mathematical modeling of laser lipolysis. Biomed Eng Online. 2008;7:10.

[21] McBean JC, Katz BE: A pilot study of the efficacy of a 1064 and 1320 nm sequentially firing Nd:YAG laser device for lipolysis and skin tightening. Lasers Surg Med. 2009;41(10):779–84.

[22] Khoury JG, Saluja R, Keel D, Detwiler S, Goldman MP: Histologic evaluation of interstitial lipolysis comparing a 1064, 1320 and 2100 nm laser in an *ex vivo* model. Lasers Surg Med. 2008;40(6):402–6.

[23] Forman Taub A, Friedman A: Laser lipolysis with a 980 nm diode laser. J Drugs Dermatol. 2010;9(5 Suppl ODAC Conf Pt 1):s58–61.

[24] Lukac M, Vizintin Z, Zabkar J, and Pirnat S. QCW Pulsed Nd:YAG 1064 nm Laser Lipolysis, J Laser Health Acad. 2009;4/1:5–17.

[25] Reynaud JP, Skibinski M, Wassmer B, Rochon P, Mordon S: Lipolysis using a 980-nm diode laser: a retrospective analysis of 534 procedures. Aesthetic Plast Surg. 2009;33(1): 28–36.

[26] Tagliolatto S, Barcellos Medeiros V, Gerin Leite O: Laserlipolysis: update and literature review. Surg Cosmet Dermatol. 2012;4(2):164–74.

[27] Badin AZ, Moraes LM, Gondek L, Chiaratti MG, Canta L: Laser lipolysis: flaccidity under control. Aesthetic Plast Surg. 2002;26(5):335–9.

[28] Ichikawa K, Miyasaka M, Tanaka R, Tanino R, Mizukami K, Wakaki M: Histologic evaluation of the pulsed Nd:YAG laser for laser lipolysis. Lasers Surg Med. 2005;36(1): 43–6.

[29] Goldman A, Wollina U, de Mundstock EC: Evaluation of tissue tightening by the subdermal Nd: YAG laser-assisted liposuction versus liposuction alone. J Cutan Aesthet Surg. 2011;4(2):122–8.

[30] Parlette EC, Kaminer ME: Laser-assisted liposuction: here's the skinny. Semin Cutan Med Surg. 2008;27(4):259–63.

[31] DiBernardo BE, Reyes J: Evaluation of skin tightening after laser-assisted liposuction. Aesthet Surg J. 2009;29(5):400–7.

[32] Dudelzak J, Hussain M, Goldberg DJ: Laser lipolysis of the arm, with and without suction aspiration: clinical and histologic changes. J Cosmet Laser Ther. 2009;11(2): 70–3.

[33] Gentileschi S, Servillo M, D'Ettorre M, Salgarello M: Abdominal subcutaneous mass after laser-assisted lipolysis and immediate multiple treatments with a dual-wavelength laser, vacuum and massage device. Aesthet Surg J. 2016;36(4):NP144–9.

[34] Bingol UA, Cinar C: Laser lipolysis without suction: reality or myth? Photomed Laser Surg. 2014;32(11):642–5.

[35] Abdelaal MM, Aboelatta YA: Comparison of Blood Loss in Laser Lipolysis vs Traditional Liposuction. Aesthet Surg J. 2014;34(6):907–12.

[36] von Drygalski A, Andris DA: Anemia after bariatric surgery: more than just iron deficiency. Nutr Clin Pract. 2009;24(2):217–26.

[37] Proebstle TM: [Cellulite]. Hautarzt. 2010;61(10):864–72.

[38] Goldman A, Gotkin RH, Sarnoff DS, Prati C, Rossato F: Cellulite: a new treatment approach combining subdermal Nd: YAG laser lipolysis and autologous fat transplantation. Aesthet Surg J. 2008;28(6):656–62.

[39] Petti C, Stoneburner J, McLaughlin L: Laser cellulite treatment and laser-assisted lipoplasty of the thighs and buttocks: combined modalities for single stage contouring of the lower body. Lasers Surg Med. 2016;48(1):14–22.

[40] McBean JC, Katz BE: Laser lipolysis: an update. J Clin Aesthet Dermatol. 2011;4(7): 25–34.

[41] Mordon S, Wassmer B, Rochon P, Desmyttere J, Grard C, Stalnikiewicz G, Reynaud JP: Serum lipid changes following laser lipolysis. J Cosmet Laser Ther. 2009;11(2):74–7.

[42] Shin JY, Chang H: Rhabdomyolysis after cosmetic laser-assisted liposuction. Aesthetic Plast Surg. 2015;39(4):635–8.

[43] Gentile RD: Laser-assisted neck-lift: high-tech contouring and tightening. Facial Plast Surg. 2011;27(4):331–45.

[44] McMenamin P: Laser face-lifts: a new paradigm in face-lift surgery. Facial Plast Surg. 2011;27(4):299–307.

Permissions

All chapters in this book were first published in BCS, by InTech Open; hereby published with permission under the Creative Commons Attribution License or equivalent. Every chapter published in this book has been scrutinized by our experts. Their significance has been extensively debated. The topics covered herein carry significant findings which will fuel the growth of the discipline. They may even be implemented as practical applications or may be referred to as a beginning point for another development.

The contributors of this book come from diverse backgrounds, making this book a truly international effort. This book will bring forth new frontiers with its revolutionizing research information and detailed analysis of the nascent developments around the world.

We would like to thank all the contributing authors for lending their expertise to make the book truly unique. They have played a crucial role in the development of this book. Without their invaluable contributions this book wouldn't have been possible. They have made vital efforts to compile up to date information on the varied aspects of this subject to make this book a valuable addition to the collection of many professionals and students.

This book was conceptualized with the vision of imparting up-to-date information and advanced data in this field. To ensure the same, a matchless editorial board was set up. Every individual on the board went through rigorous rounds of assessment to prove their worth. After which they invested a large part of their time researching and compiling the most relevant data for our readers.

The editorial board has been involved in producing this book since its inception. They have spent rigorous hours researching and exploring the diverse topics which have resulted in the successful publishing of this book. They have passed on their knowledge of decades through this book. To expedite this challenging task, the publisher supported the team at every step. A small team of assistant editors was also appointed to further simplify the editing procedure and attain best results for the readers.

Apart from the editorial board, the designing team has also invested a significant amount of their time in understanding the subject and creating the most relevant covers. They scrutinized every image to scout for the most suitable representation of the subject and create an appropriate cover for the book.

The publishing team has been an ardent support to the editorial, designing and production team. Their endless efforts to recruit the best for this project, has resulted in the accomplishment of this book. They are a veteran in the field of academics and their pool of knowledge is as vast as their experience in printing. Their expertise and guidance has proved useful at every step. Their uncompromising quality standards have made this book an exceptional effort. Their encouragement from time to time has been an inspiration for everyone.

The publisher and the editorial board hope that this book will prove to be a valuable piece of knowledge for researchers, students, practitioners and scholars across the globe.

List of Contributors

Nikolay P. Serdev
New Bulgarian University, Sofia, Bulgaria
Medical Center "Aesthetic Surgery, Aesthetic Medicine", New Bulgarian University, Sofia, Bulgaria

Hossam ElKafrawy
Department of Plastic Surgery, Alexandria University, Alexandria, Egypt

Sherif Wasief
Plastic Surgery Unit, Shark El Madina Hospital, Alexandria, Egypt

Alexandro Aguilera Salgado
National Institute of Pediatrics, Mexico City, Mexico

Johnatan Figueroa Padilla
National Institute of Cancerology, Mexico City, Mexico

José Cortés Arreguín
Moreno Valle Traumatology and Orthopedics Hospital, Mexico City, Mexico

Medha A. Bhave (Khair)
Param Hospital and ICU, Thane, Maharashtra, India

Balkovic Marija
Clinic for Plastic and Aesthetic Surgery, Medical Beauty Center, Belgrade, Serbia

Jankovic Irena
Clinic for Plastic and Reconstructive Surgery, Clinical Center Nis, Nis, Serbia

Guillermo Blugerman, Diego Schavelzon, Boris Martínez, Gabriel Wexler, Andrea Markowsky and Marcelo Lotoki
B & S Center of Excellence in Plastic Surgery, Buenos Aires, Argentina

Carlos Oaxaca
Plastic Surgeon, Torre Medica Santé, Leon, Guanajuato, México

Marcelo A. Cuadrado, Gabriel Moina and Daniel Moina
Hospital Británico de Buenos Aires, Centro de Rinología y Cirugía plástica Dr. Moina, Buenos Aires, Argentina

Javier Soto
Plastic Surgery Department, FOSCAL International, La Riviera Clinic, Aqua SPA Beauty & Health, Bucaramanga, Colombia

Hugo A. Aguilar
Plastic Surgery Department, Santander University Hospital (HUS), Bucaramanga, Colombia

Juan S. Barajas-Gamboa
Surgery Department, Autonomous University of Bucaramanga (UNAB), Bucaramanga, Colombia

Marco Romeo
University Autonoma of Madrid and Fundación Jimenez Diaz, Madrid, Spain

Ayman Elmeligy and Khalid Elsherbeny
Department of Plastic Surgery, Ain Shams University, Cairo, Egypt

Guillermo Blugerman, Diego Schavelzon Victoria Schavelzon and Guido Blugerman
Centro ByS, Buenos Aires, Argentina

Gabriel Wexler
Estetica Wexler, Cordoba, Argentina

Marcelo Lotocki
Genesis, Obera, Misiones, Argentina

Zoran Žgaljardić and Ivonne Žgaljardić
Aestehtic Surgery Center Dr. Žgaljardić Opatija, Zagreb, Croatia

Index

www.ingramcontent.com/pod-product-compliance
Lightning Source LLC
LaVergne TN
LVHW060942220926
848485LV00015B/1373